Cases on ICT Utilization, Practice and Solutions:
Tools for Managing Day–to–Day Issues

Mubarak S. Al–Mutairi
King Fahd University of Petroleum & Minerals, Saudi Arabia

Lawan A. Mohammed
King Fahd University of Petroleum & Minerals, Saudi Arabia

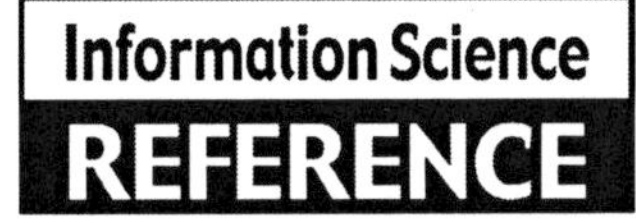

INFORMATION SCIENCE REFERENCE

Hershey · New York

Director of Editorial Content:	Kristin Klinger
Director of Book Publications:	Julia Mosemann
Acquisitions Editor:	Lindsay Johnston
Development Editor:	Michael Killian
Typesetter:	Casey Conapitski
Production Editor:	Jamie Snavely
Cover Design:	Lisa Tosheff

Published in the United States of America by
Information Science Reference (an imprint of IGI Global)
701 E. Chocolate Avenue
Hershey PA 17033
Tel: 717-533-8845
Fax: 717-533-8661
E-mail: cust@igi-global.com
Web site: http://www.igi-global.com

Library of Congress Cataloging-in-Publication Data

Cases on ICT utilization, practice and solutions : tools for managing day-to-day issues / Mubarak S. Al-Mutairi and Lawan Ahmed Mohammed, editors.
    p. cm.
  Includes bibliographical references and index.
  Summary: "This book presents in-depth insight through a case study approach into the current state of research in ICT as well as identified successful approaches, tools and methodologies in ICT research"--Provided by publisher.
  ISBN 978-1-60960-015-0 (hbk.) -- ISBN 978-1-60960-017-4 (ebook) 1. Information technology--Research. 2. Telecommunication--Research. I. Al-Mutairi, Mubarak S., 1971- II. Mohammed, Lawan Ahmed, 1968-
  T58.5.C38 2011
  658.4'038--dc22
                    2010022814

British Cataloguing in Publication Data
A Cataloguing in Publication record for this book is available from the British Library.

Table of Contents

Section 1
Fundamental Research Concepts and Methodology

Section 2
Web Services and Technologies

Section 3
Information Technology Outsourcing

Section 4
Security Issues

Section 5
Other Application Areas

Detailed Table of Contents

Section 1
Fundamental Research Concepts and Methodology

Chapter 1

Tiko Iyamu, Tshwane University of Technology, South Africa

This chapter investigates the challenges of interpretive, case study research strategy and empirical techniques applied in the information systems discipline. This chapter focuses on the realistic challenges that researchers face while conducting a qualitative, interpretive, case study, particularly during data collection.

Section 2
Web Services and Technologies

Chapter 2

Santhanamery Thominathan, Universiti Teknologi MARA Malaysia, Malaysia
Ramayah Thurasamy, Universiti Sains Malaysia, Malaysia

This case study examines the contribution of the E-filing system in Malaysia. E-filing system is a newly developed online tax submission services offered by government to the tax payers in the country to enable them to easily, quickly and safely file their tax returns.

Abad Shah, University of Engineering and Technology, Pakistan
Zafar Singhera, Oracle Corporation, USA
Syed Ahsan, University of Engineering and Technology, Pakistan

This chapter discusses the interoperability problem of databanks and tools and how web services are being used to try to solve it. Also included is a discussion on two extensively used Web Service systems for Life Sciences, myGrid and Semantic-MOBY. Further, it discusses how the state-of-art research and technological development in Semantic Web, Ontology and Database Management can help address these issues.

Nafisat Afolake Adedokun-Shittu, International Islamic University, Malaysia
Abdul Jaleel Kehinde Shittu, University Utara, Malaysia

This chapter highlights some issues that are critical in evaluating technology in education such that it will be implemented to meet educational goals and it will also serve as a spotlight for policy makers and educators to make a worthwhile return on their technology investment. Schools and institutions of learning invest heavily on technology before establishing clear plans on how it will be integrated into teaching and learning to achieve educational goal.

Tanja Arh, Jožef Stefan Institute, Slovenia
Vlado Dimovski, University of Ljubljana, Slovenia
Borka Jerman Blažič, Jožef Stefan Institute, Slovenia

This chapter provides detailed definitions of technology-enhanced learning, Web 2.0 technologies and technical terms related to it, its scope and the process of organisational learning, as well as a method for business performance assessment. Special attention is given to the findings related to the observed correlations between the aforementioned constructs.

Mubarak S. Al-Mutairi, King Fahd University of Petroleum & Minerals, Saudi Arabia

Due to high mobile phone penetration rates in developing countries, any electronic government initiatives that don't take mobile technology into account will eventually fail. While the number of landline phones and internet subscribers are growing steadily over the past few years, the number of mobile phone users and its penetration rates are skyrocketing. In the near future and with the many mobile phone features, mobile phones will remain the main media of communication and a main source for providing information to citizens and customers. This chapter discusses electronic government initiatives in Saudi Arabia.

Ġorġ Mallia, University of Malta, Malta

The case presented in this chapter revolves around the hypothesis that information processing has changed from a linear format, within a chronological progression, to a partially controlled chaotic format, with tracking achieved primarily through hypertextual nodes which goes against the enforced linearity of most institutionally imposed hierarchical learning.

Section 3
Information Technology Outsourcing

Abdul Jaleel Kehinde Shittu, University Utara, Malaysia
Nafisat Afolake Adedokun-Shittu, International Islamic University, Malaysia

This chapter took an in-depth look into various challenges facing Malaysia's ITO industry especially from suppliers' perspectives. It discusses the problems facing ITO practices in the light of government policy and ITO model. It also used qualitative research method with special reference to interpretive and exploratory approach for the analysis of relevant issues in the chapter.

Chad Lin, Curtin University, Australia
Yu-An Huang, National Chi Nan University, Taiwan
Chien-Fa Li, Puli Veterans Hospital, Taiwan
Geoffrey Jalleh, Curtin University, Australia

This chapter examines key issues surrounding the management and implementation of health information systems (HIS) outsourcing in Taiwanese hospitals and identify issues that are crucial in managing and implementing HIS outsourcing in hospitals. Four key issues and problems were identified in the HIS outsourcing process: lack of implementation in IS investment evaluation process, problems in managing HIS outsourcing contracts, lack of user involvement and participation in HIS outsourcing process, and failure to retain critical HIS contract management skills and project management capabilities in-house.

Section 4
Security Issues

Chapter 10

Dakshina Ranjan Kisku, Dr. B. C. Roy Engineering College, India
Phalguni Gupta, Indian Institute of Technology Kanpur, India
Jamuna Kanta Sing, Jadavpur University, India

As there are many graph matching techniques used to design robust and real-time biometrics systems, this chapter discusses these different types of graph matching techniques that have been successfully used in different biometric traits. This chapter makes an attempt and explain the way a graph can be used in the designing an efficient biometric system. It also deals with the problem of using wavelet decomposition and monotonic decreasing graph to fuse biometric characteristics.

Chapter 11

Neyire Deniz Sarier, Bonn-Aachen International Center for Information Technology, Germany

This chapter evaluates the security properties and different applications of Identity Based Encryption (IBE) systems. Particularly, it considers biometric identities for IBE, which is a new encryption system defined as fuzzy IBE. It also analyzes the security aspects of fuzzy IBE.

Chapter 12

Biju Issac, Swinburne University of Technology (Sarawak Campus), Malaysia

This chapter discusses on existing spam technologies and later focus on a case study. Though many anti-spam solutions have been implemented, the Bayesian spam detection approach looks quite promising. A case study for spam detection algorithm is presented and its implementation using Java is discussed, along with its performance test results on two independent spam corpuses – Ling-spam and Enron-spam.

Chapter 13

Lawan Ahmed Mohammed, King Fahd University of Petroleum & Minerals, Saudi Arabia

This chapter provides a comprehensive overview of the possible fraudulent activities that may be perpetrated against Automatic Teller Machine (ATMs) and investigates recommended approaches to prevent these types of frauds. In particular, it designed or developed a prototype model for the utilization of biometrics equipped ATM to provide security solution against must of the well-known ATM breaches.

Foreword

Information and communication technology (ICT) is one of the fastest growing areas in terms of research and development and is increasingly adopted in a wide variety of applications. As such, educators and researchers in this area need to spend extra effort to keep up with its rapid growth and to be current with its trends. Teaching methods in academia has also to adopt new ways of learning knowledge and communicating current and future trends and advances with students' expectations. Employers are expected to find university graduates well equipped with most recent ICT technologies with enough capabilities for handling and adopting the most current technologies. Textbooks play a major role in preparing graduates that meet employers' expectations. Well written text books with clear objectives of tracing most recent advances in the area supported by case studies is a scarce commodity for educators and researchers.

This book puts together the knowledge of researchers and the experience of practitioners for the benefit of researchers and developers and educators in the area of ICT. The book covers wide range of topics within the ICT area including the application of information technology in different areas such as e-business, e-commerce, e-banking and health care and bioinformatics. It also includes information security, strategic information technology and risk management in ICT. Communication technologies and networking is also covered in terms of its applications and technology development.

The effort put by the editors, Mubarak Al-Mutairi and Mohammed Lawan, into attracting authors that are quite knowledgeable and experienced in different ICT technologies and then putting them together in a manner that makes the topic coverage smooth and consistent. As a result we have a book that is comprehensive in its topic coverage and also integrated in its approach. It covers aspects of technology development as well as its adaptation strategies and practical implications in a case base approach. The book, in my opinion, can be easily adopted in ICT academic institutions in senior and graduate levels. It can also be used as a good reference for practitioners and developers in the ICT business.

Umar Al-Turki
King Fahd University of Petroleum and Minerals
College of Computer Science and Engineering, Dean

Umar Al-Turki *is an associate professor in the Department of Systems Engineering at King Fahd University of Petroleum and Minerals, Dhahran, Saudi Arabia. He Obtained his Ph.D. in Decision Sciences and Engineering Systems from Rensselaer Polytechnic Institute in 1994. He obtained an M.Sc. in Industrial Engineering and Management from Oklahoma State University in 1989. He is currently involved in conducting research in the areas of production scheduling, supply chain management and quality improvement. He authored and co-authored a large number of publications in international journal in these areas. He is also involved in consultation with local companies in quality improvement and strategic planning.*

Preface

The continuous accelerating advances in information and communication technologies (ICT) research create a necessity to possess a concise list of current research on emerging opportunities, issues, and challenges in the field. This will not only enable fresh researchers to get started with their research work but also enable instructors of ICT research courses to better prepare their students especially at postgraduate level.

This collection, entitled *Cases on ICT Utilization, Practice and Solutions: Tools for Managing Day-to-Day Issues* provides practical examples of how some researchers used different tools to solve many day-to-day computing problems, as well as covering the future research direction in the field. The book will be valuable reading material for every postgraduate student in various ICT fields. The book summarizes present past, current, and future research directions in different fields of ICT by providing in-depth insight into the current state of research; identify successful approaches, tools and methodologies in ICT research; explore points of good practices, while addressing potential pitfalls to avoid, and examining and evaluating solutions to some of ICT researchers' toughest challenges.

This book is organized in five distinct sections, providing the most wide-ranging coverage of topics such as: (1) Fundamental Research Concepts and Methodology; (2) Web Services and Technologies; (3) ICT Outsourcing; (4) Security Issues and Implications; (5) Other application areas. The following provides a summary of what is covered in each section:

Section 1, Fundamental Research Concepts and Methodology, forms the foundation of the book. The first chapter addressed crucial theories essential to the understanding of research methodology within the field of information and communication technology. The case in this section investigated the challenges of interpretive, case study research strategy and empirical techniques applied in the information systems discipline. It focuses on the realistic challenges that researchers face while conducting a qualitative, interpretive, case study, particularly during data collection.

Section 2, Web Services and Technologies, provides in-depth coverage of different web services as well as technological frameworks to provide the reader with a comprehensive understanding of the emerging technological developments within the field. The section presents an extensive coverage of various tools and technologies such as mobile, web 2.0, advances in semantic web and ontologies, e-commerce and e-filling that practioners and academicians alike can utilize to develop different techniques. The section also addresses the issue of integrating information and communication technology in teaching and learning.

Section 3, Information Technology Outsourcing (ITO), presents an in-depth look into various challenges facing ITO industries. Real case study on health information systems (HIS) outsourcing was also discussed. The section enlightens readers about fundamental research on one of the many methods used to facilitate and enhance the ITO. Through these rigorously research cases, the reader is provided with examples of research methods and the analysis of relevant issues in the field. Solutions and recommendations are provided to deal with key issues that are critical in the management and implementation of ITO.

Section 4, Security is an essential element of information technology infrastructure and applications. Concerns about security of networks and information systems have been growing along with the rapid increase in the number of ICT users and the value of their transactions. The hasty security threats have driven the development of security numerous measures to detect and protect the ICT infrastructure ahead of the threat. Though a lot of information is available on the internet about security methodologies, tools and techniques but it all is spread on so many sites and one has to spend a considerable part of his precious time to search it. In this section, a thorough survey has been made in many cases/chapters to facilitate and assist the researchers in various security issues. The issues and defend challenges in fighting with cyber attacks have also been discussed. The section provides best available up-to-date advancement in the area. The practical implementation of core tools such as biometrics, encryption, spam detection methods, and authentication systems used for protecting both wired and wireless networks were discussed.

The concluding section (5) of this book highlights research potential within the field of fiber optics, while exploring details study of erbiumdoped fiber amplifier (EDFA and erbium doped fiber laser (EDFL). In this section, research papers have been reviewed to show and clarify their strengths and weaknesses from different perspectives. It concludes by describing the future direction in optical communication particularly in EDFA and EDFL.

The second part introduces a general-purpose simulation package for power electronics. However, because of the generality of these tools and their drag-and-drop and ad-hoc features, learners usually face problems in designing a converter circuit. In this section, the problem above is addressed by introducing a design aid tool that guides the student over prescribed steps to design a power electronics circuit

Mubarak S. Al-Mutairi
King Fahd University of Petroleum & Minerals, Saudi Arabia

Lawan A. Mohammed
King Fahd University of Petroleum & Minerals, Saudi Arabia

Acknowledgment

The editors would like to acknowledge the help of all involved in the reviewing process of the chapters. We greatly appreciate individual authors of the included chapters for their thorough technical reviews, constructive criticisms, and many valuable suggestions as they served as reviewers for chapters written by others.

Special thanks go to the management and staff of IGI Global for their valuable contribution, suggestions, recommendations, and encouragements from inception of initial ideas to the final publication of the book. In particular, we would like to thanks Mike Killian for his various contributions and support. And most importantly, we are grateful to Beth Ardner for the great help initially received from her throughout the previous stages.

Deep appreciation goes to Dr. Umar Al-Turki for providing us with a constructive and comprehensive foreword.

We also thank all the people who assisted us in the reviewing process.

The editors wish to acknowledge King Fahd University of Petroleum and Minerals (KFUPM) Saudi Arabia and Hafr Al-Batin Community College for their support in providing the various facilities utilized in the process of production of this book.

This work was supported by Deanship of Scientific Research program of King Fahd University of Petroleum and Minerals (KFUPM), under Project Number: # IN101001.

Mubarak S. Al-Mutairi
King Fahd University of Petroleum & Minerals, Saudi Arabia

Lawan A. Mohammed
King Fahd University of Petroleum & Minerals, Saudi Arabia

Editors

Section 1
Fundamental Research Concepts and Methodology

Chapter 1
Qualitative Case Study Research Approach:
Empirically Unveiling the Pitfalls

Tiko Iyamu
Tshwane University of Technology, South Africa

EXECUTIVE SUMMARY

Data collection is a critical aspect of any research. To this point, it is very important that a researcher has a good understanding of why, where and how to collect data. Broadly speaking, there are two main research and data collection approaches; namely, quantitative and qualitative methodologies. These two approaches are used both in academia and professional domains. This study focuses on philosophical assumptions underpinning Information Systems (IS) research. The philosophical assumptions underlying interpretive, case study research tradition and approach implies a subjective epistemology and the ontological belief that reality is socially constructed. The study investigated the challenges of interpretive, case study research strategy and empirical techniques applied in the information systems discipline. This paper focuses on the realistic challenges that researchers face while conducting a qualitative, interpretive, case study, particularly during data collection.

INTRODUCTION

The paper is organised into four main sections. The first section is concerned with the interpretive approach as applied within information systems (IS) research. The second section discusses the case study approach, including data collection and analysis, as applied in many IS studies. The third section presents case study as an IS research

design. Finally, the paper addresses the empirical findings (challenges of qualitative, case study research approach) of the study.

Qualitative research focuses on human behaviour and the social communities inhabited by human beings. The focus is on increasing the understanding of why things are the way they are socially and why humans behave the way they do. Qualitative research is popular in the social sciences such as psychology, sociology and anthropology. On the other hand quantitative

DOI: 10.4018/978-1-60960-015-0.ch001

research approach is primarily concerned with investigating aspects which could be observed and measured in a defined pattern (Blaikie, 2003; Creswell, 1994). The observations and measurements can be made objectively and repeated by other researchers. This type of research has been applied more in the natural sciences fields. This paper focuses on qualitative, interpretive case study. It explores the challenges of case study in IS discipline. Information Systems discipline has benefited from the richness of qualitative research in the recent years – it has been applied in many works such as Galliers (1991); Hirschheim & Klein (1989); Monteiro & Hanseth (1996); Myers & Avison (2002); and Walsham (2006).

Even though a brief comparison is provided above, the aim of this paper is not to compare both approaches. The paper focuses on qualitative interpretive case study: to gain a better understanding of the challenges faced by academic IS researchers and IT practitioners such as IT Architect conducting Research & Development (R & D). Understanding of these challenges provides practitioners contemplating or undertaking interpretive case study research for the first time with guidance on the collection of data.

Qualitative research has proved to be concerned with the perceptions, opinions, experiences and feelings of individuals and groups producing subjective data. Qualitative research is argued and described as a very useful method for complex situations and theories (Boucaut, 2001). Most IS research employs a qualitative methodology mainly because it is interrogative, and allows clarification on questions such who, what, how, when, where and why. Qualitative research describes real-life experience, social phenomena as they seem to occur naturally. An attempt to manipulate the situation under study is difficult because of its natural settings. This seems to be the case with experimental quantitative research as well. Understanding of a situation is gained through a holistic perspective. We take cognisance of the difficulty of attempting to understand the situa-

tion and therefore have no intention to trivialise it. Quantitative research depends on the ability to identify a set of variables in specific context.

BACKGROUND

Interpretive Research Approach

The interpretive research approach is investigative within any social environment, including IS. In such a context, an interpretive research approach (Walsham, 1995 and 2006) is appropriate in order to understand influences on the social context of an organisation or institution. Qualitative research was more suitable for this study as it allows for clarification from respondents. Through close interaction with interviewees, research can develop a deeper understanding including that of complex situations.

In relation to research in IS, Orlikowski & Baroudi (1991) identify three philosophical perspectives: positivist, critical and interpretive research. A research method can accordingly be either positivist, interpretive or critical (Walsham, 1995). The next three paragraphs briefly discuss these research approaches:

Positivist research in information systems is based upon the assumption that reality is objectively given and that it can be described by reference to measurable properties that are independent of the researcher (Myers, 1997). The positivist approach has been criticised within the IS field, specifically in respect of its treatment of organisational reality. Also, the positivist approach has been criticised for being too deeply rooted in functionalism and too concerned with causal analysis at the expense of getting close to the phenomenon being studied (Galliers, 1991).

The critical research approach in IS research sees its main task as one of social critique, whereby the restrictive and alienating conditions of the *status quo* are shown and challenged (Klein & Myers, 1999). In critical research, the investigation is classified as emancipative if it aims to help eliminate the cause of unwarranted alienation and domination, and thereby enhance the opportunities for the realisation of human potential (Hirschheim & Klein, 1989). Critical theorists assume that people can consciously act to change their social and economic conditions. They also assume that social reality is historically constituted and that it is produced and reproduced by people. Critical research makes the assumption that people are constrained in their actions by various forms of cultural and political domination (Myers, 1997).

The interpretive approach looks at 'reality' from a different perspective to that of the positivist approach. An interpretive approach could help researchers gain knowledge of reality through social constructions such as language, shared meanings and experiences, tools, documents, etc (Walsham, 1993). In an interpretive research project, there are no predefined dependent and independent variables, but a focus on the complexity of human sense-making as the situation emerges (Kaplan & Maxwell, 1994). The interpretive researcher assumes that reality can only be accessed through social constructions such as language, consciousness and shared meanings.

According to Denzin & Lincoln (1994), qualitative research is a multi-method in focus, involving an interpretive, naturalistic approach to its subject matter. This means that qualitative researchers study things in their natural settings, attempting to make sense of or interpret phenomena in terms of the meanings people bring to them. Interpretive research involves the studied collection and use of a variety of empirical materials: personal experiences, introspective reflections, life story interviews, observation of inter-actional events, visual material and historical texts that describe routine and problematic moments and meanings in individuals' lives.

Social reality is constructed as a result of intentional and unintentional actions, which the interpretive approach assists to obtain. Interpretive approaches within IS research are particularly

aimed at producing an understanding of this social reality, the context, and the process whereby IS influences and is influenced by the context (Walsham, 1993). Orlikowski & Baroudi (1991); Walsham (1995); and Myers (1998) are some works where interpretive research was applied.

According to Walsham (1995), "interpretive methods of research adopt the position that our knowledge of reality is a social construction by human actors. In this view, value-free data cannot be obtained, since the enquirer uses his or her preconceptions in order to guide the process of enquiry, and furthermore the researcher interacts with the human subjects of the enquiry, changing the preconceptions of both parties".

Myers (1998), states that, in more traditional positivist techniques, context is treated as either a set of interfering variables that need controlling, known as noise in the data, or other controlled variables which are experimentally set up in order to seek for cause and effect relationships. The context of a situation is seen as something that can be factored out of the analysis or operationalised as a variable. In interpretive approaches, however, context is treated as the socially constructed reality of a named group, or groups, of social agents and the key task of observation and analysis is to unpack the webs of meaning transformed in the social process whereby reality is constructed.

Within interpretive research, consciously or unconsciously, hermeneutics is continuously applied. Hermeneutics provides a means of understanding and interpreting texts (Hirschheim & Klein, 1989). According to Klein & Myers (1999), the purpose of hermeneutics is to make interpretive research explicit and to demonstrate the reasons for the understanding of a text. Hermeneutics does not aim to explain and predict but to understand and to make sense of others' actions (Lee, 1994). In order to understand someone else's action, one need to be able to understand their motives, which means that there must be some common ground upon which researcher and research object can agree on meaning.

Klein & Myers (1999) therefore proposed a set of seven principles for conducting and evaluating interpretive research studies. These principles are all related and interdependent, with the hermeneutic orientation as a golden thread connecting them all. They are principles of: Hermeneutic Circle; Contextualisation; Interaction between the Researchers and the Subjects; Abstraction and Generalisation; Dialogical Reasoning; Multiple Interpretations; and Suspicion. These principles have been applied in many works such as Monteiro & Hanseth (1996); Lee (1994); and Trauth (1997). Trauth explained how her understanding improved as she became self-conscious and started to question her own assumptions.

If the set of seven principles is used, the research work is likely to become more plausible and convincing to its target audience. Hence the main aim of the set of principles is to improve the plausibility and cogency of interpretive research. According to Klein & Myers (1999), IS researchers should explore 'how' and 'which' principles may apply in any particular or different situation. The importance and relevance of each principle is partly derived from the manner in which the others are applied to the collection and interpretation of the data, which means that the set of principles may not be used mechanically.

The case study approach is the most common or popular research strategy in the IS field. Farhoomand (1992) view which is supported by Walsham (1993), argued that case studies provide the main vehicle for research conducted in the interpretive tradition.

The Case Study Strategy

According to Myers (1997), there are four qualitative traditions which are particularly significant in IS research, they include case study research, ethnography, grounded theory and action research. Orlikowski & Baroudi (1991) argue that case study research is the most commonly used qualitative approach in IS. From these traditions of qualitative research approaches, the case study approach was selected for this research. This is also, because it is the case that is been studied.

The case study approach enables in-depth exploration of complex issues such as the topic of human interaction with technology. In addition, it allows for 'thick descriptions' of the phenomena under study Yin (2003). Such thick descriptions give the researcher access to the subtleties of changing and multiple interpretations Walsham (1995), which would have been lost in other research approaches, including quantitative or experimental strategies.

Yin (2003) defines a case study as an empirical inquiry that investigates a contemporary phenomenon within its real-life context, especially when the boundaries between phenomenon and context are not clearly defined. According to Yin, the case study allows an investigation to retain the holistic and meaningful characteristics of real-life events such as individual life cycles, organisation and managerial processes, change, and the maturation of institutions. Therefore, the case study approach is especially useful in situations where contextual conditions and events being studied are critical and where the researcher has no control over the events as they unfold. The case study, as a research strategy, should encompass specific techniques for the collection and analysis of data, directed by clearly stated theoretical assumptions. Furthermore, data should be collected from different sources and its integrity should be ensured.

Stake (1994) identifies and distinguishes three types of case studies, namely intrinsic, instrumental and collective. Yin (1993) also distinguishes three types of case studies, which are exploratory, causal and descriptive case studies: Exploratory – the collection of data occurs before theories or specific research questions are formulated. Causal – looks for cause and effect relationships, and searches for explanatory theories of the phenomena. Descriptive – requires a theory to guide the collection of data and this theory should be openly stated in advance and be the subject of review and debate and later serve as the 'design' for the descriptive case study.

Case studies can be single or multiple, and can be embedded as well as holistic. An embedded case study is one in which there is more than one sub-unit, whilst in a holistic case study a global programme of organisation is investigated (Yin, 2003).

Case Study as a Research Approach in Information Systems

The use of case studies is a widely accepted research strategy in the IS field. The case study strategy has been argued to be particularly useful for practice-based problems where the experience of the actors is important and the context of action is critical (Lee, 1989; and Galliers (1991).

However, the case study research approach has been subject to criticism on the grounds of a lack of sufficient representation and a lack of statistical generalisability. Moreover, the richness and complexity of the data collected means that the data is often open to different interpretations, and potential biases (Conford & Smithson, 1996). According to Pettigrew (1985), multiple case studies are useful in developing and refining generalisable concepts and multiple case studies can lead to generalisations in terms of propositions. Importantly, Walsham (1993) makes the point, however, that generalisations can also be made from single case studies: "… the validity of an extrapolation from an individual case or cases depends not on the representativeness on such cases in the statistical sense, but on the plausibility and cogency of the logical reasoning used in describing the results from the case, and in drawing conclusions from them." Similarly, Yin (2003) argues that case studies are used for analytical generalisations, where the researcher's aim is to generalise a particular set of results, which are found to be broader than theoretical propositions.

Yin (2003) offers an approach for case studies, which emphasises field procedures and case study

questions, and this is adopted as a guide for this study. He further argued that the set of case study questions forms the heart of the method. The main function of questions is to keep the researcher focused and on track.

This clear focus led to the adoption of an interpretive stance, which seeks to uncover truth by understanding the phenomena in their real-life context (Walsham, 1995). Given the interpretive stance adopted in IS research and the nature of this research's questions, which seeks to understand the challenges of case study approach in IS, it is believed that the case study approach is the appropriate research strategy. Similar research questions could have been formulated and surveys used to examine changing patterns in organisations. However, this would not have revealed in detail the unique experiences of individuals in the organisations and the factors influencing their IT strategy. The case study method was chosen because of its advantages in creating novel and profound insights and its focus on examining the rich contextual influences.

RESEARCH METHODOLOGY

This is a qualitative study involving individuals and groups in both professional and academic domains, in South Africa. The study had two lines of investigations: it first used a social constructivist perspective to investigate why IS researchers select qualitative research method; and secondly it investigated the challenges of using case study research approach in the IS discipline.

The research strategy was to conduct the study in two different academic and professional domains. The fieldwork was conducted with both academic and professional IS researchers, including Masters & PhD students and IT R & D specialists. The main data collection techniques used were semi-structured interviews, participant observation and group discussions.

Research Design

The research design is the logical strategy to gather evidence about desired data. It provides the glue that holds the research together. It structures the research, and shows how all of the major parts fit together in order to address the research questions. The research design includes: The selection of case study sites; data sources; data collection; and sub-units of analysis of the study.

Data Sources

Data was collected from primary and secondary sources. The primary data source was interviews which were conducted with researchers, aspiring researchers (Masters and PhD candidates) and industry practitioners. The secondary data sources mainly covered literature and publications. Secondary data provided an essential preparation for the interviews and confirmation of some of the data gathered during and after the interviews. Thus data helped to cross-check formal information, learn about major events, empirical details, historical decisions and main research purposes. For this study it was possible to conduct the data collection and analysis in an iteratively managed manner.

Data Collection

The structured and semi-structured interviews were designed to elicit information on researcher's challenges and opportunities in conducting research, and why they adopt particular research methods. The study took cognisance of the fact that each research topic is unique. The interview design was based on existing work and literature (such as Walsham (2006); Myers & Avison (2002); Benamati & Lederer (1999); Klein & Myers (1999); Roode (1993); Hirschheim & Klein (1989); Kendall (1992); Galliers (1991); and Eisenhardt (1989) description of a process-based research framework for IS research was useful in generating the most appropriate questions in the semi-structured interview.

In the study, data sources included interviews, literature and theses. Semi-structured interviews, tape recordings, and documentation were used for the research data collection. A set of balanced respondent demographics was formulated and adhered to, as it was a key factor in achieving a true reflection of the situations. The demographics included academics and professionals: 5 researchers from three universities; 6 Masters and Doctoral degrees candidates from four universities; and 5 IT professionals in the Research & Development units from two professional organisations.

Criteria for selecting participants were based on the nature of the study including subject knowledge and experience. In some academic institutions, there were very few researchers. As such, the options were limited. Some of the researchers have limited knowledge and experience of qualitative case study research. The criteria for the researchers included: the size of research which adopted qualitative case study in the last three years. The number of Masters and Doctoral degrees students produced from the department of information systems in the last five years. The students were selected on the basis that they were adopting the qualitative case study approach and had or were in the process of completing data collection. The professional organisations were selected based on the volume of their research and development output.

The questions for the collection of data were grouped into three categories. The first group of questions focused on understanding the rationale for interviewees' adopting Qualitative and Case Study research approach. The second group of questions followed an inductive logic with the objective of allowing any relevant information to understand the fundamental challenges in adopting the research approach.

A set of structured guidelines was used in the interviews. This was mainly for discipline and consistency. Most importantly, it gave the researcher real-time opportunity to enrich the data. The guideline was adhered to throughout the entire process of the interviews:

i. Occasionally sought clarification, meaning of vocabulary, verified that the tape recorder was working.
ii. Asked one question at a time.
iii. Was as neutral as possible. That is, didn't show any knowledge of the topic, or emotional reactions to responses.
iv. Encouraged responses with occasional nods of the head, "uh huh"s, etc.
v. Was careful about the - manner of note-taking. That is, no sudden move to take a note, as it could have perhaps appeared as if there was surprise or satisfaction at an answer, which could influence answers to future questions.
vi. Provided transition between major topics, e.g., "we've been talking about (some topic) and now I'd like to move on to (another topic)."
vii. Didn't lose control of the interviews. This could have occurred when some respondents strayed to another topic, took too long to answer a question and time began to run out, or even asked own questions.

During and immediately after each interview, the following precautions were taken to enhance the quality of data:

i. Verified that the tape recorder was working throughout the interviews.
ii. Made notes on written notes, e.g., clarified scratches, ensured pages were numbered, filled out notes that didn't make sense, etc.
iii. Wrote down any observations made during the interview.

Unit-Based Analysis

The unit-based analysis was identified and used as the starting point for the data analysis. This allows for analysis in research study where a case-by-case basis is applied. The data from the case study were analysed at two (macro and micro) interconnected levels. The macro-level addresses issues on how qualitative, case study is applied by IS researchers. At the micro-level, the challenges of the research approach is analysed from the perspective of both academic and professional domains.

The unit-based analysis gives the researcher an opportunity to explain the objectives of the research to respondents. Participatory interest of the respondents is therefore sought and established through mutual understanding. Respondents are informed of the importance of their responses to the study, and as much openness, fairness and precision as possible were requested and appreciated by the respondents. Respondents were informed that they could obtain a copy of the research results, should they so wish.

RESULTS: SOLUTIONS AND RECOMMENDATIONS

Generally, the researchers interviewed opined that the qualitative case study approach is selected for reasons such as:

i. To observe, capture and explain participants' behaviour, which cannot be easily identified with other research approaches.
ii. To allow for a detailed view of the case studies to be presented, as factor necessary due to the nature of the topic.
iii. To study individuals in their natural settings, which involve physical interactions and gathering of materials. If participants are removed from their setting, it leads to contrived findings that are out of context.

iv. To emphasise the researcher's role as an *active learner* who can tell the story from the participants' view rather than as an "expert" who passes judgment on participants.

v. Case studies can be single or multiple and at the same time embedded as well as holistic. This is an affirmation of Yin's (2003) point.

However, the challenges as revealed in the study are first shown triangularly in a Figure 1 below. It illustrates the attributes which form the elements and these manifest themselves into the challenging factors.

The factors are not challenges by themselves in a vacuum. They include significant elements and attributes, which are informed by, among others, actors, events and situations. As depicted in Figure 1, they are interconnected as a single entity of the challenges:

i. The factor is critical in the collection of data in the qualitative case study approach. It has immersed contribution to the possibility and success of data collection as well as the quality, accuracy, less costly and timeliness of the data collection, which are vital in researches.

ii. Each Factor has collective elements which necessitate and conditionalize it to a factor in the challenging plight of individual researchers. These elements are shaped by the nature of the research. They could also be used as determining factors or criteria for data collection.

iii. The implications of the Attribute are subject to collecting quality and accurate data, which is enforced through element on the Factor. The influence of the attributes on the associated element is high.

The entity as illustrated in Figure 1 is tabulated in Table 1. The discussion that follows should be read with the Table to gain appreciation of the challenges.

Selecting Respondents

The criteria for selecting participants are based on the nature of the study. This includes demographic information, such as race, gender, skill-set, grade or level in the organisational structure, as well as the years of service at the organisation. The number of years of service is used as a criterion to ensure that the respondents understand the organisational structure and systems. This is fundamental if rich data is to be collected. According to many researchers, this has not been an easy task. Sometimes, the willing respondents have limited knowledge either of the subject or of the organisation. According to one of the researchers, "*Criteria for selecting participants were based on the nature of my study. .. this included skill-set, grade or level in the organisational structure, as well as the years of service at the organisation. This was very critical to my study. The number of years of service was used as a criterion to ensure that the respondent understands the organisational systems. Thus was fundamental to therefore provide rich data.*

Figure 1. Entity of the challenges

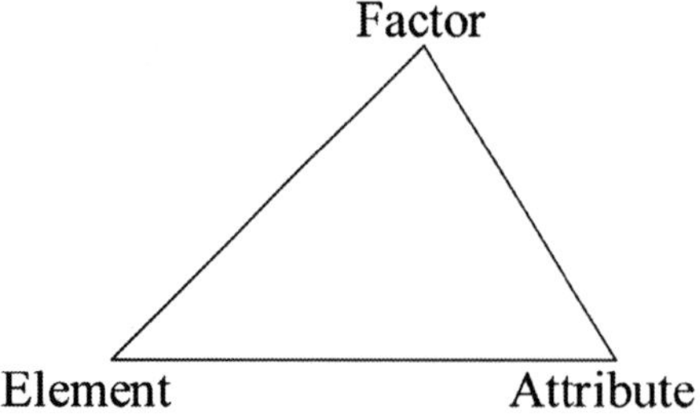

Table 1. Challenging factors

Factor	Element	Attribute
Selecting Respondents	Criteria	Subject knowledge, experience
	Number of interviewees	Point of saturation
	Participation	Demographic, Interest in the subject
Physical Presence	Prohibitive	Costs: materials, travel, interviews time
	Availability	Timing
	Spoken language	Comprehension, accent
Rehearsal (Interview Pilot)	True reflection	Subject knowledge, organisational knowledge
	Participation	Demographic, Interest, time
Observation	Cultural	Understanding cultural differences
	Analytical ability	Interaction, action, meaning
Selecting Case Study site	Distance	Travel
	Accessibility	Organisational policy, individual interest
	Objectives	Alignment with the case study

This was not an easy task – some of the identified candidates were not available for the interview, and some were not interested in the study ".

Demographic information is criteria for nominating and identifying participating respondents. Depending on the nature of the research, this could include information such as race, gender, grade or level in the organisational structure, as well as the years of service at the organisation. It is very challenging to get non-white employees, especially at senior levels in IT departments of most organisations. Also, there are many women, especially at senior levels as well, in IT department in many organisations. The demographic serves to assess the quality of the responses, to balance the responses, and to categorise the usable responses during the data analysis.

The number of respondents in the different case studies in a research normally varies, depending on the sizes of the organisation. The larger the organisation, the more different views and options the researcher gathers. It therefore takes more interviews to reach a point of saturation, which the researcher wishes to achieve. This study attributes it to the fact that the qualitative research approach encourages a point of saturation. A set of balanced respondent is a key factor in achieving a true reflection of the situations.

Physical Presence

Individuals' physical presence at the interviews is time consuming both for the researcher and respondent. However, it could be very necessary. A researcher from one of the universities expressed the following: "*In the last 4 research studies that I undertook, I adopted qualitative case study approach. Each case was unique based on their individual cultural, hierarchical and economic settings. As such, physical interaction was critical for me. Otherwise, I doubted if I had got the same quality of data that I gathered*". Travelling to the location could be prohibitive, especially for the student researchers and the experienced researchers. Furthermore, often, the identified candidates are not available (or cancel appointment when the researcher is already on site) for the interview. Some identified respondents are not interested in the study. The intensity, including travel implications and time consuming nature of data collection constrains researchers from conducting research in considerably far distances from their various locations. This, fundamentally, could necessitate smallness of data.

Spoken language is a huge challenge to many researchers, especially in diverse societies. Some respondents lack comprehension in the language of the interviewer. As a result, they are not able to express themselves in an adequate manner. Further, sometimes the accents of the researcher and the respondent are problematic, especially in the tape recording of the interviews. It becomes difficult to transcribe the texts. It is necessary that the two understand each other for more accurate data, reflection of events, and efficacy of data collection. This affects the quality of data.

Rehearsal (Interview Pilot)

Many researchers, especially aspiring (Masters and PhD degrees candidates) prefer to pilot their interviews before they undertake the actual interview. The aim of the pilot includes the adjustment of the interview guidelines. Therefore, participants should posses the same or similar level of subject and organisational knowledge as participants in the actual interviews. Otherwise, the exercise could be a wasted effort. The fact that participants in the pilot do not take part in the actual interviews makes the search for participants rigorous. A researcher from one of the professional organisations explained: *"As a result of Rehearsal practice, as well as my relationship with the interviewees, I am able to get them to feel as though we are participating in a conversation or discussion rather than in a formal question and answer situation. It gives the opportunity to express their thoughts on the topic as freely as possible. This trick always makes data very rich"*.

Some studies are too unique and as such, knowledgeable people in the subject are limited. As a result, it becomes extremely difficult to find participants for the pilot as well as for the actual interviews. It is highly essential to select ap-propriate candidates for both the pilot and actual interviews for the data to be meaningful and for the objective of the study to be met. Achieving this can be time consuming and prohibitive as well.

Observation

Not all qualitative data collection approaches require direct interaction with people. It is a technique that can be used when data collected through other means can be of limited value or is difficult to validate. Observation of the situations is reliable in that, it is possible to see actual behaviour rather than reading or being told about it. Observation can also serve as a technique for verifying or nullifying information provided in face to face encounters.

According to some respondents, observation of their research participants was often not required but observation of the environment was key because it provided valuable background information about the environment where the research project was undertaken. For example, an IS study relating to an ethnic community may need information about how people dress or about their non-verbal communication. It would be very difficult to understand or analyse what is being observed without initially understanding the cultural settings. A professional researcher explained: *"during lunch break, I see the same group of people together all the time. These people think alike – questions to them will give you same answer"*. Another researcher, also from another professional organisation stated: *I was here, I observed and I saw the impact of the reaction of some of the employees on IT services and delivering when restructuring took place in the organisation"*.

In participant and environment observation, the challenge is being able to capture "life" as it happens - because non-scheduled human activities, although exciting to observe, are very dynamic. That is, capturing data or a social phenomenon in its natural setting demands time, patience and being able to quickly react to change. Unlike in a laboratory experiment, where you can always repeat same measurements, social actions and activities cannot be altered, re-modelled or repeated.

During pilot, demographic criteria is highly taken into considerations. The researcher faces the same challenges as pointed out above in the "Selecting Respondents" section.

Selecting Case Study Site

Selection of organisations for case studies is a matter of accessibility. Many researchers emphasised the challenge of convincing organisations in order to get permission to conduct case studies on their site. The nature of some of the studies does not help matters either, as they have to do with organisational politics, which is considered a sensitive issue in many organisations.

This challenge is not new and seemingly will remain for years to come. In this regard, Buchanan, Boddy & McCalman (1988) remarked *"Research access has become more difficult to obtain"*. Even though confidentiality and anonymity are promised and potentially guaranteed in an effort to uphold research principles and to maintain respondents' rights and values, most organisations sights ethical issues as their reason for declining. Stock Exchange listed organisations are even more difficult. They are over protective of information. As a result, they decline invitation and requests to conduct research either with their employees or in their environment. According to a university researcher, *"after numerous efforts, systematically and diplomatically, two organisations, Dzuwa and Eko (both are pseudonyms) eventually agreed to participate in my study. A letter of appreciation was sent to the Heads of the IT departments of these organisations"*.

The organisations which might grant the permission may be situated far and thus not easily accessible. Also, some of the easily accessed organisations do not align with the objectives of

the study, thereby cannot provide sufficient data for the study. This limits the researcher's options for case study site.

CONCLUSION

The first contribution of this study comes from the description and analysis of the case study. The review of the theoretical concepts applied in the analysis contribute to an increased understanding of the use of qualitative case study research approach in IS environment. The other contribution arises from establishing the challenges faced by IS researchers when using qualitative case study approach. IS researchers, especially novice researchers and IT professionals need to better understand challenges for informed decision making when selecting research approaches in undertaking project or research work. The research approach through which data is collected is critical to research success or failure.

In summary, this study aimed to be of significance to IS researchers, aspiring IS researchers, including IT R & D professionals of the organisation. It is expected that the key contribution will arise from the use of qualitative case study in the different topics in IS research, to empirical analyses of the interplay between technical and non-technical factors. Through this, a better understanding of the contribution of socio-technical elements to IS will be gained.

REFERENCES

Benamati, J., & Lederer, L. (1999). An empirical study of IT management and rapid IT change, In *Proceedings of the SIGCPR conference on Computer personnel research, Communication of the ACM*, pp.144-153, New Orleans: Louisiana.

Blaikie, N. W. H. (2003). *Analyzing quantitative data*. London: Sage Publications Ltd.

Boucaut, R. (2001). Understanding workplace bullying: a practical application of Giddens' Structurational Theory. *International Education Journal, 2*(4).

Buchanan, D., Boddy, D., & McCalman, J. (1988). Getting in, getting on, getting out, and getting back. In Bryman, D. (Ed.), *Doing research in organisations* (pp. 53–67). London: Sage Publications.

Conford, T., & Smithson, S. (1996). *Project Research in Information Systems: A student's guide.* London: Macmillan Press Ltd.

Creswell, J. W. (1994). *Research design, qualitative & quantitative approaches.* Newbury Park, CA: Sage Publications Inc.

Denzin, N. K., & Lincoln, Y. S. (1994). Introduction: Entering the field of Qualitative Research. In Denzin, N. K., & Lincoln, Y. S. (Eds.), *Handbook of qualitative research* (pp. 1–17). Newbury Park, CA: Sage Publications.

Eisenhardt, K. M. (1989). Building Theories from Case Study Research. *Academy of Management Review, 14*(4), 532–550. doi:10.2307/258557

Farhoomand, A. F. (1992). Scientific Progress of Management Information Systems, Information Systems Research: Issues, Methods and Practical Guidelines. In Galliers, R. (Ed.), (pp. 93–111). Oxford, UK: Blackwell Scientific Publications.

Galliers, R. D. (1991). Choosing Information Systems Research Approaches. In Nissen, H. E., Klein, H. K., & Hirschheim, R. (Eds.), *Information Systems Research: Contemporary Approaches and Emergent Traditions.* Amsterdam: North-Holland.

Hirschheim, R., & Klein, H. (1989). Four Paradigms of Information Systems Development. *Communications of the ACM, 32*(10), 1199–1215. doi:10.1145/67933.67937

Kaplan, B., & Maxwell, J. A. (1994). Qualitative Research Methods for Evaluating Computer Information Systems. In Anderson, J. G., Aydin, C. E., & Jay, S. J. (Eds.), *Evaluating Health Care Information Systems: Methods and Applications* (pp. 45–68). Newbury Park, CA: Sage Publications.

Kendall, P. (1992). *Introduction to Systems Analysis and Design: A Structured Approach* (2nd ed.). USA: Wm. C Brown Publishers.

Klein, H., & Myers, M. (1999). A set of principles for conducting and evaluating interpretive field studies in Information Systems. *Management Information Systems Quarterly, 23*(1), 67–93. doi:10.2307/249410

Lee, A. S. (1989). A scientific methodology for MIS case studies. *Management Information Systems Quarterly, 13*(1), 33–50. doi:10.2307/248698

Lee, A. S. (1994). Electronic Mail as a Medium for Rich Communication: An Empirical Investigation Using Hermeneutic Interpretation. *Management Information Systems Quarterly, 18*(2), 143–157. doi:10.2307/249762

Monteiro, E., & Hanseth, O. (1996). Social Shaping of Information Infrastructure: On Being Specific about the Technology. In Orlikowski, W. J., Walsham, G., Jones, M. R., & DeGross, J. I. (Eds.), *Information Technology and Changes in Organizational Work* (pp. 325–343). London: Chapman and Hall.

Myers, M. (1994). Dialectical Hermeneutics: A Theoretical Framework for the Implementation of Information Systems. *Information Systems Journal, 5*(1), 51–70. doi:10.1111/j.1365-2575.1995.tb00089.x

Myers, M. (1997). Qualitative Research in Information Systems. *Management Information Systems Quarterly, 21*(2), 241–242. doi:10.2307/249422

Myers, M. (1998). Interpretive Research in Information Systems. In Mingers, M., & Stowell, F. (Eds.), *Information Systems: An Emerging Discipline? London*. Maidenhead.

Myers, M., & Avison, D. (2002). An Introduction to Qualitative Research in Information Systems. In Myers, M. D., & Avison, D. (Eds.), *Qualitative Research in Information Systems: A Reader* (pp. 3–12). London: Sage publications.

Orlikowski, W., & Baroudi, J. J. (1991). Studying Information Technology in Organizations: Research Approaches and Assumptions. *Information Systems Research*, *2*(1), 1–31. doi:10.1287/isre.2.1.1

Pettigrew, A. M. (1985). Contextualist Research and the Study of Organizational Change Processes. In Mumford, E., Hirschheim, R., Fitzgerald, G., & Wood-Harper, A. T. (Eds.), *Research Methods in Information Systems* (pp. 53–78). Amsterdam: North Holland.

Roode, D. (1993). Implications for teaching of a process-based research framework for information systems. In *Proceedings of the 8th annual conference of the International Academy for Information Management*. Orlando, FL.

Stake, E. (1994). *Handbook of Qualitative Research* (Denzin, N. K., & Lincoln, Y. S., Eds.). London: Sage Publications.

Trauth, E. M. (1997). Achieving the Research Goal with Qualitative Methods: Lessons Learned along the Way. In Lee, A. S., Liebenau, J., & DeGross, J. I. (Eds.), *Information Systems and Qualitative Research* (pp. 225–245). London: Chapman and Hall.

Walsham, G. (1993). *Interpreting information systems in organizations*. Chichester, UK: John Wiley & Sons.

Walsham, G. (1995). The Emergence of Interpretivism in IS Research. *Information Systems Research*, *6*(4), 376–394. doi:10.1287/isre.6.4.376

Walsham, G. (2006). Doing Interpretive Research. *European Journal of Information Systems*, *15*(3), 320–330. doi:10.1057/palgrave.ejis.3000589

Yin, R. K. (1993). *Applications of case study research*. Newbury Park, CA: Sage Publications.

Yin, R. K. (2003). *Case Study Research, Design and Methods* (2nd ed.). Newbury Park, CA: Sage Publications.

Section 2
Web Services and Technologies

Chapter 2
Towards a Customer Centric E-Government Application:
The Case of E-Filing in Malaysia

Santhanamery Thominathan
Universiti Teknologi MARA Malaysia, Malaysia

Ramayah Thurasamy
Universiti Sains Malaysia, Malaysia

EXECUTIVE SUMMARY

Information Communication Technology (ICT) have played an important role in today's global economy. Many countries have gained successful growth due to the implementation of ICT. In Malaysia, increased utilization of ICT has contributed significantly to the total factor productivity. One of the main contributing factors is the e-commerce and Internet based services. Therefore this case study aims to examine the contribution of the newly introduced E-government application namely E-filing system. E-filing system is a newly developed online tax submission services offered by the government to the tax payers in the country where they are able to easily, quickly and safely file their tax returns. The primary discussion in this case study concerns on the Malaysian's ICT revolution, followed by the introduction of E-Filing system, the challenges and barriers faced by the government and concluded with the future trends in the implementation of this system.

INTRODUCTION

Role of ICT

The advances in information and communication technologies (ICT) have raised new opportunities for the implementation of novel applications and the provision of high quality services over global networks. The aim is to utilize this "information society era" for improving the quality of life of all citizens, disseminating knowledge, strengthening social cohesion, generating earnings and finally ensuring that organizations and public bodies remain competitive in the global electronic marketplace (Hesson & Al-Ameed, 2007).

Developed economies are identified with countries that properly use technology for the creation of wealth and less developed economies are identified with countries lacking technological know-how necessary to create wealth (Khalil, 2000). As such,

DOI: 10.4018/978-1-60960-015-0.ch002

a proper management of technology also includes low-tech to high-tech to super-high technologies. Khalil (1993) asserted that a proper management of low or medium level technologies can still create a certain competitive advantage and be effectively used for wealth creation. This is especially evident in newly industrialized countries (NICs) such as Taiwan, Korea, Singapore and Malaysia.

In Malaysia, ICT has assimilated into people's lives in many ways such as communication, logistics or in their working environment. Malaysia has invested enormously in ICT over the years. For example in the Ninth Malaysian Plan (2006-2010), a total of US$6 billion was allocated for enhancing ICT diffusion throughout the country. This shows the importance given by the country for ICT accelerate the economic competitiveness of Malaysia (Kuppusamy et al.2009).

Impact of ICT on Economic Growth

Solow (1957) through his famous seminal research on the contribution of technology on productivity growth in the US had sparked great interest among scholars on the relationship between technology and economic progress.

Since then, various firms, industries and countries have undertaken studies to find out more on the relationship between technology and economic growth.

Based on the study of Jalava and Pohjola (2002), both the production and use of ICT have been the factors behind the improved economic performance of the United States in the 1990s. A further research done by Jalava and Pohjola (2007) proves that the ICT's contribution to the economic growth of Finland was three times larger than the contribution of electricity industry.

In relation to the study done on Korea's economic development from 1996-2001, it is proven that Korea's economic development in the 20th century are mainly due to the growth of industries related to ICT and also the government's treatment

of ICT as a strategic focus for future development (Lee, 2003)

Kuppusamy and Shanmugam (2007) examined the impact of ICT on Malaysia over the periods of 1983-2004 and reveals that ICT investment has statistically improved Malaysia's economic growth. Antonopoulos and Sakellaris (2009) investigated the impact of ICT on Greece and found that the ICT has increased the total factor productivity and also benefited the finance, real estate and business services industries and the wholesale and retail industries in Greece.

This case study sets out to describe the approach adopted by the Malaysian government in enhancing the usage of ICT in the country. In particular, this case study will focus on the success of the newly introduced E-government services in Malaysia that is the E-filing System.

Literature Review on Technology Adoption

Previous studies have proven the various reasons affecting the technology adoption. Survey done by Lai et al. (2004) on the tax practitioners and the electronic filing system in Malaysia founds that there is a strong relationship between technology readiness and intention to use E-Filing system. Technology readiness is the main motivation in using the particular system. However, the survey also reveals that perceived insecurity could be an obstacle in promoting the E-filing system.

This survey is supported by another survey done by Lai et al. (2005) which claims that tax practitioners are willing to accept a technology which is easily to be used and can enhance their job performance; however the fear of Internet security has stopped many of them on filing tax online. This is also supported by study done by Sena and Paul (2009) which finds that the main reason for the decrease in the usage of Internet banking (IB) in Turkey are due to perceived risk on security features of IB.

Ramayah et al. (2008) posit that apart from less knowledge on how to use the E-Filing system, the main reason less people engaged in the system is because they are sceptical over the security and privacy of data transmitted through the web.

Furthermore, based on a study done by Azleen et al. (2009) on taxpayers' attitude, they found that education background of taxpayers plays an important role in encouraging the attitude of taxpayers to use E-filing. Meanwhile the gender of the taxpayers does not contribute any significant differences in the usage.

Conversely, study done on the selected working women in Malaysia to identify the learning barriers in ICT adoption among them finds that ICT skills of Malaysian women are lower than expected compared to their male counterpart although they do not face any serious learning barriers. One of the possible reasons given was may be due to the attitude of the women. (Junaidah, 2008)

In addition, based on the study done by David (2008) on the adoption of e-recruitment services among job seekers in Malaysia, concluded that job seekers widely accepted the e-recruitment services despite its perceived risk due to its ease of use, usefulness, application posting speed and advantages over other job application methods.

Another study conducted by Md Nor and Pearson (2007), posit that trust is another factor that can significantly affect the attitude of users in the acceptance of Internet Banking in Malaysia. According to a survey done by Abdullatif and Philip (2009) finds that one of the criteria on winning the customers trust in adopting a particular technology is the web features particularly the utilitarian (usefulness) and hedonic (attractiveness) features. This finding is similar with the findings by Irani et al. (2008) which indicate that factors such as utilitarian outcomes, perceived resources, social influence, self-efficacy and behavioural intentions are the most important factors in determining the decision on technology adoption.

The above research findings are also supported by another group of researchers Astrid et al. (2008) whose findings reveals that hedonic features (perceived enjoyment) is more powerful determinant of intention to use a technology compared to perceived usefulness. However, according to Raman et al. (2008), their study finds that despite the attractiveness of Internet Banking (IB), the core factor for adoption of IB in Malaysia is the quality of the services provided mainly on the ease of use and reliability (less time to download).

As such we can conclude that, consumers are ever willing to adopt a technology that is useful, ease to use, has hedonic and utilitarian features, higher security or lower perceived risk, trust and quality.

BACKGROUND: INFORMATION COMMUNICATION TECHNOLOGIES (ICT) AND EMERGING TECHNOLOGIES

ICT REVOLUTION IN MALAYSIA

For the past thirty years, Malaysia has undertaken various initiatives to enhance the ICT diffusion and its' economy. The initiatives can be divided into two categories, macro level and micro level initiatives.

Macro Level ICT Initiatives: The Multimedia Super Corridor (MSC)

With the advent of the IT revolution and its positive impact on economic growth and competitiveness, many countries including Malaysia are developing their very own regional development strategies through the dynamic of a high-technology cluster. Guided by the *Vision 2020*, Malaysia has embarked on an ambitious plan by launching MSC in 1996 as the macro level initiative. *Vision 2020* is the blueprint strategy that stated that Malaysia must be a fully developed and knowledge-rich society by the year 2020, among other visions. MSC is one of the main initiatives to achieve this vision.

Figure 1. Vision 2020 (Source NEAC)

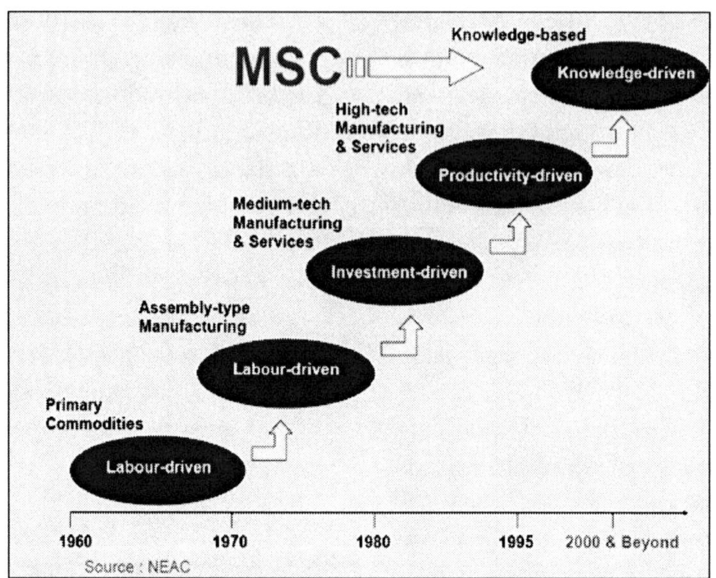

Basically, MSC is a technology park with a dedicated corridor (15 km wide and 50 km long) which stretches from the one of the world's tallest Petronas Twin Towers at the Kuala Lumpur City Centre (KLCC) in the north to the new Kuala Lumpur International Airport (KLIA) in the south.

The development of MSC is a necessity as the new engine of economic growth to ensure Malaysia is moving in the right direction in embracing the IT revolution. This huge technology park is considered as the nucleus for the concentric development of the ICT and multimedia driven industries in Malaysia. In brief, MSC is the vehicle for transforming Malaysia - social and economic development levels – in to a knowledge-based economy. There are seven key flagship applications being engineered to jumpstart in the development of MSC and also to create an ICT and multimedia utopia for producers and users of these technologies. These flagship applications are expected to expedite the diffusion of E-government and E-commerce activities in Malaysia. These applications are E-Government Flagship, Multi-Purpose card flagship, Tele-health Flagship, Smart School Flagship, R&D Cluster Flagship, E-Business flagship and Technopreneur Development Flagship.

Micro Level Initiatives: ICT Infrastructure

In order to support the ICT growth in Malaysia, the government also has concentrated on building the right and proper infrastructures to ensure speedy and efficient network of facilities and services for better transmission of ICT. During the 1980s, most of the ICT infrastructures investment went into provision of basic telephony services to rural and urban people. In the new millennium, Malaysia focused on increasing accessibility to Internet and its related services (Kuppusamy et al. 2009). As a result, there is a significant growth of the three ICT related services for the year 2000, 2005 and 2007. Based on the figure below, it can be seen that PC computers penetration rate per 100 populations was 9.4% in 2000, increased to 22.5% in 2005 and increase to 26.4% in 2007. In terms of internet access, in 2000 a total of 7.1%

of every 100 population had internet access. This figure increases over the years in 2005 to 13.9% and 14.3% in 2007. For the Internet Broadband access, there was no access to broadband during the year 2000. However the percentage has increased to 2.2% per 100 people in 2005 and 5% in 2007 and is expected to grow by 50% for household penetration by 2010.

The Development of E–Government Application

Governments around the world have developed e-commerce applications to deliver services to citizens and business, and to exchange in formations with other government agencies (Davidson et al. 2005). E-government is a term reflecting the use of information and communication technologies in public administration in an attempt to easily access to governmental information and services for citizens, businesses and government agencies. Furthermore, it is always a target to improve the quality of the services and to provide greater opportunities for participating in democratic institutions and processes (Lambrinoudakisa et al. 2003). E-Government can create significant benefits for citizens, businesses and governments around the world (Mihar & Hayder, 2007).

One of the flagships of MSC is the E- Government Flagship. This flagship seeks to improve the convenience, accessibility, and quality of interactions between citizens, the business and government sectors. It uses ICT and multimedia technologies to transform the way the government operates and improves the processes of policy development, coordination and enforcement. It includes Generic Office Environment (GOE), Electronic Procurement (eP), Project Monitoring System (SPP II), Human Resource Management System (HRMIS), Electronic delivery Services (E-services++), Electronic Labor Exchange (ELX) and E-Syariah.

Another prominent E-government application introduced in 2005 in Malaysia is the Electronic Tax- Filing (E-Filing) of income taxes. The electronic filing of income tax returns is an invaluable application that assists tax filers with the process of collecting their personal tax information and provides them the ability to electronically transmit their return. According to Fu et al. (2006) electronic filing of income taxes has the potential of improving the overall process of tax filing for the individual filer while at the same time reducing the cost to both taxpayers and tax collection agencies.

Figure 2. PC Penetration Rates (Adapted From The National ICT Association of Malaysia (PIKOM))

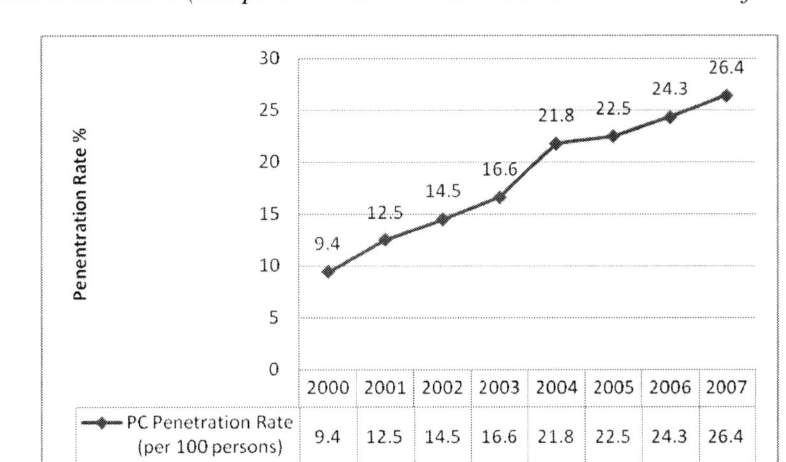

	2000	2001	2002	2003	2004	2005	2006	2007
PC Penetration Rate (per 100 persons)	9.4	12.5	14.5	16.6	21.8	22.5	24.3	26.4

Figure 3. Internet and Broadband Penetration Rates (Adapted From PIKOM 2008)

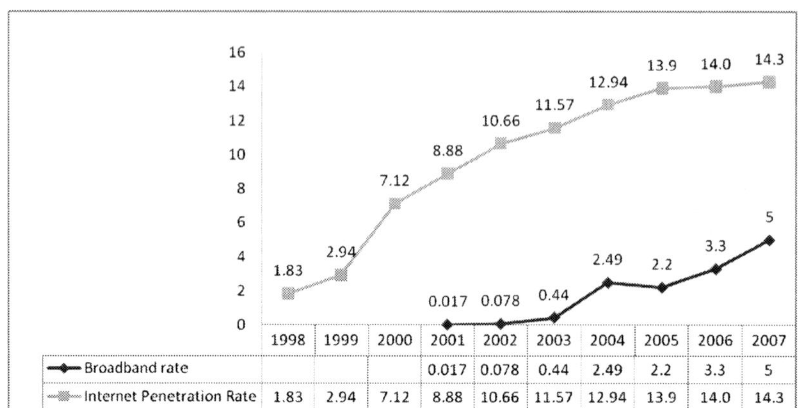

CASE DESCRIPTION: THE DEVELOPMENT OF E-FILING SYSTEM IN MALAYSIA

In Malaysia currently there are two major tax filing methods: manually and E-Filing (Internet filing). Since 2005 the Malaysian government has moved aggressively to promote the Internet filing (E-Filing) with the aim for paperless transaction, efficient process and faster refunds. Traditionally the tax payers in Malaysia have to file their tax returns manually by receiving the B (companies) or BE (individuals) forms from the Inland Revenue Board (IRB) department. Then they need to fill up the forms, do a self- calculation on their tax, attach together all the payment receipts and send it over in person or by mail to the IRB branches and later the IRB will send to them the confirmation on the tax payment amount.

However a new paradigm has taken place when the Inland Revenue Board introduces the E-Filing system. The E-Filing system developed in 2005 was one of the remarkable businesses to consumer (B2C) E-government services established by the Malaysian government. Via E-Filing and Public Key Infrastructure features, the individual tax payers in Malaysia are able to easily, quickly and safely file their tax returns.

According to Inland Revenue Board public relations officer Najlah Ishak, the electronic filing (E-Filing) of the income tax returns have increased by 30% to 1.25 million this year (2009). She stated that the number of taxpayers making E-Filing had increased gradually from 78,718 in 2006 to 538,558 (2007) and 881,387 (2008) (The Star, 01/05/2009).

Basically there are four main steps involve in filing tax electronically. The steps are:

The Advantages and Disadvantages of E- Filing System

E-filing provides many advantages to taxpayers. Among the advantages are:

(http://www.mykad.com.my/Website/secu-reefiling.php)

- **Immediate acknowledgement**
  - ○ The tax filers will get immediate acknowledgement from IRB after submission online
- **Round the clock availability and convenience**
  - ○ E-Filing is available round the clock daily. The submission work is not constrained by IRB' working hours. As long as the tax filers submit the

Figure 4. How E- Filing works (Adapted from: MSC Trustgate.com Sdn. Bhd)

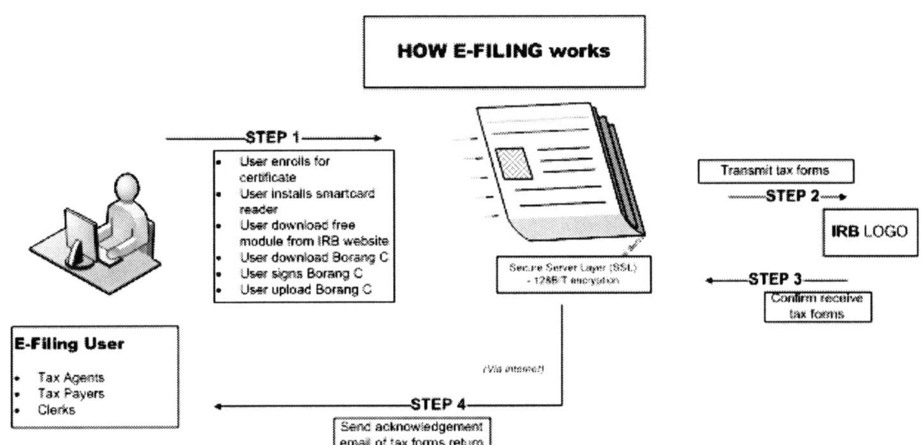

tax forms before midnight on the due date, no late penalty will be payable.

- **Immediate processing time**
  - With E-filing submissions, the tax filers can enjoy the benefits of immediacy. There is no need to physically move tax forms or wait in queues for 20 minutes or more for manual processing.
- **Cost savings**
  - There are net savings in using E-Filing system - no physical movement of tax forms, no waiting time, no transport cost and no risk of losing tax forms. Instead, tax filers enjoy convenience, 24-hour accessibility, and fast, secured and accurate tax computation.
- **User friendly**
  - The look and feel of the E-Filing-system has been designed with a user-friendly interface to allow the tax filers to easily enter or amend any information before it is submitted to IRB.
- **Security**
  - The tax filers can be assured on the security features that can prevent the hacker from altering your data as the

main key features in assessing to the system will be your password and tax file number

However, E-Filing has its disadvantages as well. Some of the disadvantages are:

- **Minimum hardware and software requirement**
  - In order for the E-Filing system to be executed at the filer's convenience the main important device is personal computer (PC). It is then must be followed by Internet access and Network configuration. The minimum requirement for the PC must also be installed with Windows XP or higher software and must have an Adobe reader application for the forms to be successfully downloaded. Failure to have all this features will enable the tax filers to access to the E-Filing website and perform the transactions.
- **Non-modification**
  - Once the forms are sent to IRB, there will be no room for modification. If the tax filers have missed any information that are supposed to be in-

cluded or excluded then they have to proceed with it manually by referring to the respective IRB branches.

- **Non-user friendly**
  - There have been a lot of complaints from the tax payers that the time allowed to do the transaction is limited. Most of the time the key-in are stopped due to time elapsed and once the system is re-entered, all the data would have to be key in once again. This has created a problem for last minute filers. (http://thestar.com.my/news/story.asp?file=/2009/3/2/focus/3380923&sec=focus)

CURRENT CHALLENGES OF E -GOVERNMENT

- **Low level of personal computer (PC), internet and broadband penetration**

It can be seen that the cellular phone growth is much more pronounced than PC or internet or broadband. This may be due to the ease of application, versatility, and convenience of anytime and everywhere usage and ongoing price reduction resulting from stiff competition among service providers. Various reasons such as poor access, lack of adequate local content, low level of awareness and motivation and lack of affordability have been cited for the low uptake of PC, Internet and Broadband (The National ICT Association of Malaysia (PIKOM), 2008)

- **Mandatory usage**

Based on survey done by Skillman (1998) in United States, the tax accountants asserted that the only way to make their tax clients to use the E-Filing is by making it a mandated usage. However, this is not the case for Malaysia where mandating electronic filing too early will attract mush resistance and criticism due to the inequality of Malaysian citizens in terms of the digital divide; income level and age factor (Lai et al. 2005). The survey also finds that the traditional channels will still need to be retained for the need of social ties, human contact and for personalization.

According to Paul and Kim (2003) quoting the articles of Wang et al., if a person is unable to use the technologies that E-government relies upon, for lack of education or limited ability, that person cannot be denied access to government information and services. "If less-advantaged segments of the population are less able to access government on the Web, their other channels to government must not be closed off or contracted."

- Availability of IT workforce

It is widely believed that with respect to IT manpower resources, the tax authority is generally suffering from a shortage IT workforce. According to IRB's Annual Report 2006, the percentage of workforce distributed for IT tasks were only 2.6%. This figure has not increased much from 2001 where the percentage of IT workforce distributed in 2001 was 2.1% (IRB Annual Report, 2001). This low distribution of workforce could dampen the effectiveness of the IT related services offered by the tax authority.

- **Digital divide**

Low ownership of PCs and disparities in internet access are among the most important challenges Malaysia faces today in implementing E-government services. Efforts to narrow the digital divide will be further intensified. For example, more Medan Info Desa and Pusat Internet Desa will continue to be built and upgraded. The government has set target to provide at least one telecentre for each mukim by 2010. (Mid Term Review, 9MP)

BARRIERS TO E-GOVERNMENT ADOPTION

• ICT infrastructure

In order for a technology to be adopted successfully, any E-government initiatives must ensure that it has sufficient resources, adequate infrastructure, management support, capable Information Technology (IT) staff and effective IT training and support. Although with the introduction of E-government services the cost will be reduced but adequate IT infrastructure still a key barrier to e- government adoption. The infrastructure is composed of hardware and software that will provide secure electronic services to citizens, businesses, and employees. For example, Local Area Network (LAN), reliable server, and internet connections are important to build a strong foundation for E-government infrastructures (Zakareya & Zahir, 2005).

• Security concerns

Another most significant barrier in implementing E-government applications is the security of the particular system. According to Lai et al. (2005), concerns over security of online tax transactions constitute a tremendous barrier to technology adoption. Sena and Paul (2009) agreed that the main reason for the decrease in the usage of Internet banking (IB) in Turkey is due to perceived risk on security features of IB. These findings is also supported by Mc Clure (2000) who finds that E-government will only succeed when all its participants including the government agencies, private business and individual citizens feel comfortable using electronic means to carry out private sensitive transactions. Stories about the hacker attack, page defacement makes the general public reluctant to do "real" business over the Internet.

• Change factor

As with E-government, public sector administrations are required to change and re-engineer their business process to adapt new strategies and culture of E-government. Government staff should be prepared for new ways of dealing with new technologies that emerge with E-government. For example, they are used in dealing with physical papers and forms, paper receipts, and traditional physical signatures, while E-government allows citizens access to the organization back-office remotely to complete the transaction processing, which emerged with new technology solutions such as electronic forms, digital signatures, electronic receipts and certificates. This reluctant to change from traditional way of doing work to a new paradigm is a major barrier to adoption (Zakareya & Zahir, 2005)

• Low confidence in the electronic administrative

According to Lai et al. (2005) one of the reasons for low usage of E-Filing system is due to low confidence in the electronic administrative capabilities of the tax authority in managing the E-Filing system successfully. The respondents perceived that the tax officers lack in the required skills, experience and competency as well as the ability in handling disaster recovery and technological crisis. Lai et al. also quoted Bird and Oldman's (2000) study which found that favourable attitude and trust in the tax authorities in managing electronic tax administration system has lead to high level of usage of E-Filing system in Singapore.

FUTURE TRENDS

Building a successful E-government adoption especially the E-Filing system may involve multiple approaches. There are general approaches and technical details. The general approaches will be first, bridging the digital divide. Government must always ensure that efforts are taken to bridge the difference in ICT supply and usage between the rural and the urban people. The Malaysian government in bridging the digital divide has constructed 108 Medan Info Desa in rural areas, 387 telecentres established, 42 Pusat Internet Desa was upgraded and targeted to provide at least one telecentre for each mukim by 2010 (PIKOM, 2008). Second approach is the IRB must create a long term marketing campaign strategy to convert reluctant taxpayers by tout that E-Filing is more convenient and less time consuming than sending paperwork via the mail, reduces preparation time, provide faster refunds, improves accuracy of returns and gives an acknowledgement-of-return receipt (Matthew, 2006). Third approach is by arranging programs such as Volunteer Income Tax Assistance and Tax Counselling for the Elderly in an effort to bring the elderly people to use the E-Filing system (Matthew, 2006). Fourth approach is on the security concerns; the normal procedure used to log in is the password and tax file number. This normal security codes are quite weak and passwords are often easy to guess, steal or crack.

In recent years, technical details approach is biometrics-based identification and authentication systems have become more widespread and have been considered for application in many application domains. Biometric techniques, such as fingerprint verification, iris or face recognition, retina analysis and hand-written signature verification, are increasingly becoming basic elements of authentication and identification systems (Zorkadis & Donos, 2004).

CONCLUSION

It is our tentative conclusion that the ICT industry in Malaysia is poised to grow positively in years to come. The role of the government in spearheading the deployment of ICT in major development corridors, continuing efforts to computerization of public services, globalization and market liberalization of financial and telecommunication verticals are among many other factors poised to contribute substantially to the economy (PIKOM 2008). The rate of increase in the number of tax filers using the E-Filing system shows the effectiveness and success of the system each year. However, for a better security, the third factor authentication process should be provided. The third authentication factor is the use of biometric such as iris or thumbprint recognition. As such, if passwords have been compromised, fraudsters need to get through another two levels of authentication to access a customer account. This would be difficult, if not, totally impossible.

REFERENCES

Abdullatif, I. A., & Philip, J. K. (2009). Rethinking Models of Technology Adoption for Internet Banking: The role of Website Features. *Journal of Financial Services Marketing*, *14*(1), 56–69. doi:10.1057/fsm.2009.4

Antonopoulos, C., & Sakellaris, P. (2009). The Contribution of Information and Communication Technology Investments to Greek Economic Growth: An Analytical Growth Accounting Framework. *Information Economics and Policy*, *21*, 171–191. doi:10.1016/j.infoecopol.2008.12.001

Astrid, D., Mitra, A., & David, M. (2008). The Role of Perceived Enjoyment and social Norm in the Adoption of Technology with Network Externalities. *European Journal of Information Systems*, *17*, 4–11. doi:10.1057/palgrave.ejis.3000726

Azleen, I., Mohd Zulkeflee, A. R., & Mohd Rushdan, Y. (2009). Taxpayers' Attitude In Using E-Filing System: Is There Any Significant Difference Among Demographic Factors? *Journal of Internet Banking and Commerce*, *14*(1), 2–13.

David, Y. K. T. (2008). A Study of e-Recruitment Technology Adoption in Malaysia. *Industrial Management & Data Systems, 109*(2), 281–300.

Davidson, R. M., Wagner, C., & Ma, L. C. K. (2005). From government to e-government: A transitional Model. *Information Technology & People, 18*(3), 280–299. doi:10.1108/09593840510615888

Economic Planning Unit (EPU). *The Mid Term Review of the Ninth Malaysian Plan*: 2006-2010.

Fu, J. R., Farn, C. K., & Chao, W. P. (2006). Acceptance of electronic tax filing: A study of taxpayers' intention. *Information & Management, 43*, 109–126. doi:10.1016/j.im.2005.04.001

Hesson, M., & Al-Ameed, H. (2007). Online security evaluation process for new e-services. *Journal of Business Process Management, 13*(2), 223–245. doi:10.1108/14637150710740473

Irani, Z., Dwivedi, Y. K., & Williams, M. D. (2008). Understanding Consumer Adoption of Broadband: An Extension of the Technology Acceptance Model. *The Journal of the Operational Research Society*, 1–13.

IRB. (2001). *Annual Report 2001*. Malaysia: Inland Revenue Board.

IRB. (2006). *Annual Report 2006*. Malaysia: Inland Revenue Board.

Jalava, J., & Pohjola, M. (2002). Economic Growth in the New Economy: evidence from advanced economies. *Information Economics and Policy, 14*, 189–210. doi:10.1016/S0167-6245(01)00066-X

Jalava, J., & Pohjola, M. (2007). The Role of Electricity and ICT in Economic Growth: Case Finland. *Explorations in Economic History, 45*, 270–287. doi:10.1016/j.eeh.2007.11.001

Junaidah, H. (2008). Learning Barriers in Adopting ICT among Selected Working Women in Malaysia. *Gender in Management: An International Journal, 23*(5), 317–336. doi:10.1108/17542410810887356

Khalil, T. M. (1993). Management of Technology and the Creation of Wealth. *Industrial Engineering (American Institute of Industrial Engineers), 25*(9), 16–17.

Khalil, T. M. (2000). *Management of Technology: The key to Competitiveness and Wealth Creation.* Singapore: McGraw Hill.

Kuppusamy, M., Raman, M., & Lee, G. (2009). Whose ICT Investment Matters To Economic Growth: Private or Public? The Malaysian Perspective. *The Electronic Journal on Information Systems in Developing Countries, 37*(7), 1–19.

Kuppusamy, M., & Shanmugam, B. (2007). Information Communication Technology and Economic Growth in Malaysia. *Review of Islamic Economics, 11*(2), 87–100.

Lai, M.L., Siti, N.S.O., & Ahamed, K.M. (2004). Towards An Electronic Filing System: A Malaysian Survey. *eJournal of Tax Research, 5*(2), 1-11.

Lai, M. L., Siti, N. S. O., & Ahamed, K. M. (2005). Tax Practitioners And The Electronic Filing System: An Empirical Analysis. *Academy of Accounting and Financial Studies Journal, 9*(1), 93–109.

Lambrinoudakisa, C., Gritzalisa, S., Dridib, F., & Pernul, G. (2003). Security requirements for e-government services: A methodological approach for developing a common PKI-based security policy. *Computer Communications, 26*, 1873–1883. doi:10.1016/S0140-3664(03)00082-3

Lee, S. M. (2003). Korea: from the land of morning calm to ICT hotbed. [Abstract]. *Journal of the Academy Management Executive (USA), 17*(2).

Matthew, W. (2006). *E-File Goals too Ambitious. FWC.COM*. Retrieved on 2/11/2009, from http://fcw.com/articles/2006/02/27 /efile-goal-too-ambitious.aspx

Mc Clure, D. L. (2000).Federal Initiatives Are Evolving Rapidly But They Face Significant Challenges. *Testimony* United States General Accounting Office, GAO/T-AIMD/GGD-00-179.

Md Nor, K., & Pearson, J. M. (2007). The Influence of Trust on Internet Banking Acceptance. *Journal of Internet Banking and Commerce, 12*(2), 2–10.

Mihyar, H., & Hayder, A. (2007). Online security evaluation process for new e-services. *Journal of Business Process Management, 13*(2), 223–246. doi:10.1108/14637150710740473

Paul, T. J., & Kim, M. T. (2003). E-government Around the World: Lessons, Challenges and Future Directions. *Government Information Quarterly, 20*, 389–394. doi:10.1016/j.giq.2003.08.001

Raman, M., Stephenaus, R., Alam, N., & Kuppusamy, M. (2008). Information Technology in Malaysia: E-Service Quality and Uptake of Internet Banking. *Journal of Internet Banking and Commerce, 13*(2), 2–17.

Ramayah, T., Ramoo, V., & Ibrahim, A. (2008). Profiling Online And Manual Tax Filers: Results from An Exploratory Study In Penang, Malaysia. *Labuan e-Journal of Muamalat and Society, 2*, 1-18.

Sena, O., & Paul, P. (2009). Exploring the adoption of a service innovation: A study of Internet banking adopters and non-adopters. *Journal of Financial Services Marketing, 13*(4), 284–299. doi:10.1057/fsm.2008.25

Skillman, B. (1998). Fired up at the IRS. *Accounting Technology, 14*, 12–20.

Solow, R. M. (1957). Technical Change and the Aggregate Production Function. *The Review of Economics and Statistics, 39*(3), 312–320. doi:10.2307/1926047

The STAR. (2009). Amount of Malaysian's choosing e-filing up by 30%. 1st May.

The, S. T. A. R. (2009). *It's Time Inland Revenue Board got Real on E-Filing*. Retrieved on June 19th, 2009. from http://thestar.com.my/news/story.asp? file=/2009/3/2/focus/3380923&sec=focus

The National ICT Association of Malaysia (PIKOM). (2008). *ICT Strategies, Societal and Market Touch*. Retrieved on June 24th, 2009. from http://www.witsa.org/news/2009-1 /html_email_newsletter_jan09_b.html

Trustgate Sdn, M. S. C. Bhd. (2009). *Secure E-Filing*. Retrieved on June 24th, 2009. from http://www.mykad.com.my /Website/secureefiling.php

Zakareya, E., & Zahir, I. (2005). E-Government Adoption: Architecture and Barriers. *Business Process Management Journal, 11*(5), 589–611. doi:10.1108/14637150510619902

Zorkadis, V., & Donos, P. (2004). On biometrics-based authentication and identification from a privacy-protection perspective deriving privacy-enhancing requirements. *Information Management & Computer Security, 12*(1), 125–137. doi:10.1108/09685220410518883

KEY TERMS AND DEFINITIONS

Information Communication Technologies: ICT covers the use of advanced technologies in private and public sectors in order to give a better service to the customers. It includes the technologies such as broadcasting information and wireless mobile telecommunications.

Economic Growth: Growth is the increase in the country's profit in terms of goods and services produced, monetary profits earned and increased in total productivity. Normally, economic growth is calculated based on the increase in Gross Domestic Product of the particular country.

E-Government: E-government refers to electronic government which means governments in a particular country use ICT or internet base to provide their services. This is done in order to improve the quality of their services, interactions and transactions with customers and businesses mainly.

E-Filing System: E-Filing system in Malaysia which is recently launched in 2006 is the way to submit the tax documents to the Inland Revenue Board through internet or online without the need to submit any paper documents. This system has provided an easy, faster and safer way of submitting the tax documents by the tax filers.

Technology Adoption: Technology Adoption refers to the rate of usage a particular technology by the consumers when it is introduced in the country either by the government or the private sectors. There are various reasons has been outline that can affect the usage or adoption of the particular system such as readiness, security concerns and level of education.

Authentication: Is the process through which an Internet merchant can be established via a trusted third party that guarantees that the merchant is indeed whom he is.

Security: In the context of E-Filing System threats can be made either through network and data filing attacks or through unauthorized access to the tax file by means of false or defective authentication.

Chapter 3
Web Services for Bioinformatics

Abad Shah
University of Engineering and Technology, Pakistan

Zafar Singhera
Oracle Corporation, USA

Syed Ahsan
University of Engineering and Technology, Pakistan

EXECUTIVE SUMMARY

A large number of tools are available to Bioinformaticians to analyze the rapidly growing databanks of molecular biological data. These databanks represent complex biological systems and in order to understand them, it is often necessary to link many disparate data sets and use more than one analysis tool. However, owing to the lack of standards for data sets and the interfaces of the tools this is not a trivial task. Over the past few years, web services has become a popular way of sharing the data and tools distributed over the web and used by different researchers all over the globe. In this chapter we discuss the interoperability problem of databanks and tools and how web services are being used to try to solve it. These efforts have resulted in the evolution of web services tools from HTML/web form-based tools not suited for automatic workflow generation to advances in Semantic Web and Ontologies that have revolutionized the role of semantics. Also included is a discussion on two extensively used Web Service systems for Life Sciences, myGrid and Semantic-MOBY. In the end we discuss how the state-of-art research and technological development in Semantic Web, Ontology and Database Management can help address these issues.

INTRODUCTION

The two major problems that biological scientists are facing are distribution and heterogeneity of the data and its analysis tools. These problems are due to autonomous, decentralized and individualistic

web based approach towards the biological research (Bodenreider & Stevens, 2006). Integration of the data and tools is a difficult task but it is vital for the integrative *insilico* experimentation and exchange of results (Lord et al., 2004). Biology has coped with this work in an effective but in ad-hoc manner. Almost all databases and tools of bioinformatics that have been made available on

DOI: 10.4018/978-1-60960-015-0.ch003

the web and the data integration techniques have been applied to the bioinformatics domain have met limited success because the data and information are made available in a non-standardized way (Lord et al., 2004; Post et al, 2007). However, unlike other domains, the bioinformatics domain on the Web has embraced the standards, such as XML and web services, and there exists a large number of bioinformatics data sources that are either accessible as web services or provide data using XML (Thakar, Ambite & Knoblock, 2005). A web service is a program/software that can be executed on a remote machine owning to the industry efforts to standardize web service description, discovery and invocation. These efforts have led to standards such as WSDL (Christenson et al, 2001), UDDI (UDDI2002), and SOAP (SOAP 2000) (Thakar, Ambite & Knoblock, 2005).

The integration of such services and their interoperability is now feasible by using web services technologies and the researchers can easily construct bioinformatics workflows and pipelines by combining two or more web services to solve their complex biological tasks such as protein function prediction, genome annotation, micro array analysis, etc (Cannta N., et al, 2008). However, these standards, in their current form, suffer from the lack of semantic representation leaving the promise of automatic integration of applications written to web services standards unfulfilled (Labarga et al., 2007).

More recently efforts have been made to populate web services with semantic metadata and semantic descriptions to enhance data exchange and integration (Lord et al., 2004; Thakar et al., 2005; Post et al., 2007). A semantic web approach provides standardized formats (such as RDF, RDF Schema (RDFS) and OWL) to achieve a formalized computational environment. The objective of Semantic Web is to bring meaning to the raw data content by defining relationships between distinct concepts using ontologies (Cabrall L. et al., 2004). The existing life sciences databanks can be built with better retrieval performance using ontological

abstractions. Fortunately, the life sciences community has realized that the semantic modeling is a necessity for the biological knowledge bases (Ruttenberg et al., 2007) and many biological ontology initiatives exist (http://obo.sourceforge. net), with Gene Ontology (GO) and it is the most widely adopted ontology ((Bodenreider O. & Stevens R., 2006; Ashburner et al., 2000).

However, a complete and seamless semantic integration of data and information sources and tools is a challenging objective that we are facing, amongst others. Problems related to the shared definitions of knowledge domains, i.e., ontologies, association of biological concepts to the existing data, semantic descriptions of services/ requirements and automatic workflow generation (Bodenreider O. & Stevens R., 2006).

We feel that for a complete understanding and appreciation of the problems faced by the integrative biology researchers, the evolution of web services tools from HTML/web form-based tools not suited for automatic workflow generation to advances in Semantic Web and Ontologies that have revolutionized the role of semantics must be traced. Also, we must examine how the state-of-art research and technological development in Semantic Web, Ontology and Database Management can help address these issues. Remainder of the chapter is organized as follows. In Section 2, we describe the special nature of the life sciences research which has led to adoption of e-science to the life science community as a necessity. In Section 3, the past efforts and solutions to cope with the problems of distribution and heterogeneity of life science resources are described. Section 4 discusses the evolution of web services for the life sciences domain. The web services architecture and its limitations are also included in this section. The role of Semantic Web for realization of semantic web services and its promising potential for the life sciences research in Section 5 and Section 6. In Section 6, we also analyze two widely used life sciences web service systems, Semantic-MOBY and myGRID.

Section 7 includes an overview of vendor web service platforms such as from Sun, IBM, SAP, Oracle and JBoss etc. We conclude this chapter in Section 8 by summarizing our contributions and future work.

NATURE OF BIOLOGICAL RESEARCH

Biological research has moved towards the post genomic era where the bottleneck has rapidly shifted to the annotation of the produced DNA sequence data, and the inter-genome research is increasingly being done (Lein et al., 2007; Souchelnytskyi, 2005; Ahsan S.& Shah A., 2008).The scientists are now able to perform complex *insilico* experiments such as characterizing a gene in terms of a sequence, its translation, expression profile, function and structure by accessing widely distributed services. Huge projects with numerous research groups collaborate to tackle complex issues such as annotating the human genome (Bodenreider O. & Stevens R., 2006). The challenge of unraveling gene functions and better understand gene regulation processes requires fast, unlimited and integrative access to the analysis tools (Labarga et al., 2007; Post et.al, 2007).

Integrating the heterogeneous data sets and tools across different databanks and the computing environments, however, is technically quite challenging due to non standardized search interfaces, web pages and APIs (Bodenreider O. & Stevens R., 2006). The difficulty is further compounded by the volatile nature of these data sets which periodically change their export formats, effectively rendering the tools useless that provide access to their data (Ahsan S. & Shah A, 2008). Most of the genomics databanks and tools do not yet provide enough standardized computer-readable metadata to facilitate the workflow automation and integration (Neerincx & Leunissen, 2005).. Hence, the bottleneck of domain-specific knowledge expert needed to interpret what the data actu-

ally represents before using it in the integration experiments cannot be removed. Because of this limitation, integrative biology experimentation is not optimal, given the variety and amount of data and tools available from distributed resources (Post et.al, 2007).

Therefore, in our opinion the life science research community should be provided with an integrated, transparent access to the analytical tools of experimentation which is necessary to achieve the following goals.

1. Support wet lab (In-silico) experiments
2. Avoid reenactment of experiments
3. Achieve interoperability of data and applications
4. Enable reusability of workflows and results
5. Share results through transparent exchange of data
6. Provide inter-application communication
7. Create, store and access experimentation procedure/methodology i.e workflows as the workflows are considered the research results in the life science research.
8. Support the autonomous development and collaborative Research

PREVIOUS EFFORTS AND EVOLVING SOLUTIONS

All the above-mentioned challenges were faced gradually by the biological research community, and the community has matured and embarked on exploring more. This resulted in continuous evolution of the bioinformatics tools. This evolution can be categorized into multiple phases. The first two of these phases used the centralized data-warehousing strategy while the remaining promoted federated or distributed strategy (Stevens R., 2003). The following paragraphs describe challenges and developments in each of those phases.

First Phase

Biological research started in silos with a few biological labs around the globe, each one was working on a specific set of problems. Each of these labs had their own data formats and analysis tools and lacked interoperability, consistency and data/results reusability features. Each lab also designed its own data formats and data analysis tools (Etzold, T. & Argos P. 1993). These tools were mostly co-located with data and were highly dependent on their execution environment and data format. This resulted not only in huge volumes of data autonomously collected by each lab, but also in equally large number of diverse data formats and analysis tools. Such tools can be categorized in the first phase.

Second Phase

With better understanding at the micro-level and increased curiosity for the data correlation across the labs, the research groups started exchanging their data and analysis tools. Moreover, instead of doing a single monolithic analysis on a data set, the scientists got interested in building analysis chains and workflows at each step in the workflow potentially involving different tool to analyze data produced by the previous step. These requirements encouraged some primitive efforts to define common data formats; developing tools to transform from one format to another; consistency among execution environments or at least efficient porting of tools and data across the environments; and analysis tools that work with common data formats and their extensions. However, tools in this phase still required to physically migrate data and tools across computing environments.

Third Phase

Moving data and tools from one environment to the other was laborious, time consuming, and error prone. Moving data across was a bigger concern because of huge data volumes, security, ownership, and consistency concerns. The third phase focused on the moving of analysis tools across system boundaries but accessing data from remote data repositories that were managed by the data owner or one of its trusted entities. Data repositories used during this phase primarily include relational database management systems (DBMS) like MySQL, PostgresSQL and Oracle; or flat-file indexing systems. One well-known such system is Sequence Retrieval System (SRS) that used flat-file indexing system (Etzold, T. & Argos P. 1993). Although not as efficient as those with co-located data, these tools however alleviated data security, consistency, and ownership concerns and saved manual data transfer efforts.

Fourth Phase

The performance of the tools in the third phase was poor because data had to be accessed remotely at a granular level during analysis. Moreover, tool consistency, update, and ownership problems were still there. This resulted in evolution to the next generation of tools that accessed a remote service where both the analysis functionality and its related data was potentially co-located in the same environment but was accessed by a client from a remote location. These tools involved in making request for a particular analysis using a specific data set, and getting the results. This approach provided a complete ownership of both data and tool to the service provider along with better performance, and allowed more manageable evolution of the tool. Early such tools were developed using distributed technologies like Remote Procedure Call (RPC), Remote Method Invocation (RMI), and Common Object Requesting Broker Architecture (CORBA). These tools still did not make the service consumer completely agnostic to the service consumer. A custom client was required for every remote service including installation of relevant distributed libraries in the client environment. There was potential for inconsistency in the request mechanism and response format. Hierarchical Access System for Sequence Libraries in Europe (HASSEL) was one of such system (Doelz R. et al., 1994). It was unfortunately ahead of its time and did not get enough attention. It was eventually abandoned in 1996.

Fifth Phase

Emergence of web caught attention of life sciences community because the autonomous, collaborative, and temporally unstable life science research mapped well with the inherently distributed, cost–effective, autonomous, easy to navigate, and volatile structure of Web (Neerincx & Leunissen, 2005). The Web and its browsers presented some features that the biological research community was eagerly looking for. Those features included a consistent client that can present a variety of diverse information by coding the appropriate web pages, a simple and friendly interface, a trusted protocol that is usually allowed to flow across network firewall boundaries and a simple enough framework that allows for efficiently building user interfaces on front-end and request-handling adapters on the back-end. A set of libraries and tools emerged to develop such interfaces and adapters, including: BioPerl, BioPython, BioJava, BioRuby, BioSQL (OpenBioInformatics Projects). Quick Web interfaces and HTTP adapters were developed and deployed in front of the existing tools so that information becomes accessible through a web browser. Primitive screen scraping tools and sophisticated scrapping and form generation tools were developed so that response from one analysis can be reformatted, can be fed as input to the next analysis in a workflow and can be automated. This provides significant advantage over the tools in the previous phases but they are inefficient because the overhead of generating a page that is only screen scraped by another tool, lack of service discovery mechanism, and complex and ad-hoc mechanisms to integrate individual tools into an integrated complex workflow. Sight

(Meskauskas, Lehmann-Horn & Kurkat-Rott 2004) and ASAP (Kossenkov et. al. 2003) were two such initiatives.

WEB SERVICES: APLICABILITY AND LIMITATIONS

Web services offer the features that were lacking in the tools described in the five (5) phases (see Section 3). As we have discussed in Section 3, the integration and interoperation of the conventional web based tools are hindered, amongst others, because of the following reasons (Knikker R. et al., 2004).

1. The applications are not language and platform independent.
2. Lack of machine friendly web interface.
3. Non-standard input and output data format of the web interfaces, application interface and message exchange protocol.
4. Transport protocols for the remote messaging are often not firewall-friendly.
5. Lack of automated service description, discovery, and integration.

Web services eliminate the need to develop and rely on ad-hoc screen scrapping mechanism that are used during the five (5) phases and offer a single uniform method for the application integration through the Internet. They provide a model for web applications in which their public interfaces and bindings are defined and described using an XML standard format (Benjamin M. & Mark D., 2006). Also, the use of XML-based messaging render the web services infrastructure platform- and language-independent and changes to the interface can immediately be detected by client software.

The basic profile of the Interoperability model (WS-I) (http://www.ws-i.org/) of Web Services describes the model as follows (Knikker R. et al., 2004; Rama A. et al., 2003):

Figure 1. Web Service architecture and service model

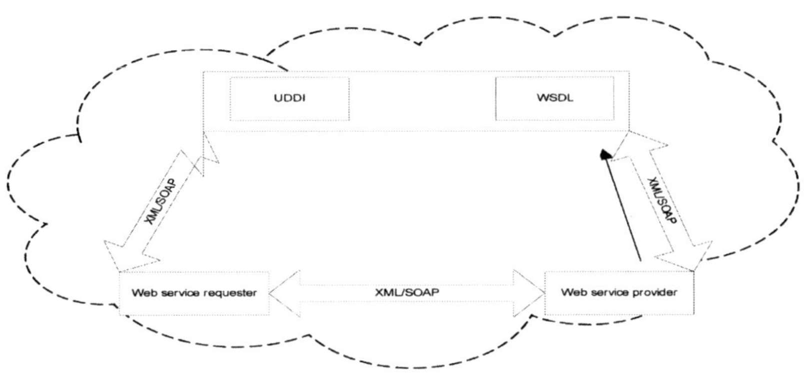

(1) The Web Service Description Language (WSDL) (http://www.w3.org/TR/wsdl) uses the XML standard format that describes a web service interface and the exchange of messages between the provider and requester in an abstract manner. Service providers are generally specialized ge-nome" centers such as National Center for Biotechnology Information (NCBI), European Bioinformatics Institute (EBI). Service consumers mostly are working in smaller laboratories and research groups with smaller, non-specialist resources (Knikker R. et al., 2004; Rama A. et al., 2003).

(2) Simple Object Access Protocol (SOAP) is an XML-based protocol for the stateless mes-sage exchange which, in general, has been developed on the top of HTTP. This makes WS -I firewall friendly as opposed to the protocols used by (CORBA) (Benjamin M. & Mark D., 2006; Knikker R. et al., 2004) (for detail see Section 3).

(3) Universal Description, Discovery and Integration (UDDI) are a standard protocol designed to publish details about an orga-nization and the web services. It provides a description and definition of web services in a central repository, which functions as yellow pages for web services. WSDL and

SOAP are the W3C standards, while UDDI is an Organization for the Advancement of Structured Information Standards (OASIS) standard. For a client to use a web service it only needs WSDL with SOAP that is com-monly being used as the default protocol (Knikker R. et al., 2004, Benjamin M. & Mark D., 2006).

Web services have been able to solve the in-teroperability problem with some success in the cases of small and well-defined domains where service provider and service requester have agreed upon the shared knowledge and semantic descrip-tions. However, web services have met with limited success to solve the most critical interoperability problems in the life sciences domain (Knikker R. et al., 2004; Lord et al., 2004). In this domain, the researchers have to construct bioinformatics workflows combining two or more web services from different locations to solve the complex biological tasks such as protein function -predic-tion, genome annotation, micro- array analysis, etc (Benjamin M. & Mark D., 2006). Discovery of a relevant and appropriate web service depends upon the ability of the service provider to provide appropriate descriptions of the web service. The service requester can then discover these services from these descriptions for composition of a workflow. However, the lack of machine readable semantic descriptions necessitates the intervention of expert biologists and bioinormaticians for the automated service discovery and composition of the complex workflows within open systems (Labarga et al., 2007). As mentioned in Section 3, this limits the practical scale and breadth of the integration, given the variety and amount of data and tools available from distributed resources (Post et al., 2007) .The primary reasons which hamper the much desired automation of the discovery, composition and invocation of web services and workflows are summarized below:

1. UDDI search capabilities in its current form are limited to the keyword-based matching. It does not capture semantic relationships between entries in its directories. (Rama A. et al., 2003).

2. UDDI supports search based on only the high-level information specified about businesses and services, i.e., the final state specification. The transitory and intermediate capabilities of the web service are not specified (Labarga et al., 2007; Rama A. et al., 2003). However, UDDI service registrations may include references to the WSDL descriptions, which may facilitate the limited automation of the discovery and invocation. But, the absence of any explicit semantic information limits the automated comprehension of the WSDL description to simple ontologies in domains without contextual and conceptual differences (Rama A. et al., 2003; Cabrall L. et al., 2004).

3. With the parameterized input invocation for filtering and delimiting the search domain is not available (Rama A. et al., 2003).

4. The search facilities in UDDI are restricted to exact matches because the search is syntax based. This discourages service composition and workflows (Rama A. et al., 2003).

5. Owning to the limitation of range imposed by non-semantic descriptions, not all WSDL documents describe the non-functional attributes such as authenticity, currency, efficiency, performance, scalability, etc. Even in the way WSDL+OWL-S, the mapping OWL-S into WSDL may lose much semantic information because WSDL can not express the abundance semantics of OWL (Knikker R. et al., 2004 ; Lord et al., 2004).

6. Both the service providers and service consumers want to remain back-ward compatible to the legacy formats. The service consumers want their data in legacy formats so that the existing tools can operate over it. The service providers are wary of changing requirements of myriad of the existing data formats. Although this is not a serious problem for the simple data types, it has serious implications for most of the biological data which is highly complex and internally structured (Cabrall L. et al., 2004).

7. Scripts which are used to compose work flows are monolithic and complex and hence lack reusability (Labarga et al., 2007; Lord et al., 2004).

Related Work

The bioinformatics research community has created thousands of web services to access several hundred databases and analysis methods (Galperin, 2005) that differ in data formats, interfaces and semantics of concepts used. Unfortunately, these differences of format, interfaces and semantics are also reflected in web services accessing them.

As of 2008, publicly accessible third party Web Services as registered by *my*Grid project number more than 1500, and still growing. Most of these web services are UDDI based, making them difficult to use as the text -based input must be provided in correct format (Cannta N., et al, 2008). Also the data at well-known sources, such as NCBI or EMBL, is not necessarily available for in-depth analysis primarily because the interfaces provided involve human interaction.

Most sites have custom query interfaces and return results through a series of HTML pages. For example, NCBI BLAST (Basic Local Alignment Search Tool) requires three or four steps to retrieve sequence homologs. Web Services such as Mat-Inspector, TRANSFAC, TRRD, or COMPEL to find the common transcription binding factors need to convert into a well-known format, such as XML (Pieter B., et al, 2005).

Several available WSDL based BioGrid middle-wares like myGrid (Stevens et al., 2003a) or BioOpera (Bausch et al., 2003), to support workflow composition through discovery and creation of services using visual builder tools like Taverna (Oinn et al., 2004), still lack suitable mechanisms for handling the issue of service interoperability because WSDL lacks semantic information about both services and data at the application level. These Web services fail to achieve semantic interoperability in bioinformatics (Wilkinson et al., 2005) as they cannot distinguish between a sequence in FASTA format or in EMBL format (both are represented as strings) nor can it distinguish between a DNA sequence and a journal article It supports mainly keyword-based retrieval that can be realized by using term frequency-inverse document frequency (TF-IDF). But UDDI can neither create new service compositions nor does it support semantic-aware service discovery (Wilkinson et al., 2005).

Services, like XEMBL service (http://www.ebi.ac.uk/xembl/) and the DDBJ BLAST service (http://xml.nig.ac.jp/wsdl/) are independently built using different data formats and semantics. Thus the service interoperability is not guaranteed as the output of one service often is in a different format than the input required by the next service. The problem of heterogeneity arises when it is needed by the scientist to replace services without affecting the entire workflow, e.g. replacing a BLAST service operating on one database with a BLAST or FASTA service operating on a different database. This happens because interfaces and data structures of the replaced and replacing services may differ in unexpected ways.

The European Bioinformatics Institute provides access to more than 200 databases and to about 150 bioinformatics applications through web services such as WSDbfetch that are described by WSDL files. EBI supports SOAP services for both database information retrieval and sequence analysis. http://www.ebi.ac.uk/Tools/webservices. It also provides several methods for retrieving information about the service (getAvailableDatabases, getAvailableFormats, and getAvailableStyles) and a fetchData operation for the actual retrieval.

The EBI also provides NCBI BLAST (including PHI-BLAST and PSI-BLAST (7)), WU-BLAST (http://blast.wustl.edu) and MPsrch (http://www.ebi.ac.uk/MPsrch/) which are protein specific search tools (Labarga et al., 2007). However these web services suffer from the limitations imposed by UDDI and WSDL as discussed above.

From the above discussion we infer the observations given in the next paragraph.

With the proliferation of web services for life sciences, the issues of relevancy and integration have become highly important in the service discovery and integration. Finding and matching of web services for the probable integration is fundamentally semantic in its nature. This lack of semantics in the current industry standards (UDDI, WSDL, SOAP) is the result of the current syntax-oriented interface representations. As a result these interface representations cannot express the context in which the services operate and also the relationships among various services in that context. Both of these challenges rely on the ability of service providers to describe the capabilities of their services and the ability of service requesters to describe their requirements in an unambiguous and machine-interpretable form.

In the next section we discus the current and the on-going efforts to populate the web services with rich semantic descriptions of their capabilities to realize the objective of Semantic Web Services

(SWS). Also, we discuss the emergence and evolution of the semantic web, which provides the infrastructure for the semantic interoperability of web services to facilitate their automated composition, discovery, dynamic binding, and invocation within an open environment.

SEMANTIC WEB: THE FOUNDATION FOR SEMANTIC WEB SERVICE

As discussed in Section 4, the lack of machine readable semantics in web services necessitates the human intervention in the automated service discovery, dynamic binding, invocation of services and workflow composition within open systems. Semantic Web Services (SWSs) overcome this shortcoming by populating web services with rich formal descriptions of their capabilities (Bodenreider O. & Stevens R., 2006). A Semantic Web Service (SWS) is defined through a service ontology, which enables the machine interpretability of its capabilities as well as the integration with domain knowledge (Lord et al., 2004). Ontology is a formalization of a domain through a common, controlled vocabulary that can be reasoned over in a well-defined manner (Labarga et al., 2007; Neerincx & Leunissen, 2005).

A prelude to realization of SWS, however, has been the emergence and evolution of Semantic Web, which provides the infrastructure for the semantic interoperability of Web Services. (Cabrall L. et al., 2004). Semantic Web is a web of data and knowledge which can be interpreted by computer programs (Cabrall L. et al, 2004; Cannata et al, 2008). The current components of the Semantic Web framework are: Resource Description Framework (RDF), RDF Schema (RDF-S) and the Web Ontology Language – OWL. RDF is a XML-based standard from W3C for describing resources on the Web (Ruttenberg et al., 2007; Post et.al, 2007). It introduces a little semantics to XML data by allowing the representation of objects and their relations through properties. RDF-

Schema is a simple type system, which provides information (metadata) for the interpretation of the statements given in RDF data. OWL (http://www.w3.org/2004/OWL/) is a W3C standard for a web based ontology language that is built upon RDF and RDF-S (Bodenreider O. & Stevens R., 2006). These standards are built upon a rich set of constructs for describing the semantics of online information sources, thus enabling the semantic interoperability of Web Services through the identification (and mapping) of semantically similar concepts. (Sheila A. et al., 2001).

In the next section we discuss the direct applicability of semantic web technologies to provide the necessary infrastructure for SWS to solve the most critical problems faced by the life sciences community.

Building Blocks for Semantics: LSID, RDF, RDF-S and Ontologies

In the previous sections, we have emphasized the inability of the conventional web services to aid in automated, integrative, *in silico* web-based biological research as a result of non existence of semantic descriptions. The main hindrance in augmenting these web services with semantic descriptions is due to the shortcomings that are listed below (Benjamin M. & Mark D., 2006):

1. Lack of globally unique and resolvable names for biological entities
2. Lack of consistent standards for data and knowledge representation
3. Lack of standard interface definitions for data retrieval and processing

SW offers solutions that address each of these shortcomings/issues through the Life Science Identifier system (LSID), RDF, Ontologies and the SWS heralding for the realization of Semantic Web for Life Sciences (SWLS) (Benjamin M. & Mark D., 2006). The deployment of SWSs, however, relies on the further development and combination of Web Services and Semantic Web enabling technologies.

Standardized Data Representation: Role of LSID and RDF

Owning the nature of biological research as discussed in Section 2, the biological entities are contextual, functional and historical meaning within the biological community (Benjamin M. & Mark D., 2006). As a result, there has been and is still a conflict in agreeing to mutual acceptable identification and naming convention for biological entities. LSID is an important first step in defining a mechanism for stable, predictable and web enabled identification and retrieval of biological entities and concepts (Pieter B., et al, 2005; Benjamin M. & Mark D., 2006).

The LSID specification includes three aspects (http://www.w3.org/TR/uri-clarification) which are given as follows:

1. Standardized identifier format, including versioning;
2. Defined protocols for the retrieval of identified data and/or metadata;
3. Customary metadata syntax.

LSIDs are location independent and extremely stable, enabling reliable generation of annotations globally. Moreover they can be used to identify not only documents but also conceptual entities such as ontologies by identifying metadata only (Benjamin M., Mark D., 2006). UniProt-RDF is the first such life sciences resource to adapt LSIDs.

The LSID metadata is, by convention, provided in the RDF format which renders it interpretable by the software that retrieves it, is referred to as the *Semantic Web Browser* (SWB). The RDF document explicitly describes the relationship between the entity named LSID and other entities on SWLS (named by LSIDs or URLs) using the subject Uniform Resource Identifier (URI) (Post et al, 2007; Cabrall L. et al., 200). The intent

(semantics) of the relationship between the two entities is thus computationally accessible through URI resolution by the LSID metadata resolution protocol. This enables the life science researchers to annotate any document or ontology on SWLS by utilizing RDF containing the same URIs, dramatically reducing the effort required to integrate distributed sources of information (Benjamin M. & Mark D., 2006; Ruttenberg et al., 2007).

In life sciences, the notable efforts to automate RDF graph interpretation using SWB has been Haystack's within the myGrid project and BioDash (Post et al, 2007; Pieter B., et al, 2005). This is an elegantly simple but incredibly powerful feature. However, it is critically dependent on the community's adoption of and adherence to consistent standards for naming such as LSID (Benjamin M. & Mark D., 2006).

Knowledge Representation Using Ontologies

In life sciences, the integrative biology scientists need to execute a single query across to multiple databases to achieve data integration. For this case, a distributed query that can handle relationships between entities (e.g., equivalency) in different databases must be formulated (Cruz, 2005). Complexity of such tasks necessitates building an ontological layer on the top of RDF and RDF-S. OWL ontologies, and this layer provide the identified entities which are unambiguously defined and the relationships between them. They can be accurately interpreted and utilized in an automated fashion by SWS (Labarga et al., 2007). By defining ontologies for a complex field such as biology, eventually a knowledge base ca be built that facilitates the exchange and interoperability of the data stored in numerous available databases using SWS. (Benjamin M. & Mark D., 2006; Post et al, 2007). Only those ontologies that can be accessed directly via URI resolution such as National Cancer Institute (NCI), Thesaurus, BioPax, Microrray Gene Expression

Data (MGED), biozen, BioMoby are actually an active part of SWLS (Bodenreider O. & Stevens R., 2006; Post et.al, 2007).

The slow and technically challenging task of the migration of non-SW ontologies such as Model of Anatomy (FMA) (http://sig.biostr.washington.edu/projects/fm/) and the Unified Medical Language System (UMLS) (www.nlm.nih.gov/research/umls/) to the SW paradigm has started (Hashmi N., 2004; Wilkinson M., 2003). These ontologies, pose a difficult challenge owning to the conflicting knowledge representation frameworks and their tremendous size (Benjamin M. & Mark D., 2006; Yang et al., 2006). Such ontologies may be broken down into semantically equivalent fragments in an open and scalable manner using LSID metadata resolution. Besides the technical challenges, there is a social issue of inability of semantic content providers to release their ontologism according to the open-access paradigm of SW and this issue must be overcome (Cannta N., et al, 2008). National Center for Biomedical Ontology (cBIO) initiative of Open Biomedical Ontologies (OBO) project for the providing OWL versions of their ontologies has been a significant step towards the realization of SWLS (Benjamin M. & Mark D., 2006; Cannata et al., 2008).

BRINGING IT ALL TOGETHER

The semantic web architecture described above enables users to automate the discovery, invocation, composition and monitoring of web resources offering particular services and having particular properties (Rama A. et al., 2003). A Semantic Web Service is defined through a service ontology, which enables machine interpretability of its capabilities as well as integration with domain knowledge (Cabrall L. et al., 2004). OWL-S (formerly DAML-S) is an OWL based Web service ontology which builds on the Semantic Web stack of standards and makes the above mentioned functionalities possible. OWL-S integrates at

the knowledge-level the information which has been defined by Web services standards, such as UDDI and WSDL with related domain knowledge (http://www.w3.org/2004/OWL/). However, its expressivity and inference power depends upon the underlying ontology language supported by the Semantic Web (Lord et al., 2004).

Since the OWL-S service ontology is public and does not prescribe a framework implementation it has been used as the building block for various bioinformatics SWS initiatives.

OWL-S describes three key aspects about a service: its profile, which describes what the service does; its process, which describes how one interacts with the service; and its grounding, which relates the ontological concepts to the implementation, usually via a mapping to the WSDL operations (Post et al., 2007). These three aspects of SWS can be abstracted into five high level architectural components (Lord et al., 2004):

1. Service Interfaces: Service providers publish interfaces to their services using some form of programming constructs.
2. Semantic Descriptions: In addition to the interface description, semantic descriptions of services are provided.
3. A Domain Ontology Terms from an ontology describing the key concepts in the domain are used within the semantic descriptions.
4. Registry/Matchmaker: A matchmaker service searches over the semantic descriptions made available to it. This may be combined with a registry such as UDDI, a service which advertises the availability of other services.

Messaging: The domain ontology is used as a controlled vocabulary that enables the service consumer to treat data from different providers in a uniform fashion.

OWL-S is the most prominent framework for supporting such architectures.

In the following paragraphs, we will discuss two important bioinformatics Web Services systems which are gradually adapting the SWS architecture. Each of these systems has adapted the SWS enabling standards at different abstract levels as illustrated in Figure 2.

The key components described above are realized within myGrid as follows (http://www.mygrid.org.uk; Lord et al., 2004):

- **Service Interfaces:** Services are published as Web services described with WSDL (Lord et al., 2004; Cabrall L. et al., 2004).
- **Semantic Descriptions:** A lightweight RDF data model is used to structure service description, with a domain ontology providing a vocabulary (Pieter B., et al, 2005; Benjamin M. & Mark D., 2006). Descriptions can be provided by third parties (Cabrall L. et al., 2004; Yang et al., 2006).
- **Domain Ontology:** The ontology is curated and stored centrally, and generated by an expert (http://www.mygrid.org.uk; Benjamin M. & Mark D., 2006).
- **Registry/Matchmaker:** A centralized UDDI registry built over a Jena back end,

augmented to enable semantic discovery (Post et al, 2007; Neerincx & Leunissen, 2005).
- **Messaging:** Pre-existing domain formats are used.

Semantic-MOBY (http://www.biomoby.org) makes extensive use of Semantic Web technology, in particular OWL-DL (Benjamin M. & Mark D., 2006). It attempts to embrace the autonomous nature of the Web wherever possible (Wilkinson M. et al., 2003). Semantic-MOBY has extensive publicly available requirements and design documentation. The key components are realized within Semantic-MOBY as follows (Lord et al., 2004):

- **Service Interfaces:** Services are simply Web resources accessible by standard protocols such as HTTP and FTP. For example, via HTTP, a simple GET returns an RDF graph that defines the underlying service interface (http://www.biomoby.org; Lord et al., 2004).
- **Semantic Descriptions:** Service descriptions are expressed in OWL-DL and con-

Figure 2. Adoption of SWS enabling standards in myGrid and Semantic-MOBY

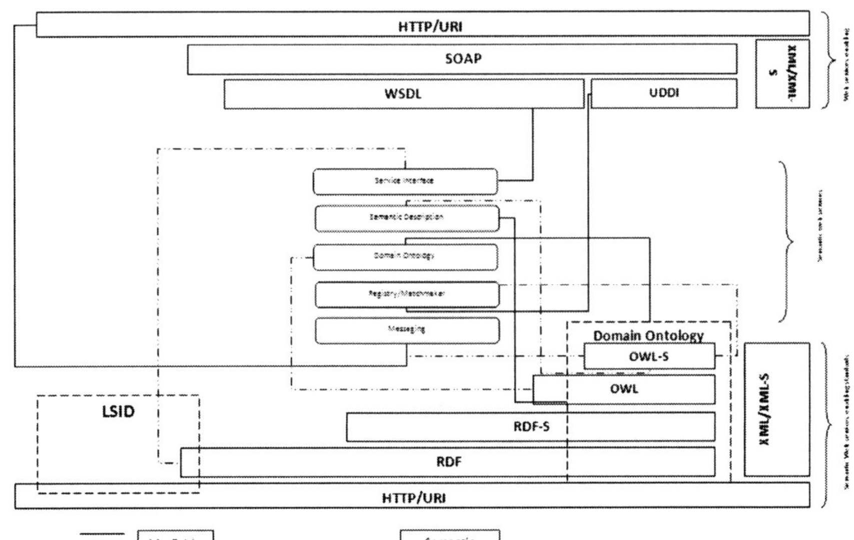

form to a canonical format, or upper ontology. This upper ontology creates the context for ontological concepts, which are resolvable into OWL-DL graphs by dereferencing their URIs. Service providers create service-specific subclasses of the ontology, grounding them with their own data-type requirements (http://www.biomoby.org; Pieter B.,et al, 2005; Lord et al., 2004).

- **Domain Ontology:** One, or several, ontologies are developed by the community, and distributed across the Web, and written in OWL-DL (Post et al, 2007; Lord et al., 2004; Neerincx & Leunissen, 2005).
- **Matchmaker:** One or more centralized search engines are provided. Service locations can be published, or semantic descriptions can be discovered by Web crawlers. Querying uses the same upper ontology as the semantic descriptions (http://www.biomoby.org; Post et al, 2007; Lord et al., 2004).
- **Messaging:** All communication uses OWL-DL and the same upper ontology (Post et al, 2007; Lord et al., 2004).

The two systems discussed above have chosen a gradual migration path to full semantic capability (http://www.biomoby.org/; http://www.mygrid.org.uk). This is because instead of providing a generic solution, they have focused on providing semantic interoperability between existing service providers and consumers. In context of five abstract levels of SWS architectural components, we also observe the following:

1. **Automated Service Composition:** Biologists and scientists are not willing to use semantic descriptions for automated service invocation and composition without establishing provenance of a service.
2. **Structured messages and middleware:** Scientists and biologists are not providing

data in XML format. This data has to be translated into required format to reduce the problem of syntactic heterogeneity.
3. **Service provision and service interfaces:** Most of the services required and used by biologists are atomic and not decomposable. As a result, nothing similar to the OWL-S process ontology has been used. For services that require complex interaction an enactment engine is used.
4. **User-Centered Service Descriptions:** Service descriptions are currently manually generated by the two projects, either by the service providers (Semantic-MOBY) or third party (myGrid).
5. **Generating an ontology for a complex domain:** Either a collaborative community style of ontology building (Semantic-MOBY) or a centralized, curated ontology building approach has been used.

The full adoption of semantic capabilities by WS is also hindered due to some of the legacy characteristics of SW. Because of evolving nature of bioinformatics research, for example, it is important for researchers and biologists to know the most recent available information (Cabrall L. et al., 2004). The static documents of SW are not able to adequately represent many semantic relationships, for example the relationship between a sequence and its homologues (Sheila A. et al., 2001). Such relationships can be dynamically calculated, by invoking the relevant SWS which establish the semantic link between the RDF triples at run time. For semantic exploration of existing static documents, the stake holders must agree to some standard of data representation such as static RDF relationships or LSID so that the distinction between Semantic Web Services and the Semantic Web can be removed (Cabrall L. et al., 2004). However, we feel that the deployment of Semantic Web Services will rely on the further development and combination of Web Services and Semantic Web enabling technologies (Cannta N., et al, 2008)

WEB SERVICES: THE ROLE OF SOFTWARE VENDORS

Biological analysis and research efforts can be treated just like another business process. Current Service Oriented Architecture (SOA) suites offer a rich set of features for Business Process Management (BPM) to define and manage a workflow, Governance tools for publishing and managing services, Enterprise Service Bus (ESB) for communication among diverse services/tools, Business Activity Monitoring (BAM) to monitor events during the execution of workflows, and Business Analytics for rule-based analysis of the business events. The next logical evolution in this area is to fully benefit from the emerging SOA suites to expedite development, evolution, and management of bioinformatics tools, facilitate easier composition of the existing tools to define complex workflows, promote better management and reuse of diverse existing tool sets from distributed remote locations, enable better monitoring during execution, and present results in a more effective and friendly fashion. We anticipate that the future developments of bioinformatics tools will fully benefit from SOA suites.

TECHNOLOGY VENDORS

The SOA market is still evolving and presents a lot of business opportunities to a diverse community of vendors. SOA involves so many diverse technologies and their integration that it becomes challenging, if not impossible, for a single vendor to excel in each aspect of SOA. The real challenge is to harness all those diverse SOA technologies in a reliable, efficient, and user-friendly environment. SOA customers prefer to have a single development, deployment, and management environment for SOA that is pretty similar to what they had for development and maintenance of their traditional monolithic applications. Instead of having diverse vendors and products that require custom/ad-hoc integration solution, the SOA customers prefer a "one-stop-shop" so that their investments, learning curves, time-to-market, and risks are minimized. This has resulted in evolution of SOA suites that support analysis, design, development, testing, deployment, monitoring, management, and maintenance of services and service composites in a well-integrated environment.

Several SOA vendors claim to have comprehensive suites of SOA products that presumably address all aspects of SOA, along with a well-integrated environment for development and deployment. However, IBM and Oracle seem to be the emerging leaders in the terms of completeness of their SOA suites. Oracle is emerging as a very strong player in this area, especially after its acquisition of BEA Systems. Microsoft is another strong player in this arena but not because of the completeness or quality of its SOA suite, but more so because of its market share, momentum, and customer loyalty. Other significant players in this market include: JBoss, Software AG (with its acquisition of WebMethods), SAP, Sun Microsystems, and TIBCO (Swanton & Finley 2007; ButlerGroup 2007). Table 1 briefly lists SOA offerings by these vendors and comments on where products from these vendors stand on most important aspects of SOA including: Business Process Management (BPM); Enterprise Service Bus; Development/Integration Environment; Service Repositories and Catalogs; and Management and Monitoring.

CONCLUSION AND FUTURE DIRECTIONS

In this chapter we traced the efforts of scientific community to solve the problems of integrative biology. These efforts have resulted in the evolution of SWS. Fortunately, Life scientists are beginning to realize the potential, possibilities and possible scenarios offered by SWS and the ongoing efforts by the Life Science community

Table 1.

Vendor	SOA offerings, strengths and weaknesses
JBoss	JBoss offers a lean, performing, and scalable SOA infrastructure (JBoss SOA) but lacks in high-level modeling, activity monitoring, and business analytics. JBoss SOA infrastructure currently includes: JBoss Application Server as deployment platform, JBoss Developer studio for IDE, JBoss jBPM for process management, JBoss Rules as rule engine, and JBoss ESB as service bus. Its SOA infrastructure is expected to gain popularity among developers and for low-cost solutions. However, a lot needs to be done before JBoss can effectively compete with major players in SOA market.
IBM	IBM has one of the most comprehensive SOA offering (IBM SOA) with a solid capability to develop for and operate in the most complex SOA environments. IBM's SOA offerings include: WebSphere Application Server for deployment; WebSphere Process Server for process management; Business Modeler and WebSphere Integration Developer for IDE; WebSphere ESB for service bus; WebSphere Service Registry and Repository for SOA governance, and WebSphere Business Monitor for activity monitoring and business analytics. It SOA tools seamlessly integrates into Rational development suite if extensive software development is required. On the flip side, IBM's product structure is somewhat complex for those unfamiliar with IBM middleware.
Microsoft	Microsoft does not offer SOA services that are as complete as those by other leading vendors. However, even with its limited offerings Microsoft appeals to organizations with .NET skills and extensive Microsoft deployments. Its SOA implementation (Microsoft SOA) is mostly around .NET/Windows, and includes: BizTalk as service bus and business process management/monitoring; Visual Studio as integrated development/composition environment; SharePoint for repositories, content management and search; and Office Business Applications for service components.
Oracle	With its acquisition of BEA Systems, Oracle has emerged as an SOA vendor with unparalleled depth and breath in its SOA offerings (Oracle SOA). Its experience in integrating its acquired applications, like those from Siebel, PeopleSoft, Retek, Demantra, G-Log, etc., has evolved into a strong Application Integration Architecture, reusable business process templates, and evolving service catalog. Its toolset is exceptional in providing round-trip capabilities with business process modeling tools upstream and with JDeveloper downstream. Oracle's SOA offerings include: Oracle WebLogic Application Server for deployment, JDeveloper for IDE, Oracle BPEL Process Manager for process management, Oracle BAM for monitoring business activity, Oracle Service Bus for service bus, and Oracle Business Rules and Oracle Complex Event Processing for business monitoring and analytics.
SAP	To cash in on its strong presence in enterprise application market, SAP has been promoting its SOA vision (SAP SOA) for years but still has not been successful in creating an integrated environment for SOA. A wide variety of stand-alone tools and their differences with operating environments make SAP offering less than desirable. SAP solution does not currently offer a business activity monitoring capability and its repositories lack behind its competitor's. However, SAP service catalog is relatively quite mature but need user friendly tools for its easy use by the development community. SAP's SOA offerings include: NetWeaver Application Server as deployment environment; NetWeaver Business Intelligence component as activity monitoring and business analytics; NetWeaver Exchange Infrastructure for messaging and service bus; NetWeaver Developer Studio, Visual Composer, and ABAP workbench as development environments, and NetWeaver Composition Environment for integration.
Sofware AG	With its own application/solutions portfolio and acquisition of WebMethods, Sofware AG has the potential to become one of the prominent players in SOA world. Inherited from WebMethods, Software AG currently has one of the best integrated SOA environments (Software AG SOA). Its scalable repository, efficient service bus, mature process management and monitoring tools have significant potential if packaged and marketed right by Software AG. Software AG's SOA offering primarily consist of WebMethod's SOA product suite, that includes modules for process management, activity monitoring, SOA governance, and service bus.
Sun	Although Sun has a strong SOA infrastructure (Sun SOA) but might have trouble becoming a major SOA player because it does not have a strong enough portfolio and experience in enterprise applications, like other leading SOA vendors. Sun's SOA offerings include GlassFish as deployment platform, NetBeans as IDE, Intelligent Event Processor (IEP) for business activity monitoring, OpenESB as service bus, and Sun Service Registry for SOA governance. Sun framework advocates Jave Business Integration (JBI) architecture (JSR 2008). In addition to being a full feature Java development environment, NetBeans also includes Composite Application Service Assembly (CASA) editor and BPEL Designer for service composition and business process management, respectively.
TIBCO	TIBCO's SOA offerings (TIBCO SOA) has always been one of the most sought out since the inception of SOA market, because of its established position in the messaging infrastructure and its early SOA offerings. Although it is still working on integrating its SOA tools into an integrated environment, but it is well respected for its high performance service bus, excellent process modeling tools, and impressive business analysis capabilities that go beyond event detection to taking automated actions to those events using an interference-based approach. TIBCO's SOA products under ActiveMatrix umbrella include: BusinessWorks for IDE, Registry for SOA governance, Policy Manager for security, Service Bus for service bus, and Service Performance Manager for activity monitoring.

for migration towards SWS can be considered as a pioneer one. Although, the realization of ontology based web surfing is technically a challenging task, the most serious impediment in its attainment, however are the social problems. In a complex and changing domain such as bioinformatics, community involvement is important as ontologies provide interoperability only so far as they are shared by members of the community.

The ontology must reflect the users' perception of the domain and enable the semantic description of services by service providers or helpful third parties, to facilitate user-oriented service discovery. The success of GO (Gene Ontology) is a good example of collaborative community style of ontology building in which familiarity is considered more important than expressivity.

The difficulties in providing domain ontology in Life Sciences are also due to complex, internally structured data types and existing legacy systems. The development of metadata for biological information, on the basis of Semantic Web standards, and its definition for all information sources is a promising approach for a semantic based integration of biological information. However, scientists should be urged to expose their data and should be instructed on how to present these to the world, and on how to identify and represent them.

Another impediment is of selection of common domain for ontology integration. The identification of common domain is still manual requiring extensive domain knowledge. Methods must be devised to automate this process. Support from SOA suites for ontology management, search, matching, and integration will be a big help to the life science community.

At present, setting-up costs of SWS systems are high, because of availability of any adequate knowledge models and those available are highly divergent. This relates to the more general problem of ontology alignment (Euzenat and Valtchev, 2003). BioMOBY has taken the initiative to merge MOBY-S and Semantic-MOBY with subsequent ontology alignment with myGrid. Another related issue is of keeping the separation of Ontology from RDF representation to preserve data independence. This may be achieved with an explicit mapping in the form of the linking statements.

Research in related technologies such as knowledge engineering and technologies to support friendly insertion of semantics in web pages is important. At present, for example, the common usage of ontologies in biology is limited to annotation purposes. Instead, their use for the interpretation of high throughput biological data can benefit from knowledge inference, thus allowing using ontologies as knowledge bases from which new information can be derived.

To establish trust within the Life Sciences community for SWS usage, it is imperative that semantic descriptions should emphasize non functional parameters such as provenance and performance metrics such as scalability, response time, reliability, availability. We are currently extending our work on Data Provenance to incorporate SWS (Ahsan S. & Shah A., 2008).

In our opinion, it will significantly help to have more extensive support for ontologies in SOA suites. Moreover adoption of SOA suites, that have well-integrated environment, easy to learn, and cost-effective, by life science communities will significantly enhance productivity, reliability, presentation, and reuse.

We feel that with the emerging W3C standards and their adoption, the distinction between SW and SWS will disappear. With its most promising standards, technologies and tools, the objective of semantics interconnection and interlinking can be achieved and ontology driven browsing will finally be achieved.

REFERENCES

W3C. (n.d.). *URIs, URLs, and URNs: Clarifications and Recommendations 1.0*. Retrieved June 14, 2006, from http://www.w3.org/TR/uri-clarification/

W3C. (n.d.). *Web Services Description Language (WSDL) 1.1*. Retrieved October 7, 2008, from http://www.w3.org/TR/wsdl

W3C. (n.d.). *Web Services Interoperability Organization*. Retrieved October 15, 2008, from http://www.ws-i.org/)

Ahsan, S., & Shah, A. (2008). A Framework for Agile Methodologies for Development of Bioinformatics. *The Journal of American Science, 4*, 15–21.

Ahsan, S., & Shah, A. (2008). *Quality Metrics For Evaluating Data Provenance, Designing Software Intensive Systems-Methods and Principles* (pp. 455–473). Hershey, PA: IGI Global.

Allan, R., & Ed, S. Lein. (2007). Genome-wide atlas of gene expression in the adult mouse brain. *Nature, 445*, 168–176.

Bada, M., Stevens, R., Goble, C., Gil, Y., Ashburner, M., & Blake, J. (2004). *A Short Study on the Success of Gene Ontology*. Accepted for Publication in Journal of Web Semantics.

Bodenreider, O., & Stevens, R. (2006). *Bio-ontologies: current trends and future directions, Briefings in Bioinformatics Advance Access*. Oxford, UK: Oxford University Journals.

ButlerGroup. (2007). *SOA Platforms – Software Infrastructure Requirements for Successful SOA Deployments*. Ferensway Hull, UK: Butler Direct Ltd.

Cabral, L., Domingue, J., Motta, E., Payne, T., & Hakimpour, F. (2004). *Approaches to Semantic Web Services: An Overview and Comparisons*. Berlin/Heidelberg, Germany: Springer.

Cannta, N., et al. (2008). A semantic web for bioinformatics: goals, tools, systems and applications, BMC Bioinformatics. In *Proceedings of the Seventh International Workshop on Network Tools and Applications in Biology*, Pisa, Italy

Cruz, S. M. S. D. (2005). Mining and Visualization of Logs of Bioinformatics Web Services in silico Experiments. In *Proceedings of the Brazilian Symposium on Computer Graphics and Image Processing*.

Doelz, R. (1994). Hierarchical Access System for Sequence Libraries in Europe (HASSEL): A Tool to Access Sequence Database Remotely. *Computer Applications in the Biosciences, 10*, 31–34.

Etzold, T., & Argos, P. (1993). SRS – An Indexing and Retrieval Tool for Flat-File Data Libraries. *Computer Applications in the Biosciences, 9*, 49–57.

Good, B., & Wilkinson, M. (2006). The Life Sciences Semantic Web is Full of Creeps! *Briefings in Bioinformatics, 7*(3), 275–286.

Hashmi, N., et al. (2004). Abstracting Workflows: Unifying Bioinformatics Task Conceptualization and Specification through Semantic Web Services. In *Proceedings of the W3C Workshop on Semantic Web for Life Sciences*, Cambridge, MA.

IBM SOA. (n.d.). *IBM - Service-Oriented Architecture (SOA)*. Retrieved September 15, 2008, from http://www-01.ibm.com/ software/ solutions/soa/

JBoss SOA. (n.d.). *JBoss – SOA Resource Center*. Retrieved September 5, 2008, from http://www.jboss.com/resources/soa

JSR 208. (n.d.). *JSR 000208 java Business Integration 1.0*. Retrieved August 25, 2008, from http://jcp.org/aboutJava/communityprocess/final/jsr208/index.html

Knikker R., Guo, Y., Li1, J., Kwan, A., Yip, K.,Cheung, D., & Cheung, K. (2004). A web services choreography scenario for interoperating bioinformatics applications. *BMC Bioinformatics*.

Kossenkov, A., Manion, F., & Korotkov, E. (2003). ASAP: Automated Sequence Annotation Pipeline for Web-based Updating of Sequence Information with a Local Database. *Bioinformatics (Oxford, England)*, *19*, 675–676.

Labarga, A., Valentin, F., Anderson, M., & Lopez, R. (2007). *Web Services at the European Bioinformatics*, EMBL-EBI, European Bioinformatics Institute, Wellcome Trust Genome Campus, Hinxton, CB10 1SD, Cambridge, UK.

Lord, P. W., Bechhofer, S., Wilkinson, M. D., Schiltz, G., Gessler, D., Hull, D., et al. (2004). Applying semantic Web services to bioinformatics: Experiences gained, lessons learned. In *Proceedings of the 3rd International Semantic Web Conference*, Springer

Meskauskas, A., Lehmann-Horn, F., & Jurkat-Rott, K. (2004). Sight: Autmating Genomic Data-mining without Programming Skills. *Bioinformatics (Oxford, England)*, *20*, 1718–1720.

Microsoft, S. O. A. (n.d.). *Microsoft – SOA and Business Process*. Retrieved September 9, 2008, http://www.microsoft.com/SOA.

Neerincx Pieter, B. T., & Leunissen, J. A. (2005). Evolution of web services in bioinformatics. *Briefings in Bioinformatics*, *6*(2), 178–188.

OpenBioInformatics Projects. (n.d.). *Open BioInformatics Foundation – Projects*. Retrieved from http://www.open-bio.org/wiki/Projects

Oracle, S. O. A. (n.d.). *Oracle - Service-Oriented Architecture (SOA)*. Retrieved September 20, 2008, from http://www.oracle.com/tec hnologies/soa/index.html

Pieter, B., Neerincx, T., & Leunissen, J. A. M. (2005). Evolution of Web Services In Bioinformatics. *Briefings in Bioinformatics*, *6*(2), 178–188.

Post, L. J. G., Roos, M., Marshall, M. S., Driel, R. V., & Breit, T. M. (2007). A semantic web approach applied to integrative bioinformatics experimentation: a biological use case with genomics data. *Bioinformatics (Oxford, England)*, *23*(22), 3080–3087.

Rama, A., Goodwin, R., Doshi, P., & Roeder, S. (2003). A Method For Semantically Enhancing the Service Discovery Capabilities of UDDI, In *Proceedings of the Workshop on Information Integration on the Web, IJCAI 2003*, Mexico, Aug 9-10, 2003

Redaschi, N., Doelz, R., & Eggenberger, F. (1995). *HASSEL v5*. Advanced Computer Network Communications: Hierarchical Access System for Sequence Libraries in Europe.

SAP SOA. (n.d.). *SAP – Service-Oriented Architecture (SOA)*. Retrieved August 26, 2008, from http://www.sap.com/ platform/soa/index.epx

Sheila, A., McIlraith, T. C. S., & Zeng, H. (2001). *Semantic Web Services*. IEEE Educational Activities Department.

Software, A. G. SOA. (n.d.). *Software AG – Service-Oriented Architecture (SOA)*. Retrieved September 11, 2008, from http://www.softwareag.com/ Corporate/products/wm/default.asp

Souchelnytskyi, S. (2005). Proteomics of TGFbeta signaling and its impact on breast cancer. *Expert Review of Proteomics*, *2*, 925–935.

Stevens, R., Robinson, A., & Goble, C. (2003). myGrid: Personalized BioInformatics on the Information Grid. *Bioinformatics (Oxford, England)*, *19*(90001), 302–304.

Sun, S. O. A. (n.d.). *Sun Service-Oriented Architecture (SOA)*. Retrieved August 28, 2008, from http://www.sun.com/ products/soa/index.jsp

Swanton, B., & Finley, I. (2007). *SOA and BPM for Enterprise Applications: A Dose of Reality*, Report #: AMR-R-20372, AMR Research Inc., 125 Summer Street, 4th floor, Boston, MA 02110-1616.

Thakar, S., Ambite, J. L., & Knoblock, C. A. (2005, September). Composing, Optimizing, and Executing Plans for bioinformatics Web services. *VLDB Journal, Special Issue on Data Management. Analysis and Mining for Life Sciences, 14*(3), 330–353.

TIBCO SOA. (n.d.). *TIBCO – Service-Oriented Architecture (SOA) Resource Center*. Retrieved September 1, 2008, from http://www.tibco.com/solution s/soa/default.jsp

Wilkinson, M., Gossler, D., Farmer, A., & Stein, L. (2003). A Bio-Moby Project Explores Open-Source, Simple, Extensible Protocols for Enabling Biological Database Interoperability. In *Proceedings of Virt. Conference Genom and Bioinformatics, 3*, 16-26.

Yang, B., Xue, T., Zhao, J., Kommidi, C., Soneja, J., Li, J., et al. (2006). Bioinformatics web services, In *Proceedings of The 2006 International Conference on Bioinformatics & Computational Biology (BIOCOMP)*, June 2006, Las Vegas, NV.

Chapter 4
Critical Issues in Evaluating Education Technology

Nafisat Afolake Adedokun-Shittu
International Islamic University, Malaysia

Abdul Jaleel Kehinde Shittu
University Utara, Malaysia

EXECUTIVE SUMMARY

This chapter highlights some issues that are critical in evaluating technology in education such that it will be implemented to meet educational goals and it will also serve as a spotlight for policy makers and educators to make a worthwhile return on their technology investment. Schools and institutions of learning invest heavily on technology before establishing clear plans on how it will be integrated into teaching and learning to achieve educational goals. Even though many studies have reported positive impact of technology on students' learning yet; not much of studies have been carried out to investigate whether the investment on technology in schools have been commensurate with the investment. Particularly needs assessment on both students and teachers' technology needs is often ignored before technology implementation. Educators and policy makers need to consider certain evaluation issues before committing huge budgets into technology. It is crucial to ask what can technology do that cannot be done without it, what percentage of the institution's budget should be invested on technology, how should technology be integrated in the curriculum to achieve educational goals and lots more before investing on educational technology to avoid resource wastage. Thus, this chapter highlights these critical issues in the light of a study conducted on the integration of information and communication technology (ICT) in the teaching and learning of science and mathematics in Malaysian secondary school (Adedokun, 2008). The research investigated some concerns that culminated from the integration of ICT in the instruction of English, mathematics and science in Malaysia among which are: Can the teachers deliver? Do they have the strong will to deliver? Are there adequate facilities for them to carry out this new task? Do they possess the necessary skills for them to be able to deliver? Does the government provide adequate training on the integration of ICT in subject content? Are the students prepared for the change in the medium of instruction? What is the present situation in schools with regards to the use of ICT? And is better teaching and learning achieved with the integration of ICT?

DOI: 10.4018/978-1-60960-015-0.ch004

INTRODUCTION

Technology in Education is seen as a tool for achieving instructional goals, not a goal in itself. Yet, many institutions are putting the cart before the horse by investing in educational technology before establishing clear plans on how to deploy it. Education technology is not just an ornament for school design, but an important component of the curriculum. Education researchers (QED, 2004) have observed that government and institutions are expending huge sum of money on technology in education as an indication of development and improvement in schools. However, studies observed that these funds will amount to wastage if not properly expended. Thus, policy makers and educational administrators need insight into how to deploy the technology expenditures and maximize its positive impact on education.

Educational technology has greatly impacted on teaching and learning and grossly increased improvement on students' achievement. Internet technology helps students become independent, critical thinkers, able to find information, organize and evaluate it, and then effectively express their new knowledge and ideas in compelling ways.

Similarly, technology acts as a catalyst for fundamental change in the way students learn and teachers teach, and it revolutionizes the traditional methods of teaching and learning. Educational technology has a significant positive impact on achievements in subject areas, across all levels of school, and in regular classrooms as well as those for special-needs students. Most of these reported effects of technology integration occur with peculiar conditions that worked in those situations and may not necessarily result in positive effect in other situations if the right conditions are not in place. Issues like teacher readiness, training, student attitude and access to proper technology infrastructure are the right conditions for successful technology integration.

In like manners, the onus of the positive acknowledgements in education does not go to technology alone. The extent of this effectiveness is influenced by several other factors such as; the instructional design, the teacher's role, the student population, students grouping, and the levels of student access to technology. Adedokun & Hashim, (2008) reported that teachers believed that ICT can only be useful when complemented with other instructional materials. This indicates that technology alone cannot do the trick but with an interconnected system in place and a judicious use of technology in teaching and learning.

THE CASE STUDY

Malaysia identifies ICT as one of the most important factors in achieving the aims of Education Development thus; ICT was integrated in secondary schools across the country especially in the teaching of English, Science and Mathematics (Ministry of Education, 2004). This swift change in the Malaysian Education policy raised several concerns from the teachers, parents, students and other concerned stakeholders. Hence, studies on the success of the policy, the policy implementation process, teachers' and students' perception of the policy and many other relevant issues become prominent. This study under discourse in this chapter (Adedokun, 2008) investigate the teachers' and students' perception on the ICT integration in the teaching and learning of science and mathematics with respect to its use, ease of use, adequacy, problems encountered and students' learning. A mixed method approach was devised to gather comprehensive data for the study. A 20-item questionnaire was designed to analyze students' perception of the use of ICT in the teaching and learning of both science and mathematics.

Similarly, a 20-item interview question was developed to examine the perception of science and mathematics teachers on ICT integration in their respective subjects. Lastly, two science classes and one mathematics class were observed and video-recorded to triangulate and validate the study. The sample of this study includes 100 students to whom questionnaires were distributed, 10 science and mathematics teachers interviewed and 3 science and mathematics classes observed. The strength of this study is in its combination of varying research methods to offset the weaknesses inherent in each of the methods when applied singly. This study (Adedokun, 2008) is discussed in this chapter in the light of some crucial issues that have been identified by researches as success factors in technology integration in education.

ISSUES IN SUCCESSFUL TECHNOLOGY INTEGRATION

Embracing technology requires complete integration throughout the curriculum, the delivery of instruction, the preparation of teachers and their professional development such that learning objectives such as: increased student engagement, student achievement test scores, assessments and development of critical, higher-order thinking skills can be achieved. Integrating technology into instruction is a complex, fund-gulping and time-consuming process; thus it requires proper planning and involvement of all stakeholders in education. Policy makers, parents, curriculum developers, and especially the teachers and students must be involved in any successful integration. In contrast to this critical success factor, this study (Adedokun, 2008) reveals that neither the students nor the teachers who are the primary users of the ICT facilities integrated in the schools were consulted before the implementation. Both the science and mathematics teachers in the study were blunt when commenting on government's policy. The Science teachers all identified lack of consultation as a prime factor that contributes to less use of ICT in teaching by science teachers because of their non-preparedness.

One of them, (SR1) hit the nail on the head when she said; *"The process is top down and we have to follow no objection if we object, no point. The*

government is too egoistic and business minded." Similarly, all the mathematics teachers did not mince words when commenting on the government's policy on ICT. One of them, (MR3) said: *"the government just introduced ICT in a drastic and sudden manner without proper consideration for the teachers who are the real implementers, the situation on ground and the students who are at the receiving end. Most probably that is why I don't use it and some other problems associated with it."* Another (MR1) acknowledged; *"Normally they will not consult us they use experts and direct us to use".* Scholars of instructional technology like: (Lee & Owens, 2004; Dick & Carey, 2001) all reiterated the essence of needs assessment for any policy implementation in education to achieve an effective and workable result. Teachers and students' feelings ought to be analyzed to ensure acceptable and successful implementation.

Similar to the teachers and students' involvement is the issue of teachers' training and knowledge about technology integration into curriculum. Coppola (2004) indicates that the single most important factor in the effective use of technology is the quality of the teacher knowledge of effective technology uses in instruction. Coppola also noted that the effect of technology on students' access to knowledge is determined by the pedagogical knowledge and skill of teachers. Teachers need to be taught how to use technology to deliver instruction. Helping teachers to learn to integrate technology into curriculum is a critical factor in the successful implementation of technology in schools (Sivin-Kachala & Bialo, 2000), but most teachers have not had training in using technology effectively in teaching (Silverstein et al., 2000). Most of the teachers interviewed in this study identified inadequate ICT skills and insufficient training on how to integrate ICT into the subject they teach as part of the initial obstacles they face in the use of ICT in teaching. One of the mathematics teachers (MR1) asserted; *"The beginning part of it is always the toughest part we need time to adjust ourselves…"*. Another (MR2) commented; *"Training! not really enough but at least I know some things like searching the internet…."* It was observed that most of the mathematics teachers who claimed to possess inadequate skills are those with more than 20 years of teaching experience.

The science teachers on the other hand possess a better ICT skill but described it as insufficient. One of them (SR5) described their skills thus; *"Not enough. We need to know more about how to use it to teach the subject, how to use it to do some other things like preparing exam, recording result etc"*. Many studies (Bransford, Darling-Hammond, & Page, 2005; Fishman & Davis, 2006) have also identified that teacher training is a key element to education reform, particularly training that focuses on classroom practices and engages teachers in a community of professional practice and development.

Recurring technical faults, and the expectation of faults occurring during teaching sessions, are likely to reduce teacher confidence and cause teachers to avoid using the technology in future lessons (BECTA, 2003). This issue was also found to be a hindrance in the use of ICT both in the Science and mathematics classes observed in our study (Adedokun, 2008). In the second science class observed, *the lesson time was short of the 10 minutes (12.5%) spent on the installation of the courseware. The teacher has no problem with setting up the ICT facilities, but she encountered technical problem in the installation of the courseware, which was intended for visual enhancement of the topic. She later gave up on that and turned to the PowerPoint presentation she had prepared that contained, the human growth pattern, effects of nutrition on growth, the growth curve, stages of growth and a review of the lesson.* Likewise in the mathematics class observed, though *there was no technical hitch but the setting up of the ICT facilities took almost 15minutes which was equivalent to 25% of the class time because of the slow pace of the system and the CD-ROM* (see Table 1).

The first science class however did not encounter any of these problems. To substantiate the class findings, teachers interviewed (both science and mathematics) have experienced technical problems of some sort while using ICT to teach. A mathematics teacher (MR4) explains; *"… sometimes but it doesn't happen every time because I don't use always"*. A science teacher (SR1) says; *"Technical problem, yes but not much. Maybe software problem"*. The students' response on the presence of technical problems during ICT-related classes also show 90% agreement indicating that they experienced technical problems both hardware and software related in class.

Another issue of concern in technology integration is the fact that students sometimes focus too heavily on the technology-related aspects of assignments (Henriquez & Riconscente, 1999), teachers also can be distracted by the "glitz" of technologically sophisticated student work and lose sight of the "guts" or content. The goal of technology is to improve student achievement through enhanced delivery of curriculum and instruction; imaginations of teachers and students are the only limitations. Thus varying methods and styles of delivering lessons in a dynamic manner should be used to stimulate the classroom environment. A blended approach should also be employed to use technology in conjunction with well-defined curriculum objectives in order to reshape and improve the method and style of traditional curriculum delivery. This study as observed in the classes and responses of most of the teachers interviewed shows a blended approach is employed. A mathematics teacher (MR4) affirms that; *"ICT cannot help students 100%, it depends on the teachers. ICT is quite good to make the subject attractive, it helps but I cannot depend 100% just 20%. If I want to start a new chapter I use it"*. She argues that mathematics needs a lot of calculation and exercises that can only be done on the whiteboard. She believes that mathematics cannot be understood using only ICT but a large part of the lesson has to be taught by the teacher

Table 1.

Theme	Issues	Maths Observed	1st science observed	2nd science observed
Class description	Population	Large	Large	Large
	Class control	Easy	Difficult	Easy
Subject	Topic	Coordinates: Plotting Points and Stating the Co-ordinates of the Plotting	Reaction between Metals and Non-metals	Human growth pattern
	Content	Explanation on the topic, examples of plotting coordinates on a graph, examples of writing out coordinates of a plotted graph, exercises on plotting and writing out coordinates.	Definition of terms, explanation of concept, example, summary	Effects of nutrition on growth, graph, chart, stages of growth, review of lesson
	Lesson outcome	Write the coordinates of the points shown on the graph; drag the correct coordinates to their points on the chart.	Describe what a mineral is; describe properties of mineral; write equation in words to show the effects of heat on mineral	State the stages of human growth; state the nutrients necessary for human growth and their impor-tance; draw the human growth curve
Instructional aids	Types	Textbook, laptop, LCD, software	Textbook, laptop, LCD, software, PowerPoint, whiteboard	Textbook, laptop, LCD, software, PowerPoint
	Usage	75% ICT usage, 6.25% Textbook, 12.5% Setting up, 18.75% Teacher explanation	62.5% ICT usage, 25% Textbook and whiteboard usage & 12.5% setting up time	62.5% ICT usage, 18.75% Textbook, 12.5% instal-lation
Teacher	ICT skill	Good	Good	Good
	Mastery of subject	Good	Good	Good
	Teaching strategy	Blends ICT with textbook	Blends ICT with other instructional aids	Blends ICT with textbook
Students	Attitude	Attentive & participatory	Noisy but participatory	Attentive & participatory
	Attention	On teacher, LCD, text-book as directed by the teacher	On teacher	On teacher, LCD, text-book as directed by the teacher
	Reaction	To teacher: attentive To content: understand To ICT: Normal, not strange To question: answer all correctly Students ask questions	To teacher: attentive To content: understand To ICT: Normal, not strange To question: answer all correctly Students ask questions	To teacher: attentive To content: understand To ICT: Normal, not strange To question: answer all correctly Students ask questions
Technical issues	Technical Problem Technical Assistant	Yes – Initial setting up problem No	No No	Yes – courseware instal-lation Yes – colleague

using the textbook and whiteboard. (SR4) stresses that; *"ICT can't cover all; we need reference books, articles. It's ok for teaching but teachers have to put more effort"*. (SR1) declares; *"I use it to summarize after I teach the topic, we cannot use every time we teach"*.

Similarly from all the classes observed, more than half of the lesson time was expended on the

ICT enabled instruction and other instructional aids such as textbooks and whiteboard were used to support the ICT. In the mathematics class, half of the session (40 minutes) was used on teaching with ICT, students spent 20 minutes working exercises on the CD-ROM, 15 minutes was spent on teacher's self explanation and correction to the students' exercises and 5 minutes on textbook exercises resulting in 75% ICT usage, 18.75% teacher explanation and 6.25% textbook usage. In the first science class, more than half of the lesson time (25 minutes) was expended on teaching with ICT, 10 minutes doing exercises from the textbook and 5 minutes for setting up ICT facilities amounting to 62.5% ICT usage, 25% textbook and whiteboard usage and 12.5% setting up time. In the second science class, more than half of the lesson time (50 minutes) was spent on teaching with ICT and 15 minutes doing textbook exercises this culminated into 62.5% ICT and 18.75% textbook usage (see Table 1).

A statement by (MR3) indicates that; *"Students are carried away by ICT sometimes they don't concentrate on what the teacher is teaching"*, supporting the claim by (Henriquez & Riconscente, 1999) that students could be distracted by the glitz of technology. MR3 also agreed with this saying; *"Students are carried away by ICT sometimes they don't concentrate on what the teacher is teaching."* However, another mathematics teacher, (MR2) explains that; *"ICT is interesting and very useful especially for weak students but for good students, they don't really like it because it is too slow for them; they understand quickly and prefer working more exercises"*. This could be further confirmed from the students survey in which more than half (60%) of them disagreed they could learn more from a computer (multimedia, internet) than from books; they believed they learn better from books than from multimedia.

Access to technology is equally important when assessing the success of technology integration. Research (BECTA, 2003) reveals that students and teachers are best served if they have convenient, consistent, and frequent access to technology. All the teachers in this study expressed inadequacy of the facilities especially the unavailability of internet and hands-on opportunity for students. MR3 complains thus; *"For mathematics not enough room we only have one multimedia room. I have to carry my laptop always but if facilities are improved it can help a lot"*. MR2 recommends; *"government has to spend more money, provide us rooms for mathematics like the science they have lab we share multimedia room with other subject"*. SR2 complained that; *"ICT facilities are not really adequate because we don't have internet..."*. The teachers all believe that an improved access to ICT facilities will lead to effective ICT use. *"I foresee a brighter future in teaching with ICT if facilities are improved, with more software introduced, enrichment materials, backups..."* R1 remarked.

Pedagogical and curricular change is an especially important component of operational policies, particularly for strategic policies that promote education reform (Kozma, 2005). Content development is also emphasized because of the need to develop digital content as part of the operational policy. This study (Adedokun, 2008) revealed that both the science and mathematics CD-ROM/software provided for teaching cover and enhance the curriculum. SR1 expresses thus; *"CD covers the topics in the curriculum, it enhances the curriculum because of visual representation"*. MR5 supported this by saying; *"Yes with the software, it is integrated into the curriculum"*. However to ensure effective ICT integration in teaching and learning, policy makers should train teachers more on how to integrate ICT into curriculum. Responses of the teachers interviewed in this study (Adedokun, 2008) disclosed that the training they received was primarily on the basic use of some application programs like Microsoft Words, Excel, and PowerPoint etc. They were not trained on how to use it to reshape lesson content and how to integrate the CD-ROM in instruction. MR1 details the training she received thus; *"I attended only once it's only a 1 day course about 3 to 4 hrs; it's not really helpful because they taught us very general thing…*". SR4 lists the skills she acquired through the training as; "*we have the basic skills in computer like Microsoft word and PowerPoint*". SR5 explains; "*…We need to know more about how to use it to teach the subject, how to use it to do some other things like preparing exam, recording result etc*"

Summarily, this research offers some recommendations that will be useful to the policy makers, the school and the teachers on possible ways of successful technology integration. Future technology integration in the school should involve teachers in the implementation process such that their feelings and confidence about the technology integration will be part of the implementation considerations. This is important because this research discovers that some teachers were reluctant to use the ICT for teaching and some of them resisted to maximize its use because their views were not sought before the implementation. ICT facilities should also be enriched so that the students will have hands-on opportunity and the teachers will have improved access to the ICT facilities. Likewise, the internet should be incorporated in the school and integrated in classroom lessons to facilitate teaching and to enhance students use for information search. This study reveals that if facilities are improved and hands-on opportunities are created for students, it will improve students' learning. Moreover the science and mathematics CD-ROM should be designed to fit in with the curriculum and students' pace. It was gathered from this study that the CD-ROM provided for both mathematics and science are designed at a rather slow pace for students to follow and for teachers to use within the limited class time to be able to complete the syllabus. Effective ICT integration in teaching and learning also requires that teachers be trained more on how to integrate ICT into curriculum. It was observed from the response of the teachers that the training they received was primarily on the basic use of some application programs like

Microsoft Words, Excel, and PowerPoint etc. They were not trained on how to use it to reshape lesson content and how to integrate the CD-ROM in instruction. Likewise both students and teachers complained that there is no technical assistant to help with ICT technical problems in class. As such mentors and technical assistant should be provided in schools to help with any technical problem arising during the course of the lesson to avoid waste of lesson time.

Conclusively, the Ministry of Education should ensure that the situation of ICT in schools be reviewed periodically in order to sustain teachers' utilization of the facilities, make up for the lapses in the implementation program and correct any problem encountered with ICT use in schools. This research therefore suggests for further research to delve into areas that this study could not cover. Other researches can study ICT integration on a wider scale than the scope of this study especially evaluation of students' outcome as a result of a blended approach of both technology and traditional instructional strategies.

ISSUES IN EVALUATION

The study reported in this chapter (Adedokun, 2008) does not include evaluation in its scope because it did not evaluate the Malaysian ICT integration in education as a whole but the study itself is evaluative in nature because it assesses teachers' and students' perception on the use of ICT in teaching and learning. The nature of this study and the fact that proper evaluation of a program or policy is one of the success factors of such policy thus give an avenue for us to discuss issues in evaluation in this chapter.

There is no magic formula that educators and policymakers can use to determine if the return on the investment is actually worth it. Perhaps, rather than asking, "Is technology worth the cost?" the more important question is, "Under what conditions do technology has the most benefits for students?" Investments in technology, in terms of fiscal and time expenditures, can have substantial return when trade-offs and relative benefits have been considered and accounted for. Rather than comparing the effectiveness of varying technologies and instructional media, efforts would be better spent in determining the optimal combinations of instructional strategies and delivery media that would best produce the best learning outcomes for a particular audience (Joy, 2002) as cited in Greenberg, 2004).

We discovered that most researchers fail to control for essential factors such as prior student knowledge, pedagogical methods techniques, and teachers' and students' ability for it. Learning should drive the use of technology rather than technology driving education. Choosing technology first and then trying to fit ourselves, our pedagogies, and our learning goals in it is a great mistake educators make and this has led to numerous false-starts and failures. If we can understand which technologies are best for accomplishing which kinds of cognitive or affective goals, then we can make well-informed decisions and increase the probability of deploying technology successfully.

Researchers should also intensify on a more complicated task of investigating the impact of technology use on higher order thinking skills, problem-solving and analytical skills that can not be measured through standardized tests. Students' ability to understand complex phenomena, analyze and synthesize multiple sources of information, and build representations of their own knowledge should be captured by teachers. Similarly, standardized assessments that emphasize the ability to access, interpret, and synthesize information must be developed. Education stakeholders like parents, teachers, policy makers, and even students themselves should be braced up for the challenges that standardized test scores will not only signify the improvement in students' learning brought

about by technology; they all should contribute and express their expectation of technology in education so that it could be put into measurable form. There is need for continuous assessment that is integrated into regular, ongoing instructional activity and involvement of new assessment methods that include performance tasks and portfolio assessments (Mislevy, et al., 2007). Thus stressing the need for new forms of assessment that will measure the impact of ICT in learning which transcends standardized test scores and evaluate other skills that ICT pedagogy instills in students.

Research efforts should be geared towards investigating what kind of technologies used in under what conditions and what benefits do they give rather than assessing the impact of all technologies as the same. Each technology is likely to play a different role in students' learning. Two general distinctions can be made. Students can learn "from" computers where technology used essentially as tutors and serves to increase students basic skills and knowledge; and can learn "with" computers—where technology is used as a tool that can be applied to a variety of goals in the learning process and can serve as a resource to help develop higher order thinking, creativity and research skills (Ringstaff & Kelley, 2002).

When students are learning "from" computers, the computers are essentially tutors. In this capacity, the technology primarily serves the goal of increasing students' basic skills and knowledge. In learning "with," by contrast, students use technology as a tool that can be applied to a variety of goals in the learning process, rather than serving simply as an instructional delivery system. Students use the technology as a resource to help them develop higher order thinking, creativity and research skills. Learning with technology involves students using technology to gather, organize, and analyze information, and using this information to solve problems. In this manner, the technology is used as a tool, and teachers and students (not the technology) control the curriculum and instruction. Generally, more advanced technology is involved in learning "with." Technology used in these ways leads to outcomes that tend to be difficult to measure. The difficulty results not only from rapid changes in technology, but also because many existing assessments do not adequately capture the skills that this technology enhances, such as critical thinking, higher order thinking skills, writing, and problem solving (Critical Issue, 1999).

Russell, et al. (2003) concludes that if we accept "the good news" that technology does not hurt education; then efforts could be shifted to employing technologies properly and effectively. Also Greenberg (2004) expresses that: "When we accept that technology, suitably and properly deployed; yields no significant difference for learning outcomes, we can stop expecting it to be the be-all, end-all to education". At this juncture we can propose that, rather than comparing the effectiveness of varying technologies and instructional media, efforts would be better spent in determining the optimal combinations of instructional strategies and delivery media that would best produce the best learning outcomes for a particular audience.

One of the problems with evaluation in general is getting its findings used (McLemore, 2009). Often times evaluation results and recommendations are not implemented but evaluation data only become meaningful to stakeholders when they are transformed into information, and ultimately into usable or actionable knowledge (Mandinach & Honey, 2005). Therefore, an effective means of convincing parents, the business community, and taxpayers that teaching with technology complemented with other useful instructional approaches result in better learning outcome is to involve them in students' education. A concerted partnership between schools and communities leads to ample opportunities to develop students' educational outcomes that can result from educational technology.

It is equally important to evaluate properly how education technology funds are being expended. Findings have reported that collecting, allotting, and using technology fees is disjointed and disconnected. It should be noted that, spending massively on hardwares and softwares is merely a partial investment, other aspects include infrastructural refurbishment and the "useware" of the technology itself. Continuous and up-to-date professional development in the integration of teaching and learning should be given a reasonable budget, maintained and sustained. The issue is building teachers' knowledge and skills in alternative types of pedagogy and content, and such an increase in human capabilities requires substantial funding that will be unavailable if almost all resources are put into hardware.

To conclude this write-up, it must be noted that much research has not been carried out on a comprehensive evaluation measure that covers the impact of technology in education, as such, researchers should concentrate efforts on this area of research. The Secretary's Conference on Educational Technology (1999) proposes the following submission that may be useful for researchers:

- The effectiveness of technology is embedded in the effectiveness of other school improvement efforts.
- Current practices for evaluating the impact of technology in education need broadening.
- Standardized test scores offer limited formative information with which to drive the development of a school's technology program.
- Schools must document and report their evaluation findings in ways that satisfy what diverse stakeholders' need to know
- In order for evaluation efforts to provide stakeholders with answers everyone must agree on a common language and standards of practice for measuring how schools achieve that end.

- The role of teachers is crucial in evaluating the effectiveness of technology in schools
- Implementing an innovation in schools can result in practice running before policy. Some existing policies need to be "transformed" to match the new needs of schools using technology.

Similarly, in a review of studies of ICT impact on schools in Europe conducted by (Balanskat, et al., 2006) they recommend the following on research and development on ICT in education:

a. Consider context-sensitive and process-oriented research methods
b. create a closer link between research and practice
c. encourage more qualitative transnational research into ICT impact
d. make national research into impact accessible
e. rethink the approach to evidence and its relation to decision making
f. ICT impact studies based on both quantitative and qualitative evidence

CONCLUSION

This chapter discusses findings of a study conducted by Adedokun, (2008) on ICT integration in the teaching and learning of science and mathematics in secondary school in Malaysia in the light of some success factors in technology integration. We therefore conclude that positive changes in the learning environment evolve over time and do not occur quickly. Steadiness and consistency in the use of technology in education, positive attitude on the part of teachers towards infusion of technology in their classrooms, readiness of the government to invest in the right technology and retraining of teachers and facilitators as new educational technology evolves are possible means of successfully integrating Information and Communication Technology into education.

REFERENCES

Adedokun, N. A. S. (2008). *Integration of ICT into Instruction of Science and Mathematics: A Case Study of Sekolah Menengah Kebangsaan Gombak Setia, Malaysia*. (M.ed Thesis – copyright International Islamic University, Malaysia.)

Adedokun, N. A. S., & Hashim, R. (2008). Integration of Information and Communication Technology (ICT) in the Teaching and Learning of Science: Teachers' and Students' Perception. In *Proceedings of the Conference of Asian Science Education* (CASE 2008) http://case2008.nknu.edu.tw/

Balanskat, A., Blamire, R., & Kefala, S. (2006). *The ICT impact report: A review of studies of ICT impact on schools in Europe*. n.p.: European Schoolnet. Retrieved September 7, 2009, from http://ec.europa.eu/education/pdf/doc254_en.pdf

Becta (2003). *Using ICT to Enhance Home-school Links – an Evaluation of Current Practice in England*, Becta, UK. http://partners.becta.org.uk/index. php?section=rh&&catcode =&rid=13639-2006, *The Becta Review 2006: Evidence on the Progress of ICT in Education*, Becta, UK. http://becta.org.uk/corporate/publications/ documents/The_Becta_Review_2006.pdf 2007, *What Is a Learning Platform?* http://schools.becta.org.uk/index .php?section=re&&catcode =&rid=12887

Bransford, J., Darling-Hammond, L., & LePage, P. (2005). Introduction. In Bransford, J., & Darling-Hammond, L. (Eds.), *Preparing teachers for a changing world: What teachers should learn and be able to do* (pp. 1–39). San Francisco: Jossey-Bass.

CGD. (2006). *When Will We Ever Learn? Improving Lives Through Impact Evaluation*. Washington, DC: Center for Global Development.

Coppola, E. M. (2004). *Powering up: Learning to teach well with technology*. New York: Teachers College Press.

Fishman, B., & Davis, E. (2006). Teacher learning research and the learning sciences. In Sawyer, R. K. (Ed.), *Cambridge Handbook of the Learning Sciences* (pp. 535–550). Cambridge, UK: Cambridge University Press.

Greenberg, A. D. (2004). *Navigating the sea of research on videoconferencing-based distance education: A platform for understanding research into technology's effectiveness and value.* Retrieved from http://www.wainhouse.com/files / papers/wr-navseadistedu.pdf

Henriquez, A., & Riconscente, M. (1999). *Rhode Island Teachers and Technology Initiative: Program evaluation final report.* New York: Education Development Center, Center for Children and Technology.

Higgins, C. (2005). Primary school students' perceptions of interactive whiteboards'. *Journal of Computer Assisted Learning*, 21.

Higgins, C., Falzon, C., Hall, I., Moseley, D., Smith, F., Smith, H., & Wall, K. (2005). *Embedding ICT in the Literacy and Numeracy Strategies: Final Report.* UK: University of Newcastle.

Hofer, L. (2003). *Critical issues in evaluating the effectiveness of technology. Critical Review CET 720.* New York: Springer.

IEG. (2006). *Impact Evaluation Experience of the Independent Evaluation Group of the World Bank.* Washington, DC: World Bank.

Jones, R. (2003). Local and national ICT policies. In R. Kozma (Ed.) *Technology, innovation, and educational change: A global perspective* (pp. 163-194). Eugene, Kelley, L. (2002). *A Review of Findings from Research By: Cathy Ringstaff.* Retrieved October 13, 2009, from http://www.wested.org/ cs/we/view/rs/619

Kozma, R. (2005). National policies that connect ICT-based *education* reform to economic and social development. *Human Technology, 1*(2), 117–156.

Krajcik, J., & Blumenfeld, P. (2006). Project-based learning. In Sawyer, R. K. (Ed.), *Cambridge Handbook of the Learning Sciences* (pp. 317–334). Cambridge, UK: Cambridge University Press.

Machin, S. (2006). *New Technologies in Schools: Is There a Pay Off?* Germany: Institute for the Study of Labour.

Mandinach, E. B., & Honey, M. (2005). *A theoretical framework for data-driven decision making.* Paper presented at the Wingspread Conference on data-driven decision making, October 30-November 1, Racine, WI.

McLemore, A. (2009). *Advantages and disadvantages of online instruction.* Retrieved 12 August, 2009 from http://www.americanchronicle.com

Means, B. (2006). Prospects for transforming schools with technology-supported assessment. In Sawyer, R. K. (Ed.), *Cambridge Handbook of the Learning Sciences* (pp. 505–520). Cambridge, UK: Cambridge University Press.

Means, B., Roschelle, R., Penuel, W., Sabelli, N., & Haertel, G. (2004). Technology's contribution to teaching and policy: Efficiency, standardization, or transformation? In Floden, R. E. (Ed.), *Review of Research in Education* (*Vol. 27*). Washington, DC: American Educational Research Association.

Mislevy, R. J., Behrens, J. T., Bennett, R. E., Demark, S. F., Frezzo, D. C., Levy, R., Robinson, D.H., Rutstein D. W., & Valerie J. (2007). *On The Roles of External Knowledge Representations in Assessment Design.* CSE Report 722.

Norris, C., Sullivan, T., Poirot, J., & Soloway, E. (2003). No Access, No Use, No Impact: Snapshot Surveys of Educational Technology in K-12. *Journal of Research on Technology in Education, ISTE, 36*(1), 15–28.

OECD. (2004). *Are Pupils Ready for a Technology-rich World? What PISA Studies Tell Us*. France: OECD.

OECD. (2005). E-learning in tertiary education: where do we stand? *Evaluation & Skills, 4*(1), 1–293.

Pittard, V., Bannister, P., & Dunn, J. (2003). *The Big pICTure: The Impact of ICT on Attainment, Motivation and Learning,* DfES Publications, UK. http://www.dfes.gov.uk/research/ data/up-loadfiles/ThebigpICTure.pdf

Quale, A. (2003). Trends in instructional ICT infrastructure. In Plomp, T., Anderson, R., Law, N., & Quale, A. (Eds.), *Cross-national information and communication technology policies and practices in education* (pp. 31–42). Greenwich, CT: IPA.

Quality Education Data (QED). (2004). *Technology Purchasing Forecast, 2003-2004*. Denver, CO: Scholastic, Inc.

Ringstaff, C., & Kelley, L. (2002). *The Learning Return on our Educational Investment*. Retrieved October 6, 2009 from http://www.westedrtec.org.

Russell, M., Bebell, D., O'Dwyer, L., & O'Connor, K. (2003). Examining Teacher Technology Use Implications for Preservice and Inservice Teacher Preparation. *Journal of Teacher Education, 54*(4), 297–310. doi:10.1177/0022487103255985

Sandholtz, J. H. (2001). Learning to teach with technology: A comparison of teacher development programs. *Journal of Technology and Teacher Education, 9*(3), 349–374.

Sivin-Kachala, J., & Bialo, E. (2000). *2000 research report on the effectiveness of technology in schools* (7th ed.). Washington, DC: Software and Information Industry Association.

Underwood, J., et al (2005). *Impact of Broadband in Schools,* Nottingham Trent University, Becta, June 2005.

Underwood, J., et al. (2006). *ICT Test Bed Evaluation-Evaluation of the ICT Test Bed Project,* Nottingham Trent University, UK. Retrieved from http://www.evaluation.ictte stbed.org.uk/about

Wagner, D., Day, R., James, T., Kozma, R., Miller, J., & Unnwin, T. (2005). *Monitoring and evaluation of ICT in education projects: A handbook for developing countries*. Washington: infoDev, World Bank.

Chapter 5
ICT and Web 2.0 Technologies as a Determinant of Business Performance

Tanja Arh
Jožef Stefan Institute, Slovenia

Vlado Dimovski
University of Ljubljana, Slovenia

Borka Jerman Blažič
Jožef Stefan Institute, Slovenia

EXCUTIVE SUMMARY

This chapter aims at presenting the results of an empirical study, linking the fields of technology-enhanced learning (TEL), Web 2.0 technologies and organizational learning, and their impact on the financial and non-financial business performance. The chapter focuses on the presentation of the conceptualization of a structural model that was developed to test the impact of technology-enhanced learning and Web 2.0 technologies on the organizational learning and business performance of companies with more than 50 employees. The paper provides detailed definitions of technology-enhanced learning, Web 2.0 technologies and technical terms related to it, its scope and the process of organisational learning, as well as a method for business performance assessment. Special attention is given to the findings related to the observed correlations between the aforementioned constructs. The results of the study indicate a strong impact of ICT and technology-enhanced learning on organizational learning and the non-financial business performance.

INTRODUCTION AND BACKGROUND

Success in a highly dynamic environment requires a more efficient response to customers from the side of the companies, more flexible approaches in facing their business circle and more focus on their core competencies (Smith, 2008). What are companies expected to do in order to introduce the necessary changes in the whole business circle? The answer definitely lies in people. The employees' knowledge and competencies significantly contribute to the company's ability to react to the

DOI: 10.4018/978-1-60960-015-0.ch005

requirements of the fast changes markets, customer needs and successful business processes. With this in view, companies are obliged to manage and maintain the knowledge of their employees. Maintaining the knowledge means to evaluate the employees' tacit and explicit knowledge, and provide knowledge within the company with the suitable tools (Reychav & Weisberg, 2009).

To perform this approach effectively, employees and all members of the company are expected to continuously refresh and enhance their skills and knowledge (Collins & Smith, 2006). As the human capital replacing the physical capital as the source of competitive advantage, organizational learning emerges as a key element for success (Varney, 2008). Only by making learning a truly strategic investment we can ensure an organization in which every person within the company is fully enabled to perform effectively and meet the ever changing demands.

When companies devise their strategies for the employee knowledge acquisition, they can find the most suitable solutions among the methods based on information and communication technologies (ICT), Web 2.0 technologies and technology-enhanced learning (TEL). Technology-enhanced learning as a way of acquiring knowledge and competences has been adopted by many companies as a promising time and cost saving solution providing learn-on-demand opportunities to individual employees, TEL enables workers to access various on-line databases, tools and e-services that help them find solutions for work-related problems (Zhang, 2002; 2003). The term Web 2.0 was coined by O'Reilly (2005) as a common denominator for recent trends heading towards the 'Read-Write Web', allowing everyone to publish resources on the web using simple and open, personal and collaborative publishing tools, known as the social software: blogs, wikis, social bookmarking systems, podcasts, etc. The main features of these tools are dynamism, openness and free availability. According to MacManus and Porter (2005), the power of social software

lies in the content personalization and remixing with the other data to create much more useful information and knowledge. The continuously growing dissemination of social and open software in technology-enhanced learning is expected to reshape the technology-enhanced learning landscapes that are currently based on closed, proprietary, institutionalized systems. Thanks to the web evolution, the use of social and open software for learning is becoming an increasingly feasible alternative to these closed, proprietary, institutionalized systems.

However, earlier authors (Roach, 1987) argued that ICT still had not paid off in terms of the required productivity growth. The phenomenon was called the 'productivity paradox' and it asserted that the ICT investments did not result in productivity gains (Navarette & Pick, 2002). Carr (2003) believes that 'ICT may not help a company gain a strategic advantage, but it could easily put a company at a cost disadvantage.' Indeed, the latest empirical studies (Dewan & Kraemer 1998; Navarette & Pick 2002; Dimovski & Škerlavaj 2003) tend to reject the productivity paradox thesis – the phenomenon of organisational learning can be seen as a way out of the dilemma called the productivity paradox. In the last few decades the field of organisational learning has attracted a lot of interest from academics as well as practitioners. A key question in this context is the connection between ICT and organisational learning, and the impact they both have on the business performance (Škerlavaj & Dimovski, 2006).

In the past decade, quite a lot of research studies dealt with the influence of ICT (investments, usage, etc.) on (mainly financial) business performance. We can divide them into four streams of research based on the observed units: business, industry, national and international levels. The results were mixed. Some recent studies in our context (Dimovski & Škerlavaj, 2003) that analysed the influence of hardware, software, telecommunications and knowledge investments on value added per industry in Slovenia for the period 1996-2000, demonstrated a statistically significant, positive influence of hardware and telecommunication investments on value added (Škerlavaj & Dimovski, 2006). Dimovski (1994) confirmed the positive impact on both – the financial and non-financial performance aspects, using a one-industry research design and a stratified sample of 200 credit unions in Ohio, based on the asset size criterion (Škerlavaj & Dimovski, 2006). This study investigated the determinants, processes and outcomes of organisational learning, as well as the relationship between organisational learning and performance. Sloan et al. (2002), Lam (1998) and Figueireido (2003) also arrived at similar conclusions. Simonin (1997) found strong effects of learning on the financial and non-financial performance in the context of strategic alliances.

This chapter has four parts. The first section provides definitions of technology-enhanced learning and Web 2.0 technologies, technical terms related to it, its scope and the process of organisational learning, as well as a method for the business performance assessment in order to develop a set of constructs and an empirical basis for the relationships among them. In the second part, the model's operationalisation through the development of a measurement sub-model is presented. In the third section, the model is tested using a structural linear modelling technique. We conclude with a discussion on the implications of the results and offer some guidelines for future research.

CONCEPTUALISATION OF STRUCTURAL SUB-MODEL

A complete research model normally consists of two sub-models: measurement and structural (Jöreskog, Sörbrom, 1993). The measurement sub-model shows how each latent variable is operationalised through observations of corresponding indicators, and also provides data on validity and reliability of the variables observed. The structural sub-model describes relationships between the latent variables, indicating the amount of unexplained variance. Development of a quality model requires first to establish a structural framework, which is usually implemented in two steps: presentation of fundamental constructs and review of potential correlations between them. Results of the final analysis greatly depend on good conceptualisation of a research model (Jöreskog, Sörbrom, 1993).

Technology-Enhanced Leaning and Web 2.0 Technologies

Technology-enhanced learning is a term introduced along with the introduction of information and communication technology for educational purposes. Up to date companies have widely used this term as a synonym for e-learning (Arh, Pipan & Jerman-Blažič, 2006). Definitions of technology-enhanced learning are various, diverse and lack unity, consequently, it is of outmost importance to provide precise definitions of technology-enhanced learning and related notions. Hereby we refer to the process of studying and teaching as technology-enhanced learning when it includes information and communication technology, regardless of the mode or the scope of its use (Henry, 2001).

Kirschner and Paas (2001) defined technology-enhanced learning as a learning process in which the Internet plays the key role in the presentation, support, management and assessment of learning. Rosenberg (2001) defines technology-enhanced learning as a learning process in which information technology partially or fully undertakes the role of a mediator between different stakeholders involved in the learning process. We refer to the process of studying and teaching as technology-enhanced learning when it includes information and communication technology, regardless of the mode or the scope of its use (Henry, 2001; Dinevski & Plenković, 2002). Technology-enhanced learning extends the company out to ever-widening circles of impact. The companies are participating in a radical redefinition of industries, markets and the global economy itself. Today, organizations are investing great efforts into the making of proper adjustments to the changing business environment in order to enhance their competitiveness. In an attempt to keep up with the development of information technology and the Internet, many businesses are replacing traditional vocational training with e-learning to better manage their workforce. However, it is questionable whether training programs actually change employee behaviour after the implementation. In the case of the US companies, only 10-15% of training is applied to work (Sevilla & Wells, 1988).

When we talk about technology-enhanced learning we cannot overlook the impact of the Web 2.0 technologies on the process of technology-enhanced learning. The Web 2.0 technologies are changing the way messages spread across the web. A number of online tools and platforms are now defining how people share their perspectives, opinions, thoughts and experiences. The Web 2.0 tools, such as instant messaging systems, blogs, RSS, video casting, social bookmarking, social networking, podcasts and picture sharing sites are becoming more and more popular. One major advantage of the Web 2.0 tools is that the majority of them are free. There is a large number of the Web 2.0 tools, some of the more popular ones are: instant messaging systems, blogs, video-wiki and xo-wiki, Doodle, podcasting, RSS, etc.

Instant Messaging Systems (IMS)

The need for communication tools in the learning process is often underestimated by educators, especially those who feel comfortable with the traditional, instructive way of teaching. However, even with their 'traditional' approach learners need to communicate with each other when working together. At the beginning of the 90s, digital communication tools were rather limited: apart from the direct face-to-face meetings, the main way to communicate was through the plain old telephone. Sharing course materials was only enabled by a copy or a fax machine. However, these devices were rarely available in ordinary households. The only barriers to communication that exist today are the lack of skills needed to operate the new technologies. This barrier goes mostly unnoticed with the younger generations that have grown up as digital 'natives', rarely pulling themselves away from their computers (even out on the street they keep the mobile phones in their pockets), but it is definitely still a serious obstacle for many educators. However, the new technologies are inevitably permeating our everyday lives, and it is probably not necessary to explain the purpose of instant messaging to anyone in 2009. The number of users of the world top 10 instant messaging systems is counted in hundreds of millions according to the Wikipedia (2008) statistics, e.g. QQ 783 million total, 317.9 million active, 40.3 million peak online (mostly in China), MSN 294 million active, Yahoo 248 million active, Skype 309 million total, 12 million speak online, etc. The decisive factor for choosing an instant messaging system by an ordinary user is a friend recommendation (most people start using the same system the majority of their friends are already using). The IMS are used for any kind of information exchange including communication between employees or students regarding their study or learning environment. This is the reason this practice is included in the technology that contributes to the personalized learning environment.

Blogs

A blog is a type of a web site in which entries are made as in a journal or a diary and are displayed in reverse chronological order. Basically, an individual maintains his or her own weblog and it functions as a sort of a personal online diary. Regular entries such as comments, descriptions of events, or other types of materials combined with text, images, and links to other weblogs and web sites are the typical weblog ingredients. Blogs have attracted a lot of attention within the educational circles, where they are experienced as the tools that support several pedagogical aims and scenarios, ranging from an individual knowledge management and competence development to group-based learning activities. Therefore, blogs have become an important educational tool in recent years, providing an opportunity for both facilitators and employees to publish their ideas, essays, or simply providing a space to reflect upon their particular learning processes and reading materials. In the context of teaching and learning, blogs can do much more than just deliver instructions or course news items to employees. They can be an interesting collaboration tool for employees who can join relevant community and find people to collaborate with, give feedback to the management and others. In a learning environment blogs are most frequently used for content publishing and sharing. The blog technology can be improved by plug-ins such as the FeedBack tool used to track and integrate the content of other authors within one blog. FeedBack is a standard plug-in piece of code developed within the framework of the iCamp project (www.icamp-project.eu). In a simple way it is used to enable blog users to subscribe to each others' blogs. The blogging technology, in combination with innovations such as the FeedBack specification, has definitely a high potential to be considered a powerful tool for learning with others.

Video-Wiki and Xo-Wiki

Publishing or presenting someone's thoughts online usually means writing some text and illustrating it with pictures. Still, the most natural form of communication for humans is face to face, and for most people the majority of information is presented orally, directly facing the presenter, whose non-verbally communicated information is often even more important than the words they

utter. Video could serve as a replacement for the face-to-face presentation, since it can convey the visible behaviour and important non-verbal information. In the past, recording a video and making sure it reached the target audience was quite a big challenge. Depending on the number of intended users, TV broadcasts or video tapes could be used. Employees taking part in an e-learning course work in groups, and are suggested to form groups by getting to know each other and discover some common topics. The mentor/tutor usually uses VideoWiki to record for ex. short self-introduction videos in which employees present their background, or explain their expectations regarding some specific topic for the group assignment. VideoWiki is based on the Red5 open-source Flash server written in Java and Flash. It allows video recording, searching and playback through the main system web page or via the standard URL links. VideoWiki also provides RSS feeds for each name, space or author, and videos can be embedded on any web page using special code snippets. Collaborative creation and maintenance of knowledge artefacts is one of the emerging phenomena of the online Internet communities, such as Wikipedia.org, MediaWiki.org, LyricWiki.org, Microformats. org and Wikitravel.org. A collection of web pages (a so-called wiki) can also be very useful for the teaching and learning purposes; for instance if learners need to collaborate to work on certain topics, or if facilitators wish to develop and share their learning content with others. Consequently, a contemporary approach to technology-enhanced learning requires tools which can enable learners to work on artefacts collaboratively, either by allowing them to publish small posts which can be reused and combined with others (see the blog-based solution presented in the previous section) or by providing real wiki functionality. XoWiki is one such wiki implementation, realized as a component of OpenACS (Open Architecture Community System), a framework for building scalable, community-oriented web applications.

XoWiki includes a rich text editor for easy creation and editing of wiki pages, and provides features for structuring, commenting, tagging and visualisation of the wiki-based content.

Doodle

When employees work on a group project they need to divide tasks among the members of the group and monitor the progress of work. This requires the employees to engage in collaboration, discussion and decision making processes. In the context of bringing different cultures, educational systems, levels of teaching, languages and technology skills into a common virtual learning space, planning a series of meetings several weeks in advance may simply not work. Taking this into account, employees must adopt simple solutions to meet their needs. There are plenty of solutions which can help make a project run smoothly. One of them is Doodle. Doodle can be described simply as a web-based tool for finding suitable appointment dates. Doodle allows employees to plan their meetings with partners, suppliers and other employees. In addition to time management, it can be used as a voting tool for any other issue that arises as a part of the distance learning process; for example, the literature that needs to be selected and analysed in order to complete a particular task.

Searching the Net: ObjectSpot

ObjectSpot is a meta-search engine designed to facilitate different types of research. It can be used to find publications and other learning resources on the web. ObjectSpot realizes federated searches over an ever-increasing number of digital libraries and learning object repositories. It provides access to more than 10 million learning objects spread across famous libraries such as the Directory of Open Access Journals (DOAJ), OAIster, EBSCO, ACM, CiteBase and IEEE. Some of these repositories are open access, whilst others require registration or subscription.

Organisational Learning

In recent years, the concept of organizational learning has enjoyed a renaissance among both academics and practitioners seeking to improve organizations. Early proponents (e.g. Argyris & Schön, 1978) found their ideas largely confined to the periphery of management thought during the 1980s, but the 1990s witnessed a rebirth of interest. The current renaissance is evident in the creation of a journal about organizational learning (*The Learning Organization*) as well as in the devotion of special issues of several journals to the topic (e.g., *Organization Science*, 1991; *Organizational Dynamics*, 1993; *Accounting, Management and Information Technologies,* 1995; *Journal of Organizational Change Management*, 1996). The appearance of several major review articles is testimony to organizational learning's growing stature in the research community (see Crossan, Lane & White, 1999; Dodgson, 1993; Fiol & Lyles, 1985; Huber, 1991; Jones, 2000; Levitt & March, 1998; Miner & Mezias, 1996). Moreover, a large number of articles in professional periodicals describing the design and management of learning organizations attest to the popularity of organizational learning and knowledge management among practitioners. New theories of knowledge creation have become prominent (Nonaka, 1994; Raelin, 1997), and formal knowledge management programs have been undertaken in many companies (Davenport, De Long & Beers, 1998). As we head into the twenty-first century, therefore, organizational learning promises to be a dominant perspective with influence on both organizational research and management practice (Argyris & Schön, 1996).

Defining Organizational Learning

Organisational learning is defined in numerous ways and approached from different perspectives. The pioneers (Argyris, & Schön, 1996; Senge, 1990) defined organisational learning as an individual's acquisition of information and knowledge, and development of analytical and communicational skills. Understanding organisational learning as a process, which can take up different levels of development, makes the learning organisational structure an ideal form of organisation, which can only be achieved once the process of organisational learning is fully optimised and the organisation is viewed as a system (Senge, 1990). Jones (2000) emphasizes the importance of organizational learning for the organizational performance, defining it as "a process through which managers try to increase organizational members' capabilities in order to better understand and manage the organization and its environment and accept the decisions that would increase organizational performance on a continuous basis." The aforementioned statements regarding the lack of unity of organisational learning definitions are also supported by the findings of Shrivastava, 1983 and Dimovski, 1994. The former states that extensive research carried out in the field of organisational learning has mostly been fragmented, while the latter adds the fragmentation lead to the multitude of definitions (for ex. Nonaka & Takeuchi, 1996 and Wall, 1998), differing according to the criteria of inclusion, scope and focus (Škerlavaj, 2003). Dimovski (1994) and Dimovski & Colnar (1999) provided an overview of previous research and identified four varying perspectives on organizational learning. Dimovski's model managed to merge informational, interpretational, strategic and behavioural approaches to organizational learning, and defined it as a process of information acquisition, information interpretation and the resulting behavioural and cognitive changes which should, in turn, have an impact on the company performance.

Development of our research model is based on DiBella and Nevis' model (DiBella & Nevis, 1998) of integrated approach, according to which the organisational learning factors are divided into study guidelines and study promoters, and on the Dimovski approach (Dimovski, 1994), which combines the aforementioned four aspects of organisational learning.

In this sense the organisational learning can be defined as a dynamic process of the acquisition, transfer and use of knowledge (Crossan, Lane & White, 1999; Dibella & Nevis, 1998), which starts at the core of the organisation – related to individual and team performance – and enable companies to strengthen the efficiency of the financial and non-profit (non-financial?) business achievements (Tippins & Sohi, 2003).

Business Performance

Business performance assessments have advanced over the past years, and developed from traditional, exclusively financial criteria, to modern criteria, which include also the non-financial indicators. Due to numerous disadvantages of the classical accounts and the growing need for quality information on company performance, the theory of economics started developing improved models for performance assessment, taking into account all shareholders: employees, customers, supplier employees and the wider community, also advocated by the Freeman's shareholders theory (Freeman, 1994; 1984). There are several approaches to the non-financial indicator selection, the most established of which is the Balanced Scorecard – BSC (Kaplan & Norton, 1992). The existing models, based on the accounting categories, combine with the non-financial data and the assessment of the so called 'soft' business areas, which mostly improve the assessment of companies' perspective possibilities. For a good performance of a modern company we need to introduce the non-financial indicators along with the financial ones.

Relationship among Constructs

Findings based on a rather wide overview and systematisation of literature has shown that we can expect positive impact of ICT and technology-enhanced learning on organisational learning and business performance. Robey et al. (2000) do warn that technology-enhanced learning and relative ICT may take either the role of a promoter or the role of an inhibitor of organisational learning, so the following hypothesis can be posed:

H1: *Technology-enhanced learning has positive impact on organisational learning.*

H2: *Technology-enhanced learning has positive impact on financial performance.*

H3: *Technology-enhanced learning has positive impact on non-financial performance.*

Correlation between organisational learning and business success is often a controversial issue when we begin to deal with the company management (Inkpen & Crossan, 1995). Some authors believe better performance is related to organisational learning, though their definitions of business results differ greatly. In relation to this we can mention the capacity of organisational learning to have a positive impact on the financial results (Lei et al., 1999; Slater & Narver, 1995), on the results related to shareholders (Goh & Richards, 1997; Ulrich et al., 1993) and on the business results, such as innovativeness and greater productivity (Leonard-Barton, 1992). Mintzberg (1990) says the company performance is an important piece of feedback information on effectiveness and efficiency of the learning process. The study of Perez et al. (2004) has shown organisational learning has a significant impact on the company performance. On this basis, the following hypotheses can be put forward:

H4: *Organisational learning leads to improved financial results.*

H5: *Organisational learning leads to improved non-financial results.*

CONCEPTUALISATION OF MEASUREMENT SUB-MODEL

Having understood the hypothesized correlations between the latent variables, the following question is logically raised: 'How should these four constructs be operationalised and measured?' There are certainly various approaches available, since the number and the type of indicators to be used for the assessment of a certain construct, the number and the type of items to be included under an indicator and the methods for their integration are decided on the basis of validity and variability of specific measuring instruments. Table 1 presents constructs, indicators used for construct assessment, number of items summed up to give the value of an indicator and the theory or empirical research on the basis of which the measurement items were developed.

In short, the hypothesized model shall be composed of four constructs and 13 indicators, and will be of recursive nature, meaning that there shall be no cases of two variables appearing simultaneously, i.e. as a cause and a consequence to one another.

Development of Research Instrument

The questionnaire used has been under constant development and validation for more than 10 years. Dimovski (1994) used it on a sample of Ohio credit unions in order to measure the organizational learning process as a source of competitive advantage. Škerlavaj (2003) upgraded it to include the measures of non-financial performance, while he replaced the industry-specific measures of financial performance with two measures valid for

Table 1. Specification of constructs

Latent Variables	Indicators and Number of Items from Questionnaire
Technology-Enhanced Learning	Information and communication infrastructure (ICI) – 9 items Education technology (ET) – 10 items Learning contents (LC) – 3 items
Organisational Learning	Knowledge acquisition (KAc) – 9 items Knowledge transmission (KTt) – 10 items Use of knowledge (UoK) – 10 items
Financial Performance	Return on assets (FP1) – 1 item Return on capital (FP2) – 1 item Value added per employee (FP3) – 1 item
Non-Financial Performance	Employee fluctuation (NFP1) – 1 item Share of loyal customers (NFP2) – 1 item Number of customer complaints (NFP3) – 1 item Supplier relations (NFP4) – 1 item

all companies. For this study the operationalisation of all four constructs involved was improved and applied on a sample of Slovenian companies with more than 50 employees in 2007. The reason to include smaller companies is to improve the generalizability of the research findings. The measurement instrument used in this study has 22 items for the technology-enhanced learning construct, 29 items for the organizational learning construct, 3 items for the financial and 4 items for the non-financial performance. The pre-testing procedures were conducted in the form of interviews and studies with managers and focus groups of research and academic colleagues.

RESEARCH HYPOTHESES AND MODEL

Once the theoretical frame of the model is devised, illustration of conceptualisation by the means of a flow chart is to be tackled (Arh, Dimovski & Jerman-Blažič, 2008). Flow chart is a graphical representation of interrelations between various elements of a model. Measurement variables belonging to exogenous latent variables are marked with an x, while their measurement deviations are marked with a δ. Endogenous latent variable indicators are marked with a y, and measurement deviations with an ε. Structural equation deviations are ζ, exogenous latent variables are ξ, endogenous constructs are η, and one-way influence of exogenous latent variables on exogenous are γ. To describe relations between latent variables and their indicators (measurement variables) we use λ. The Figure 1 below is showing a conceptualised research model, presenting all basic constructs and hypothesized correlations between them. We aim at proving: (1) that the latent variable of technology-enhanced learning (TEL) has positive impact on organisational learning (OL), (2) financial (FP) and (3) non-financial performance (NFP); (4) that the latent variable of organisational learning (OL) as a process of knowledge creation leads to improved financial results (FP), as well as to (5) improved non-financial results (NFP); (6) that it is impossible to expect significant statistical correlations between financial performance (FP) and non-financial (NFP) performance.

RESEARCH PROCEDURE

The methodology applied to test our research model was structural equation modelling (SEM). This involves a combination of confirmatory factor analysis (CFA) and econometric modelling, which aims to analyse hypothesised relationships

Figure 1. Conceptualised research model

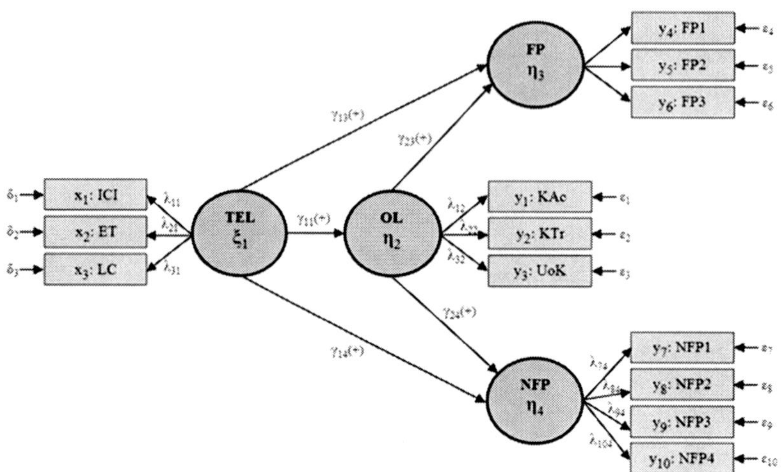

among the latent constructs, measured with observed indicators (measurement variables). Table 2 provides the procedure for data analysis.

First, the item analysis was performed to describe the sample characteristics, to investigate the item means, and to assess item-to-total correlations. Second, exploratory factor analysis was performed to explore whether the items load highly on their intended latent construct, and have low cross-loadings. After the exploratory factor analysis, reliability of the underlying factors was discussed in terms of Cronbach's alphas. Third, confirmatory analysis (CFA) was performed to ensure that the constructs are valid and reliable; this refers to the measurement part of the model. Consequently, CFAs (without any structural relationships) were performed with LISREL 8.80 to check whether the items meet the criteria for convergent and discriminant validity, as well as construct reliability. Properties of the four research constructs in the proposed model (Figure 1) and the five hypotheses were tested using LISREL 8.80 and PRELIS 2.30 packages for structural equation analysis and procedures. As estimation

Table 2. Research pocedure

Stage	Analysis	Purpose
1.	Item Analysis	Investigation of sample characteristics Investigation of item means Investigation of item-to-total correlations
2.	Exploratory Factor Analysis	Exploration of loadings; removal of items with low loadings and high cross-loadings; Assessment of number of latent factors Assessment of reliability (Cronbach's alpha)
3.	Confirmatory Factor Analysis	Assessment of convergent validity Assessment of discriminant validity Assessment of construct reliability Assessment of correlations and multicollinearity
4.	Testing Hypothesis	Assessment of structural relationship (H1-H5) Parameter Estimates for Overall Measurement Model Convergent and Discriminant Validity
5.	Presentation of Results	Discussion of findings

method for model evaluation and procedures, the maximum likelihood (ML) method was utilized. Structural equation modelling (SEM) is designed to evaluate how well a proposed conceptual model that contains observed indicators and hypothetical constructs explains or fits the collected data. It also provides the ability to measure or specify the structural relationships among the sets of unobserved (latent) variables, while describing the amount of unexplained variance. Clearly, the hypothetical model in this study was designed to measure structural relationships among the unobserved constructs that are set up on the basis of relevant theories, and prior empirical research and results. Therefore, the SEM procedure is an appropriate solution for testing the proposed structural model and hypotheses for this study.

Data Gathering and Sample

Based on the model's conceptualisation, a measurement instrument (questionnaire) was developed and sent in June 2007 to the CEOs or board members of all Slovenian companies with more than 50 employees, which accounted for 1215 companies. In the first three weeks 356 completed questionnaires were returned, five out of which were excluded from further analysis due to missing values. The response rate was 29.7%, which can be considered successful in the Slovenian context (using our primary data collection technique and no call backs). It is an indication that, beside academia, managers are also interested to know whether and in which circumstances investments in ICT and technology-enhanced learning pay off. We aimed at an audience of top and middle managers bearing in mind the idea of a strategic and to some degree even an interdisciplinary perspective of the companies in question, although there is some discrepancy between the desired and the actual structure of respondents. Based on the criterion of the average number of employees, in 2006 73.88% of the selected companies had between 50 and 249 employees, followed by 14.61%

with 250 to 499 employees, while 11.51% of the companies had 500 to 999 employees. According to the company revenues in 2006, 33.15% of the Slovenian companies had the annual revenue of 2 to 7.3 million EUR. A somewhat smaller proportion (32.87%) of companies had the net income of 7.3 to 29.2 million EUR in this same period, 19.94% had the annual turnover of more than 29.2 million euro, and only 14.04% have not reached the annual revenue threshold of 2 million euro. The questionnaire was mostly completed by middle management respondents (directors of functional departments). The top and middle management were almost equally represented within the sample.

Table 3 demonstrates the industry structure of the companies in question. Our respondents reported in almost half of all cases that their main industry was manufacturing, followed by 13.8% of companies in the construction business and 11.5% in the wholesale & retail, repair of motor vehicles, personal & household goods. One out of fifteen industries have only one company representative, there was no company from the fishery sector and only two companies working the field of education. This is logical since we excluded the non-profit and small businesses from our analysis.

Parameter Value Estimates

The results of structural equation analysis by LISREL were utilized to test the hypotheses proposed in this study. As discussed in the previous section, the relationships between the constructs were examined based on t-values associated with path coefficients between the constructs. If an estimated t-value was greater than a certain critical value (p < .05, t-value = 1.96) (Mueller, 1996), the null hypothesis that the associated estimated parameter is equal to 0 was rejected. Subsequently, the hypothesized relationship was supported.

The maximum likelihood (ML) method was used to estimate the parameter values. In this phase,

Table 3. Structure of respondents (by industry)

Industry (EU NACE Rev.1)	Frequency	Percent (%)
A Agriculture, hunting and forestry	7	2
B Fishing	0	0
C Mining and quarrying	7	2
D Manufacturing	158	44.4
E Electricity, gas and water supply	15	4.2
F Construction	49	13.8
G Wholesale & retail, repair of motor vehicles, personal & household goods	41	11.5
H Hotels and restaurants	12	3.4
I Transport, storage and communication	14	3.9
J Financial intermediation	7	2
K Real estate, renting and business activities	16	4.5
M Education	2	0.6
N Health and social work	1	0.3
O Other community, social and personal services	27	7.6

the hypotheses posed in the conceptualisation phase are tested. Even though several methods can be used for this purpose, ML is the one most often used and has the advantage of being statistically efficient and at the same time specification-error sensitive because it demands only complete data and does not allow for missing values. All methods will, however, lead to similar parameter estimates on the condition that the sample is large enough and that the model is correct (Jöreskog & Sörbrom, 1993). Figure 2 shows a path diagram of our model (with completely standardised parameter estimates).

The Tpu construct demonstrated a statistically significant, positive and strong impact on the Ou. Namely, the value of the completely standardised parameter almost equals the margin of 0.70. However, Tpu did not exhibit any statistically significant impact on the Fp, meaning that the hypothesis 2 must be rejected. The Ol construct demonstrated a statistically significant positive and strong impact on the Fp and an even stronger one on the Nfp. This means that the hypotheses 4 and 5 can be considered empirically supported by the data at hand.

Global Fit Assessment

Bollen (1989) explained that the model fit relates to the degree to which a hypothesised model is consistent with the available data – the degree to which the implicit matrix of covariances (based on the hypothesised model) and the sample covariance matrix (based on the data) fit. The aim of the global fit assessment is to determine to what degree is the model as a whole consistent with the data gathered. Over the years numerous global fit indices have been developed. To every researcher's regret, none of them is superior to the others. Different authors favour different measures. Diamantopoulos and Siguaw (2000) recommend using several measures and at the same time provide reference values for every one of them (Table 4).

The most traditional value is χ^2 statistics. Using this fit indicator we test the hypothesis that the implicit covariance matrix equals the sample covariance matrix. Our goal was not to reject this hypothesis, however, in our case this hypothesis must be rejected (at a 5% level of significance). Nonetheless, quantifying the degree of misfit is

*Figure 2. Research model (completely standardised parameter values, *significant at p > 0.05)*

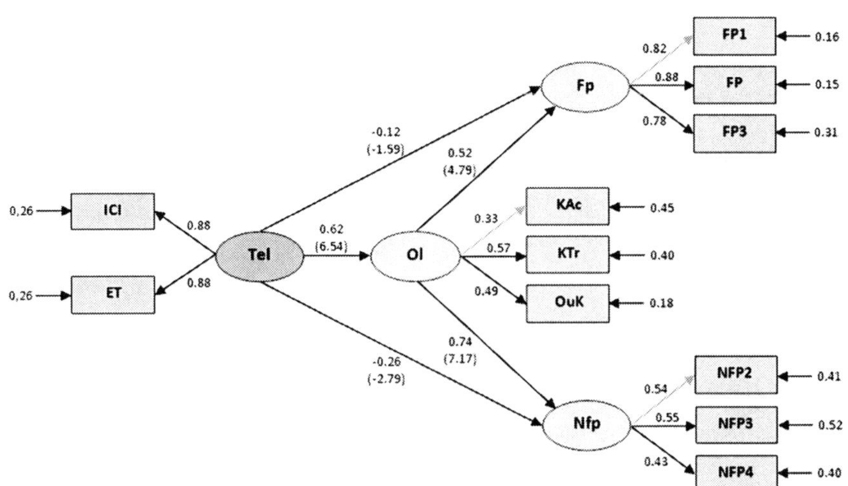

often more useful than testing the hypothesis of exact fit, which χ^2 statistics are designed for. All other indices lead to the conclusion that the model is an appropriate representation of reality. The root means square error of approximation (RMSEA) is the most widespread measure of the global fit and in our case points to the acceptable fitness of the model. The consistent Akaike information criteria (CAIC) of the model needs to be compared against the CAIC of the saturated and independent model, where smaller values represent a better fit. Standardised root mean square residual (standardised RMR) is a fit index calculated on the basis of standardised residuals (differences between elements of the sample and implicit covariance matrixes). The goodness-of-fit (GFI) index and the adjusted goodness-of-fit (AGFI) index are absolute fit indices which di-

Table 4. Fit indices

Fit Indices	Reference Value	Model Value	Global Fit
Chi-square ($\chi2$) of estimate model	(χ^2/df < 2)	89.29 (df = 38) = 2.34	No
Goodness-of-fit index (GFI)	$\geq .90$	.96	Yes
Root mean square residual (RMR)	< .05	.023	Yes
Root mean square error of approximation (RMSEA)	$\leq .05$	.062	Yes
CAIC	CAIC saturated model CAIC independent model	281.79	Yes
Adjusted goodness-of-fit index (AGFI)	$\geq .90$	.92	Yes
Non-normed fit index (NNFI)	$\geq .95$	.97	Yes
Normed fit index (NFI)	$\geq .90$	.96	Yes
Parsimony goodness-of-fit index(PGFI)	$\geq.50$	.55	Yes
Comparative fit index (CFI)	$\geq .90$	.98	Yes
Critical (CN)	N = 248.77	356	Yes

rectly assess how well the covariances based on the parameter estimates reproduce the sample covariances (Gebring &Anderson, 1993). All of the indices described above lead to the conclusion that the model can be regarded as an appropriate approximation of reality (at a global level).

SOLUTIONS AND RECOMMENDATIONS

The aim of this paper was to present the conceptualisation of a model for the assessment of the impact of technology-enhanced learning, and the respective information and communication technology on the business performance of Slovene companies with more than 50 employees. The theoretical and empirical grounds were studied in order to demonstrate the correlations between the aforementioned constructs with the basic aim to present a hypothesized research model as a concrete result.

The study focuses on the findings achieved through the estimation of the relations between information and communication technology and technology-enhanced learning, organizational learning and business performance, and their operationalisation. In accordance with stakeholder theory and balanced scorecard, both the financial and non-financial aspects of business performance are considered. Within this approach, a structural equation model was conceptualised based on the prior theoretical and empirical foundations.

In the study, five hypothesis were tested: (1) technology-enhanced learning has a positive impact on organizational learning, (2) technology-enhanced learning has a positive impact on the financial business results, (3) technology-enhanced learning has a positive impact on the non-financial business results, (4) organizational learning as a process of knowledge creation has a positive impact on the financial performance, and (5) organizational learning has a positive effect on the non-financial performance. A sample of data collected was used through the survey question-

naire, which was circulated among the CEOs and presidents of the management boards of Slovenian companies with more than 50 employees in June 2007. Out of a total of 1215 questionnaires sent, 356 correctly completed questionnaires were returned, which means that the response rate was 29.7%. The questionnaire was structured in four parts. The first construct (technology-enhanced learning) was based on 22 measurement variables, the second construct (organizational learning) on 29 measurement variables related to the acquisition of knowledge, knowledge transfer and the use of knowledge. The third and the fourth constructs were designed with the intention of measuring the financial and non-financial company results (three measurement variables for the financial and four measurement variables for the non-financial results). Equation modelling methodology was used for the analysis in the empirical part of the study. The methodology of structural equation modelling enabled us to concretely determine whether the hypothetical links between the constructs or latent variables are valid or not.

The results of the survey prove a statistically significant, strong and positive impact of ICT and technology-enhanced learning on organizational learning, and a decisive influence of organizational learning on the financial and non-financial business results. The companies which systematically incorporated various advanced educational tools and systems into their daily work, and ensured high quality information and communication technology equipment recognized the importance of organizational learning as the most effective process for the production, dissemination and application of knowledge. Furthermore, the positive effects of organizational learning on the financial and non-financial business results confirm that this concept really guarantees the achievement of higher performance both in financial and non-financial terms. Knowledge is definitely one of the most important criteria of the competitive advantage, which is confirmed by the results of the study.

The study contributes to the technology-enhanced learning and organizational learning base of knowledge in the following three dimensions: (1) theoretical, (2) methodological, and (3) practical. Technology-enhanced learning contributes to sustainable competitive advantage through its interaction with other resources. Recent literature suggests that organizational learning is a process that plays an important role in enhancing company's competitive advantage (Lei, Slocum & Pitts, 1999), which may benefit from the judicious application of technology-enhanced learning. It has also been argued that a prerequisite for the firms to be successful is the completion of Tel with Ol. Within the broader conceptual framework, this study focuses on the relationship between technology-enhanced learning, organizational learning and business performance. As such, the conceptual model offers several research opportunities and provides a solid base for further empirical testing of hypotheses related to technology-enhanced learning and organizational learning.

REFERENCES

Argyris, C., & Schön, D. A. (1978). *Organizational Learning: A Theory of Action Perspective*. Reading, MA: Addison-Wesley.

Argyris, C., & Schön, D. A. (1996). *Organizational Learning II: Theory, Method and Practice*. Reading, MA: Addison-Wesley.

Arh, T., Dimovski, V., & Jerman-Blažič, B. (2008). *Model of impact of technology-enhanced organizational learning on business performance. V P. Cunningham, M. Cunningham (ur.), Collaboration and the knowledge economy: issues, applications, case studies, (str. 1521–1528)*. Netherlands: IOS Press.

Arh, T., Pipan, M., Jerman-Blažič, B. (2006). Virtual learning environment for the support of life-long learning initiative. *WSEAS transactions on advances in engineering education*, 4(4), str. 737–743.

Bollen, K. A. (1989). *Structural equations with latent variables*. New York: Wiley.

Carr, N. G. (2003). IT doesn't matter. *Harvard Business Review, 81*(5), 41.

Collins, C. J., & Smith, K. G. (2006). Knowledge exchange and combination: the role of human resource practices in the performance of high-technology firms. *Academy of Management Journal, 49*(3), 544–560.

Crossan, M., Lane, H. W., & White, R. E. (1999). An organizational learning framework: from intuition to institution. *Academy of Management Review, 24*(3), 522–537. doi:10.2307/259140

Davenport, T. H., De Long, D. W., & Beers, M. C. (1998). Successful knowledge management projects. *Sloan Management Review, 39*(2), 43–57.

Dewan, S., & Kraemer, K. L. (1998). International dimensions of the productivity paradox. *Communications of the ACM, 41*(8), 56–62. doi:10.1145/280324.280333

Diamantopoulos, A., & Siguaw, J. A. (2000). *Introducing LISREL*. London: SAGE Publications.

DiBella, J. A., & Nevis, E. C. (1998). *How Organizations Learn – An Integrated Strategy for Building Learning Capability*. San Francisco, CA: Jossey-Bass.

Dimovski, V. (1994). *Organisational learning and competitive advantage*. Unpublished doctoral dissertation, Cleveland State University.

Dimovski, V., & Colnar, T. (1999). Organizacijsko učenje. *Teorija in Praksa, 5*(36), 701–722.

Dinevski, D., & Plenković, M. (2002). Modern University and e-learning. *Media, culture and public relations, 2*, 137–146.

Dodgson, M. (1993). Organizational learning: a review of some literatures. *Organization Studies, 14*(3), 375–394. doi:10.1177/017084069301400303

Figueiredo, P. N. (2003). Learning processes features: How do they influence inter-firm differences in technological capability - Accumulation paths and operational performance improvement? *International Journal of Technology Management, 26*(7), 655–689. doi:10.1504/IJTM.2003.003451

Fiol, C. M., & Lyles, M. A. (1985). Organizational learning. *Academy of Management Review, 10*(4), 803–813. doi:10.2307/258048

Freeman, E. R. (1984). *Strategic Management – A Stakeholder Approach*. London: Pitman.

Freeman, E. R. (1994). Politics of Stakeholder Theory: Some Future Directions. *Business Ethics Quarterly, 4*, 409–422. doi:10.2307/3857340

Gerbing, D. W., & Anderson, J. C. (1988). An updated paradigm for scale development incorporating unidimensionality and measurement error. *JMR, Journal of Marketing Research, 25*, 186–192. doi:10.2307/3172650

Goh, S., & Richards, G. (1997). Benchmarking the learning capability of organizations. *European Management Journal, 15*(5), 575–583. doi:10.1016/S0263-2373(97)00036-4

Henry, P (2001). E-learning technology, content and services. *Education + Training, 43*(4), 251–259.

Huber, G. P. (1991). Organizational Learning: The Contributing Processes and the Literatures. *Organization Science, 2*(1), 88–115. doi:10.1287/orsc.2.1.88

Inkpen, A., & Crossan, M. M. (1995). Believing is seeing: Organizational learning in joint ventures. *Journal of Management Studies, 32*(5), 595–618. doi:10.1111/j.1467-6486.1995.tb00790.x

Jones, G. R. (2000). *Organizational Theory* (3rd ed.). New York: Prentice Hall.

Jöreskog, K. G., & Sörbrom, D. (1993). *LISREL 8: Structural Equation Modelling with the SIMPLIS Command Language*. London: Lawrence Erlbaum Associates Publishers.

Kaplan, R. S., & Norton, D. P. (1992). Balanced Scorecard – Measures That Drive Performance. *Harvard Business Review, 1–2*, 71–79.

Kirchner, P. A., & Pass, F. (2001). Web enhanced higher education: a Tower of Babel. *Computers in Human Behavior, 17*(4), 347–353. doi:10.1016/S0747-5632(01)00009-7

Lam, S. S. K. (1998). Organizational performance and learning styles in Hong Kong. *The Journal of Social Psychology, 138*(3), 401–403. doi:10.1080/00224549809600392

Lei, D., Hitt, M. A., & Bettis, R. (1996). Dynamic core competencies through meta-learning and strategic context. *Journal of Management, 22*(4), 549–569. doi:10.1177/014920639602200402

Lei, D., Slocum, J. W., & Pitts, R. A. (1999). Designing organizations for competitive advantage: The power of unlearning and learning. *Organizational Dynamics, 27*(3), 24–38. doi:10.1016/S0090-2616(99)90019-0

Leonard-Barton, D. (1992). The factory as a learning laboratory. *Sloan Management Review, 34*(1), 23–38.

Levitt, B., & March, J. G. (1998). Organizational learning. *Annual Review of Sociology, 14*, 319–340. doi:10.1146/annurev.so.14.080188.001535

MacManus, R., & Porter, J. (2005): *Web 2.0 for design: bootstrapping the social web*. Retrieved April 15th 2008, from: http://www.digital-web.com/articles/ web_2_for_designers

Miner, A. S., & Mezias, S. J. (1996). Ugly duckling no more: pasts and futures of organizational learning research. *Organization Science, 7*(1), 88–99. doi:10.1287/orsc.7.1.88

Mintzberg, H. (1990). Strategy formation: Schools of thought. In Frederickson, J. W. (Ed.), *Perspectives of strategic management* (pp. 105–235). New York: Harper Business.

Mueller, R. O. (1996). *Basic Principles of Structural Equation Modelling: An Introduction to Lisrel and EQS*. New York: Springer.

Navarette, C. J., & Pick, J. B. (2002). Information technology expenditure and industry performance: The case of the Mexican banking industry. *Journal of Global Information Technology Management, 5*(2), 7–28.

Nonaka, I. (1994). A dynamic theory of organizational knowledge creation. *Organization Science, 5*(1), 14–37. doi:10.1287/orsc.5.1.14

Nonaka, I., & Takeuchi, H. (1996). A Theory of Organizational Knowledge Creation. *International Journal of Technology Management, 11*(7/8), 833–846.

O'Reilly, T. (2005). *What Is Web 2.0. Design Patterns and Business Models for the Next Generation of Software*. Retrieved November 10, 2009, from http://oreilly.com/web2 /archive/what-is-web-20.html

Péréz López, S., Montes Peón, J. M., & Vázquez Ordás, C. Managing knowledge: The link between culture and organizational learning. *Journal of Knowledge Management, 8*(6), 93–104. doi:10.1108/13673270410567657

Raelin, J. A. (1997). A model of work-based learning. *Organization Science, 8*(6), 563–578. doi:10.1287/orsc.8.6.563

Reychav, I., & Weisberg, J. (2009). Good for workers, good for companies: How knowledge sharing benefits individual employees. *Knowledge and Process Management, 16*(4), 186–197. doi:10.1002/kpm.335

Roach, S. (1987). *America's technology dilemma: A profile of the information economy. Economics Newsletter Series*. New York: Morgan Stanley.

Robey, D., Boudreau, M., & Rose, G. M. (2000). Information Technology and Organizational Learning: a Review and Assessment of Research. *Accounting. Management and Information Technologies, 10*, 125–155. doi:10.1016/S0959-8022(99)00017-X

Rosenberg, M. (2001). *E-Learning, Strategies for Developing Knowledge in the Digital Age. New York*. McGraw-Hill.

Senge, P. M. (1990). *The fifth discipline: art and practice of the learning organization*. New York: Doubleday.

Sevilla, C., & Wells, T. D. (1988). Contracting to ensure training transfer. *Training & Development, 6*(1), 10–11.

Shrivastava, P. A. (1983). Typology of Organizational Learning Systems. *Journal of Management Studies, 20*, 1–28. doi:10.1111/j.1467-6486.1983.tb00195.x

Simonin, B. L. (1997). The importance of collaborative know-how: An empirical test of the learning organization. *Academy of Management Journal, 40*(5), 1150–1173. doi:10.2307/256930

Škerlavaj, M. (2003). *Vpliv informacijsko-komunikacijskih tehnologij in organizacijskega učenja na uspešnost poslovanja: teoretična in empirična analiza*. Unpublished Master's theses. Ljubljana: Ekonomska fakulteta.

Škerlavaj, M., & Dimovski, V. (2006). Study of the Mutual Connections among Information-communication Technologies, Organisational Learning and Business Performance. *Journal for East European Management Studies, 11*(1), 9–29.

Slater, S. F., & Narver, J. C. (1995). Market orientation and the learning organization. *Journal of Marketing, 59*(3), 63–74. doi:10.2307/1252120

Sloan, T. R., Hyland, P. W. B., & Beckett, R. C. (2002). Learning as a competitive advantage: Innovative training in the Australian aerospace industry. *International Journal of Technology Management, 23*(4), 341–352. doi:10.1504/IJTM.2002.003014

Smith, R. (2008). Aligning Competencies, Capabilities and Resources. *Research Technology Management: The Journal of the Industrial Research Institute*, September-October.

Tippins, M. J., & Sohi, R. S. (2003). IT competency and firm performance: Is organizational learning a missing link? *Strategic Management Journal, 24*(8), 745–761. doi:10.1002/smj.337

Ulrich, D., Jick, T., & von Glinow, M. A. (1993). High-impact learning: Building and diffusing learning capability. *Organizational Dynamics, 22*(2), 52–66. doi:10.1016/0090-2616(93)90053-4

Varney, S. (2008). Leadership learning: key to organizational transformation. *Strategic HR Review, 7*(1), 5–10. doi:10.1108/14754390810880471

Wall, B. (1998). Measuring the Right Stuff: Identifying and Applying the Right Knowledge. *Knowledge Management Review, 1*(4), 20–24.

Zhang, D. *Media structuration – Towards an integrated approach to interactive multimedia-based E-Learning*. (Ph.D. dissertation, The University of Arizona, 2002. Zhang, D., & Nunamaker, J. F. (2003). Powering e-learning in the new millennium: an overview of e-learning and enabling technology. *Information Systems Frontiers, 5*(2), 207–218.

KEY TERMS AND DEFINITIONS

Technology Enhanced Learning: Technology-enhanced learning (TEL) refers to any learning activity supported by technology. TEL is often used as a synonym for e-learning, however, there are significant differences between the two; namely, TEL focuses on the technological support of any pedagogical approach that utilizes technology. However, it rarely includes the print technology or developments related to libraries, books and journals occurring in the centuries before computers.

Web 2.0: Web 2.0 is a category of new Internet tools and technologies created around the idea that those who consume the media, access the Internet, and use the web should not just passively absorb what is available; they should be rather active contributors, helping customize the media and technology for their own purposes, as well as those of their communities. Web 2.0 marks the beginning of a new era in technology – one that promises to help the nonprofits operate more efficiently, generate more funding, and affect more lives. These new tools include blogs, social networking applications, RSS, social networking tools, and wikis.

Organizational Learning: Organizational learning is an area of knowledge within the organizational theory that studies models and theories about the ways an organization learns and adapts. Argyris and Schön (1978) were the first to propose models that facilitate organizational learning; others have followed in the tradition of their work. They distinguished between the single- and double-loop learning. In the single-loop learning, individuals, groups, or organizations modify their actions according to the difference between the expected and obtained outcomes. In the double-loop learning, entities (individuals, groups or organizations) question the values, assumptions and policies that led to the actions in the first place; if they are able to view and modify those, then the second-order or the double-loop learning has taken place. The double-loop learning is the process of learning about the single-loop learning.

Balanced Scorecard (BSC): The balanced scorecard (BSC) is a strategic performance management tool – a semi-standard structured report supported by proven design methods and automation tools that can be used by managers to keep track of the execution of activities of staff within their control, and monitor the consequences arising from these actions. It is perhaps the best known of several such frameworks, and was widely adopted in the English speaking western countries and Scandinavia in the early 1990s. The BCS based on the use of three non-financial topic areas as prompts to aid the identification of the non-financial measures in addition to the one looking at the financial measures. The four perspectives are: financial, customer, internal business, and innovation and learning.

LISREL: LISREL is the pioneering software for structural equation modelling which includes statistical methods for complex data survey. LIS-REL was developed in 1970s by Karl Jöreskog and Dag Sörbom, both professors at the Uppsala University, Sweden.

Structural Equation Modelling: Structural equation modelling, or in short SEM, is a statistical technique for testing and estimating causal relationships using a combination of statistical data and qualitative causal assumptions. SEM allows both confirmatory and exploratory modelling, meaning it suits both theory testing and theory development. Factor analysis, path analysis and regression all represent special cases of SEM.

Confirmatory Factor Analysis: Confirmatory factor analysis (CFA) is a powerful statistical technique. CFA allows researchers to test the hypothesis of the existence of a relationship between the observed variables and their underlying latent construct(s).Researchers apply their theoretical knowledge, empirical research, or both, postulate the relationship pattern a priori and then tests the hypothesis statistically.

Chapter 6

M–Government:
Challenges and Key Success Factors – Saudi Arabia Case Study

Mubarak S. Al-Mutairi
King Fahd University of Petroleum & Minerals, Saudi Arabia

EXECUTIVE SUMMARY

In developing countries like the Saudi Arabia, due to high mobile phone penetration rates, any electronic government initiatives that don't take mobile technology into account will eventually fail. While the number of landline phones and internet subscribers are growing steadily over the past few years, the number of mobile phone users and its penetration rates are skyrocketing. In the near future and with the many mobile phone features, mobile phones will remain the main media of communication and a main source for providing information to citizens and customers.

A BRIEF HISTORY

The development in the telecommunications industry came along way and in different phases until it became what we see today. In the mid 19s, so many technologies were introduced and faded away shortly or got replaced with newer ones. In 1971, Advanced Mobile Phone Service (AMPS) was introduced by AT&T in USA. Later that year, ARP (Autoradiopuhelin or car radio phone) was launched in Finland. ARP was the first commercially operated public mobile phone network in Finland

The first generation (1G) of commercial cell phones (uses radio analog signals) was introduced in the late 1980s. The Nordic Mobile Telephone (NMT) is one of the earliest 1G-standards. NMT was developed jointly in Denmark, Finland, Iceland, Norway and Sweden. In Japan, the first commercial 1G service was provided by Nippon Telegraph and Telephone Public Corporation (NTTPC) in 1979, where they introduced the 'automobile telephone'. Soon the device became detached from automobiles and was called 'shoulder phone'. Between 1985 and 1988 a number of new carriers entered the market.

The second generation (2G) which is the well known technology today (GSM) was launched in

DOI: 10.4018/978-1-60960-015-0.ch006

Finland in the 1990s. Later, the mobile technology development rhythm speeded up drastically. High speed services were being developed as an extension to 2G networks, also known as 2.5G, such as the General Packet Radio Service (GPRS) and Enhanced Data rates for Global Evolution (EDGE), both GPRS and EDGE allow improved data transmission rates.

According to some statistics, there were 295 million subscribers on 3G networks worldwide by the end of the year 2007. During that year, the 3G mobile services generated over 120 billion USD in net profit. The top 10 telecom companies in the world made over $600 billion in revenue and over $70 billion in net income at the end of 2007. As for Saudi Arabia, telecom companies generated $27 billion in revenues and $7.4 billion in net income. With the expansion of networks and the emergence of the latest technologies used to develop 3.5G network, it's viewed easier to use high-speed broadband for internet use and web-based applications for consumers. High speed bandwidth such as WAP, GPRS and EDGE allowed mobile operators to provide services such as Multimedia Messaging, Video calls and much more. The evolved version of the 3.5G systems will be 4G. It will be based on cellular systems but will require very small cells (Yuan & Zhang, 2003). There are some indicators that the 4G systems could expanded to included machine to machine interactions rather than just simply human to human or human to machine (Turban et al., 2004; Siau & Shen, 2003; Varshney, 2002; Varshney & Vetter, 2000)

MOBILE PHONE MARKET

According to Wireless Intelligence, the Middle East has surged to become the second-fastest growing mobile phone market in the world. With penetration set to cross the 50% mark, over 150 million handsets in circulation and a 30% growth rate in 2006, the Middle East is now only trailing Africa as the fastest-growing market. Turkey, Iran and Saudi Arabia represent almost 70% of total connections in the Middle East. In these markets, the average market penetration is around 67%, which is above the average market penetration rate for the region (50%). Saudi Arabia is the second biggest market in the Middle East; it represents about 15% of total connections in the region. At the end of 2006, Saudi Arabia passed the 20 million connections mark, and the market is expected to grow by almost 30% each year.

Saudi Arabia with a population of 23 million already comprises the largest telecommunications markets in the Arabian Gulf and is one of the fastest growing in the Middle East. The sector which has some 4 million fixed lines and 20 million mobile lines has been expanding at a rate of 30% a year.

The acceleration in services has been boosted by deregulation and partial privatization of the national telecoms provider Saudi Telecommunications Company. This was sealed in a 2003 initial public offering of 30% of the latter's shares. Prior to this the government had liberalized the sector and opened it up to foreign investment and competition.

A regulator was established and designated the Saudi Telecommunications and Information Technology Commission (STITC) in April 2003. The STITC is responsible for awarding licenses to investors and for the regulation of telephone and Internet services as well as other media in addition to tariffs, competition, interconnectivity and equipment standards. The total number of users of the three mobile service providers is shown in Figure 1. This number is compared to the land lines (fixed phone line) and internet users in Figure 2.

E-GOVERNMENT VS. M-GOVERNMENT

The use ICT applications have changed the way governments function. It brought in drastic changes in terms of the functions and relations of G2G,

Figure 1. Mobile phone subscribers in Saudi Arabia

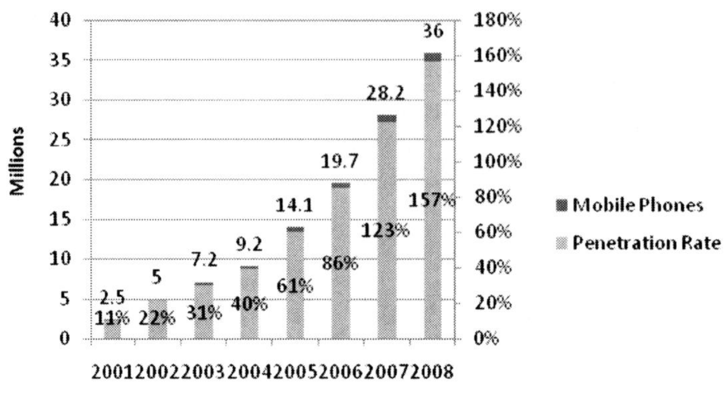

G2C, G2B, B2C, and B2B. Over the past couple of years, internet (e-government in particular) was the most promising technology to increase the government's efficiency and effectiveness (Layne & Lee, 2001). The rapid advances in mobile devices and wireless technologies opened new opportunities for further developments in public sector services (Kakihara & Sorensen, 2002). As per the UN website, "the e-government refers to the use of information and communication technologies (ICT) - such as Wide Area Networks, the Internet, and mobile computing - by government agencies".

For so many years, the focus was mainly on internet to deliver the governmental services to its citizens in a more effective and efficient way.

Due to low internet penetration rates in some countries, new means have to be investigated to make sure that all services are accessible by all citizens (Odedra, 1991; Roggenkamp, 2004; West, 2002). Internet enabled mobile devices such as cell phones, PDAs, Laptops, WiFi, and Wireless networks created opportunities to develop mobile government and business models (ESCWA, 2005; Kristoffersen & Ljungberg, 1999; Sadeh, 2002). Mobile technology represents a relatively cheaper and a more convenient way for delivering government services especially in remote and less developed areas. Such services are usually referred to as Mobile Government or m-government for

Figure 2. Mobile, land line, and internet subscribers in Saudi Arabia

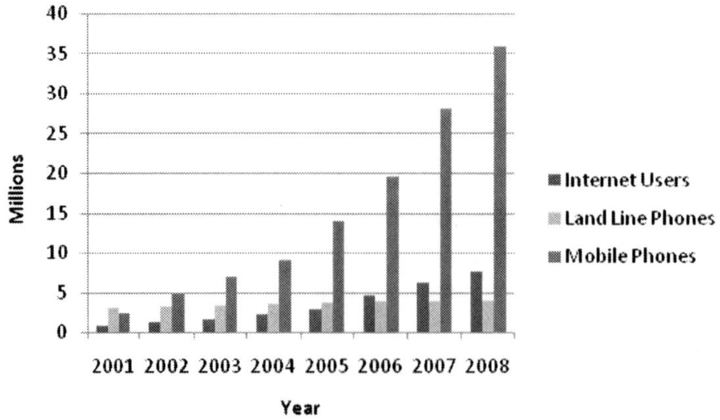

short (Chang & Kannan, 2002; Ghyasi & Kushchu, 2004; Tachikawa, 2003; Senn, 2000).

M-government is not to be looked at as replacement for the existing well known e-government scheme but rather a complimentary subset of e-government utilizing ICTs to improve and provide the "anytime, anywhere" promised functionality (Easton, 2002). M-government is defined as a strategy utilizing all kind of mobile and wireless technology when compared to the traditional wire-connected e-government services (Kushchu & Kuscu, 2003). Simply speaking, m-government is tended to deliver the services to the users at their locations rather than bringing them to a specific location (Goldstuck, 2004). The m-government is distinguished from the traditional e-government in terms of:

- Personalized information: while computers often are used by different users, mobile devices are being used by a specific user. As such, personalized information could be delivered to that specific user anytime anywhere using the mobile technology.
- Always on: unlike computers, mobile devices usually are on all the time. This ensures delivering the required information on a timely manner.
- Mobility: from its name, a mobile device is designed to be carried around. Services are designed to be delivered to the users regardless of their physical location.

SUCCESS FACTORS

Unlike e-government initiatives, m-government projects depend on some factors that individually or collectively contribute to the success of such projects. Each of these factors will be discussed briefly in the following sections (Kushchu & Kuscu, 2003; May, 2001).

Cost

Providing enough funding for the m-government was and will be always a major issue for government providing electronic services to its citizens. Upgrading and renewing the current outdated or deteriorated infrastructure to provide quality reliable services in a timely manner often requires huge investments. Justifying those huge investments to the decision maker is one issue. Calculating the expected return on investment (ROI) and making it attractive for the private sector to invest, operate, and maintain it wholly or as partners is another issue (Banister & Remenyi, 2000, 2004). From the private sector's point of view, they want to invest in profitable projects that guarantee them the highest ROI. The decision to invest or not is driven by several factors. These factors include: local and regional markets' accessibility, availability of skilled taskforce to support the business and ensure its continuity, partnerships with local industry, R&D institutions and academia, and the right political and economic environment. Once all or most of these factors are satisfied, it will create an attractive investment opportunity for the private sector (Banister & Remenyi, 2005).

Business Processes Re-Engineering

Most if not all business processes are not ready to be digitized or mobilized as is. The entire process procedure needs to be re-engineered. The process needs to be simplified and shortened. This will eventually create some resistance among the old school management people who will look at it from a different angle (Devadoss, 2002, O'Hara, 2006). They will see it as:

- Lose of centralized management control (lose of something of value to some individuals). This is quite usual and expected in strong control cultures.
- Reduction in their power and direct responsibilities.

- Fear of being overcome by the new generation who is more comfortable using computers.
- Misunderstanding the change and its implications.
- Change rejection due to a belief that it will not add anything to the organization or just simply because some people have a low tolerance for a change of any type.
- nExternal resistance where people like to stick to the way things being done before. This is due to either their fear of using the technology or the removal / introduction of some requirements that was not in the original process before the re-engineering stage.

Usability

Any m-government application designed for public users needs to take into consideration the end-user during the design stage. When designing an application for public use, we are talking about a wide range of users. Among them, old, young, educated, illiterate, male, females, people living in big cities with good telecom infrastructure, and people living in small remote areas with less telecom facilities. At the end, the application needs to be user-friendly with error detection and correction techniques (Zalesak, 2003). Though this issue is subjective and vary widely from one user to another, some of the important issues that need to be taken into consideration are (Bias, 1994; Ehrlich, 1994; Muller, 1993; Nielsen, 1993a,b, 1994; Shackel, 1971; Wasserman, 1989; Lewis, 1991a,b,c, 1992a,b; Dumas, 1994; Gould, 1985):

- Friendly user interface.
- Smooth and easy navigation scheme.
- Error detection and correction mechanisms.
- Grouping of relevant information (personal data, education, social, income, etc).
- Clear and complete content.

- Help menus (explain terms or show examples).

The lack of usability is more noticeable than usability itself. As a result, one can define usability as: a user friendly interface with no more space for improvements.

Accessibility

The issues of usability and accessibility are closely related. When making the design for usability, it is important to make sure that no one is lift behind. In other words, the design should be made in a way that makes it accessible by almost everyone including those with certain disability or challenged by a way or another. The advances in technology made it easier to imbed certain technologies for people with certain disabilities. This includes:

- Screen readers (text into voice for blind people).
- Refrain from using colors not visible to some users (color blindness).
- When the use of video / audio is required, provide sign language for deaf users.

Accessibility is not just an issue of people with disabilities but even for normal people. Viewing a video or animation on slow connections can be very annoying if not difficult in the first place. This could be easily solved using an alternative of a simple text for users with slow connections. To ensure compliance with the usability and accessibility, strict rules need to be put in place from the initial design throughout the production and implementation. This is will be reflected by a better user satisfaction and a broader reach to more customers.

Acceptance

Regardless of the technology being used to deliver the m-government services, it has to be accepted by the user. In other words, the user needs to be assured that it worth the effort. Yet there are other factors affecting the ICT acceptance level. Some of these are social and others are cultural. Users need to be assured that the service is secured, efficient, and easy to use. The main factors affecting the ICT acceptance and use are:

- System usefulness. This is achieved through:
  - Reducing transaction time.
  - More availability (24/7).
  - Additional mobility (anywhere anytime).
- Process simplification.
- System usability.
- System reliability.
- System technical support.

Without the proper awareness program about the benefits of accepting and using such programs, people will be always reluctant to use them. In some societies, word of mouth and others experiences works like magic. In those societies, people tend to build high expectations on others experience even though they have different skills and circumstances. The role of the government is to foster an awareness program and in other situations, they need to impose some regulations on using technological channels for processing some transactions. Going with the saying "you will not realize its benefits until you try it", the government can gradually force the use of its e/m-transactions by offering it only over this channels and refraining from the usual face to face transactions. This will eventually raise the public level of ICT acceptance and usage.

Security

Changing the transaction media from the regular face-to-face way to an electronic form bring in another variable in the transaction equation; more specifically the issue of security. With the skyrocketing number of electronic media users and transactions, so does the threat to those transactions. Fear of intrusion and identity thefts are two major issues. Users need to assured that their transaction media is secured and that their real identity will be authenticated before processing any transaction.

In general, Information security is achieved by adopting and implementing the appropriate set of quality controls, whether they are policies, procedures, standards, practices, awareness programs or organizational structures and ethics (Gandon & Sadeh, 2004; Head & Yuan, 2001; Ives & Learmonth, 1984). Information security is an integral and essential element of business today (Schwiderski-Grosche & Knospe, 2002).

The main goal of the information security process is to protect information confidentiality, integrity and availability. A comprehensive security process encapsulates and consolidates the three main processes of prevention, detection and recovery (see Figure 3) (Smith et al., 2000).

Whether they are providing a service or offering a commodity, online businesses have some assets that need to be protected. The main focus of a secure e/m-service (like other distributed systems) depends mainly on protecting communications between the trading parties (Voydock & Kent, 1983), and controlling the system access and any other resources involved in providing the service (Tanenbaum & Van Steen, 2002). Using secured channels for communication protects the confidentiality, integrity, and authenticity of the information it carries. Access control verifies that only authorized parties have access to the resources and prevents any unauthorized users from accessing the system (Nichols & Lekkas, 2002).

Figure 3. Main processes of a security system

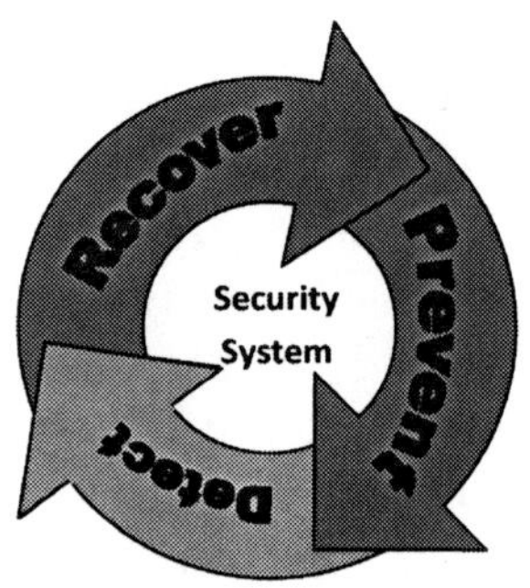

In conclusion, no matter how much we invest in security systems, security will remain a subjective issue. There is no such 100% secured system. Depending on the source of the threat, security needs to be tackled at three different levels: business environment and physical security, front-end security, and back-end security. This will be reflected on the system complexity and usability levels (see Figure 4).

Privacy

Privacy is usually mistakenly used interchangeably with security. While security is primarily concerned with verifying the identity and protecting the transaction channel, privacy is more directed towards protecting the personal information of users. Information like, names, addresses, e-mails, phone numbers, social security numbers, credit cards' numbers, etc. are not to be shared with other organizations or misused on the personal level. Privacy legislations need to be enforced to protect the personal information of users. The legislations need to address the following issues:

- Users' data collected need to be protected from public disclosure. Recent public surveys have shown that selling users' information for commercial purposes is becoming a profitable business.
- Current data management policies in government agencies undermine the privacy laws currently in place. There are no assurances that data collected by one government agency will not be disclosed for another one. In addition, filtering techniques need to be implemented to allow only relevant information to be released by a specific government agency rather than releasing the entire record.
- Collecting or browsing users' data is to be done for legitimate reasons (update of information or providing a service to the user).
- Establishing a commission or a national center to issue the privacy bylaws to protect the users' data and to enforce them. This will help protecting the available online data.

Figure 4. Multilayered security system model

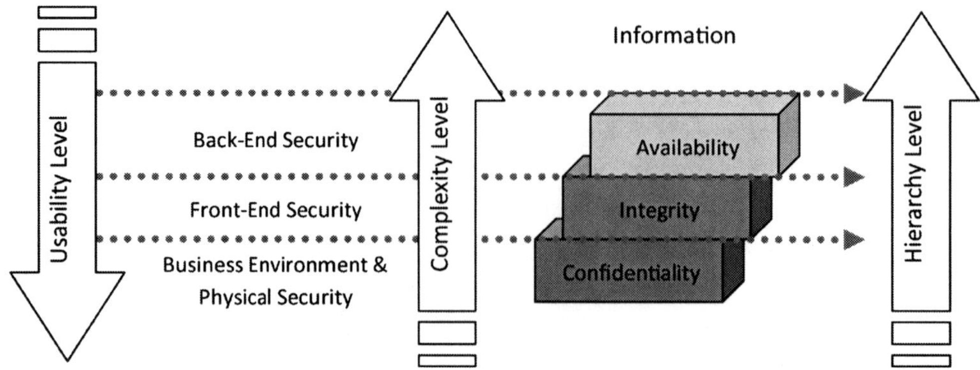

- Educating the public on how to protect their private and personal information.

The security and the privacy issues are not to be overlooked or compromised just for the sake of providing online services. Once some personal or sensitive information are released or breached online, there are no assurances on the abuse of these data. Once the government passes legislations on the protection of all users' private information, people will be more comfortable using online services.

High Rates of Technology Adoption

Before implementing an electronic or mobile government project, certain factors are needed to be considered in advance. These include but not limited to:

- The country's most popular technology. i.e. internet, mobile phones, landline telephones, or any other wired / wireless technology.
- The adoption rate among the majority of the population.
- Future trends in that technology and in that country in particular.
- The availability of skilled workforce that support the investment in that technology.

It is not always the case that the financial resources are the only determent factor for technology adoption in a particular country. Other factors may include: the country's area, geographical nature, and the level of coordination between the different government bodies.

Yet the adoption of technology is highly linked to the community cultural and social aspects. The biggest challenge is that even though the same technology is being used when used by different users, it could produce different results. The claim that this is to do with the level of the user's education is not always true. Users' technology ac-

ceptance has been noticed since the early seventies and still persists even with our increasing level of knowledge (Benjamin & Blunt, 1992; Keen, 1981; Lucas, 1975; Markus, 1983; Markus & Benjamin, 1996). Government agencies and decision maker need to be aware of the human behavioral aspects and the different stages of technology adoption when planning to implement an online or mobile governmental service.

Strong Political Will

A strong political will is needed to plan, implement, and monitor action plans for digitizing the society. The government involvement will include:

- Updating the countries ICT infrastructure in a rate that can support the government's digital initiatives and support any future technological changes or expansions.
- Open the market for foreign investments.
- Motivating the private sector to invest in the country's ICT infrastructure as a partner rather than a user. The private sector can build, run, and maintain major parts of the country's network.
- Issuing or modifying the existing legislation to protect the rights of both the investor and the end-users at the same time.
- Adopting a national campaign to market those digital services and aware the user of the benefits of using such channels.
- Investing in the training of a technical taskforce to support these technologies and maintain them.
- Forcing some transaction to be only available through electronic or mobile technology.
- Introducing IT programs in the countries educational system.

The presence of a strong political will in addition legislations to support the ICT development will eventually create a healthy atmosphere towards a digital society. The digitization process will not happen overnight but in the usual circumstances will take five to ten years to elapse. In other cases, it may even take a longer time.

DIFFICULTIES FACING M-GOVERNMENT INITIATIVES

Most of the m-government initiatives face difficulties that need to be analyzed and addressed. Some of these issues are technology related while other are countries specific issues and mostly has something to do with the country's culture as will explained shortly (Heeks, 2003; Heeks & Lallana, 2004).

One-Stop Portal

According to some estimates, the US government global spending on IT sector is around USD 3 Trillion (excluding health, education, utility sectors). The European countries, Canada, and the United States are competing to have the most advanced e-government capabilities. The adoption of e/m-government is a major administrative and political priority in the European Union since the 1990s (research funds, seed funds, competitions, benchmarking and awards). However, it is estimated that 60-80% of the e/m-government projects have failed or are still in its early stages. In other words, the e/m-government transformation is slow and superficial and far below the expectations. This is due mostly to the fact that each government body is developing its own services in isolation of the other government bodies. As a result, the end user needs to visit different sites or SMS different numbers for different services (see Figure 5). There is no single one-stop portal where the user can access all governmental services. More attention needs to be given to developing a unified framework to implement e/m-government that includes cross-governmental integration that enables data sharing and G2G transactions.

The concept of connected government is derived from the whole-of-government approach which is increasingly using technology as a strategic tool and as an enabler for public service innovation and productivity growth. The e/m-government interoperability can be defined as the ability of constituencies to work together. At a technical level, it is the ability of a system or process to use information and/or functionality of another system or process by adhering to common underlying framework or standards. Having a single government portal will provide the end users with a single, reliable, secure and consistent

Figure 5. Different government bodies with different service channels

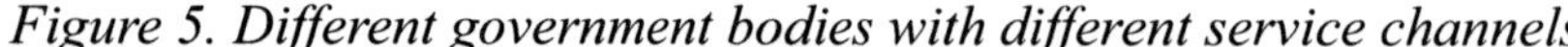

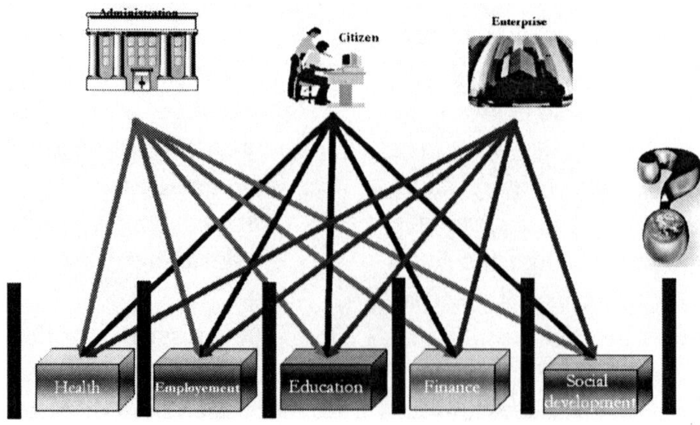

route for secure, authenticated messages into and out of their backend systems (see Figure 6).

Incomplete ICT Infrastructure

The main three pillars of electronic initiatives are the service provider, the end user, and the transaction media (available ICT infrastructure). The pace of the provided service is determined by the slowest of the three. When having the well to provide the service and the end users are equipped with the right skills to use it, all what is left is the good ICT infrastructure to support it. In 2007, the Saudi government dedicated one billion US dollars to complete the ICT infrastructure to support its electronic and mobile transactions over the coming five years. The expected outcomes include:

- Increasing the efficiency of the public sector.
- Better services to all citizens and businesses anywhere anytime.
- Increasing the ROI for public and private sectors.
- Making all the necessary information available and accessible in timely secured manner.

Low-Level of IT Skilled Staff

The development of the ICT infrastructure and the offering of many electronic services need to be supported by adequate IT skill level both on the user level and the institution or the government level. Working on the two axioms (IT skills and the services being provided) in parallel will help reduce the IT skill deficiency. The Saudi government has taken some preliminarily steps in order to bridge the gap between the national advancement in technology application and the public level of IT skills. In 2007, the Saudi government announced its initiative to provide one million Saudi homes with one million computers. Later in the same year, it dedicated three billion US dollars to build its new "computer-based" educational system. Parents, students, and teachers alike can access the information from anywhere anytime they need. In the late 2009, the Saudi government spent over five billion US dollars to send 50,000 Saudi students studying in more than 30 countries (20,000 students in the US alone) and mostly in technology related fields.

Figure 6. Single government service portal

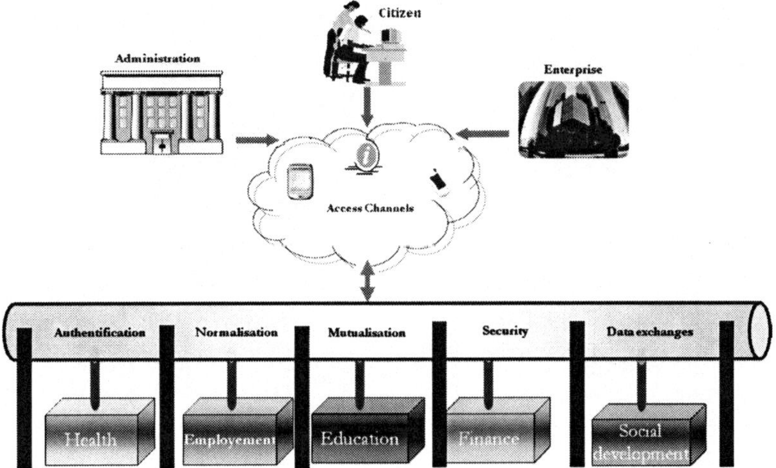

Public Awareness and ICT Supporting Legislation

As mentioned earlier, the main three pillars of any digital initiative are the service provider, the end user, and the transaction media. Public needs to be aware of the different electronic services and the ease and advantageous of using them. A public awareness campaign is an integral part of any digital initiative. Without it, the project is most likely to fail because we will be lacking the anticipated cooperation and the participation of the intended users. This could be done through:

- Specialized workshops, sessions, and conferences.
- Public media awareness campaign.
- Recognition of government and businesses achieving high rates of users and better customer satisfaction.

At the other end, the government needs to issue and maintain ICT supporting legislations. The users need to assured about the security, privacy, and the confidentiality of their transactions and personal information. They need to know their rights and obligations in advance. Some of the issues to be considered:

- Legislations to govern the online transactions.
- Standards for what to be considered secured or non-secured transactions. Based on meeting a minimum standard, they will be awarded a certificate or issued a logo that can be included in their web sites.
- Public Key Infrastructure (PKI) to secure and protect all transactions.
- Mechanisms for identity verification.
- Digital Certificates and Signatures.
- Centralized body for document verification and certification.
- Developing a fast and secured payment system.

- Standards for personal information security and privacy protection.
- A centralized body to make sure that all legislations governing the electronic transactions are being implemented and contracts are being executed as agreed upon.

This will help spreading the awareness about the concepts of electronic transactions and their applications which will encourage more businesses and government agencies to join in. indirectly, supporting services like mail and package delivery will improve too.

Technology Selection

The interoperability is defined as the set of policies to be adopted by government institutions that standardize the way the information is being exchanged and shared services are being used. The interoperability framework will define:

- Data types and schemas
- Metadata element and dictionaries
- Technical policies like:
  - Integration approach and standards
  - Connectivity standards
  - Security standards
  - Information access and delivery standards

If adopted properly, interoperability framework will decrease the time and cost required for developing the electronic exchange of information between government institutions which is a core requirement for successful e-government implementation. The interoperability framework covers the exchange of information and governs the interactions between:

- Government and Citizens
- Government and foreign workers/expats with work permit

- Government and local and foreign businesses
- Organization/ministries/institutes of the government
- Government to other governments

The technology selection should be driven by interoperability, market support, scalability, openness, and international standards.

- *Interoperability:* only specifications that are relevant to systems interconnectivity, data integration and service access are specified.
- *Market support:* the specifications selected are widely supported by the market in order to reduce cost and risk of the government systems.
- *Scalability:* the specifications selected have the capacity to be scaled to satisfy changed demands made on the systems (e.g., data volume, number of transactions, number of users).
- *Openness:* the specifications are documented and available to the public.
- *International standards:* preference will be given to standards with the broadest remit

FUTURE TRENDS AND CHALLENGES

The future of m-government and business applications seems promising and offers a good complement for the traditional e-applications in some situations. Despite the numerous advantages of m-applications, it presents some challenges like, mobile authentication, mobile payment, location-aware applications, and the content display management.

Mobile Authentication

When using mobile devices for business transactions, the biggest concern is the mobile device loss or theft. Logging in using usernames and passwords has been a staple option on desktops and laptops. To limit the unauthorized use of lost or stolen mobile devices all popular mobile operating systems now support power-on passwords. A password policy (length and complexity) should be implemented to reduce the chances of guessing the password. Even more, the mobile device could be locked in case of repeated login failures. Increasing the security options will reduce the usability. A trade off point is required where the device offers a reasonable usability with an acceptable security.

Mobile Payments

In order to facilitate m-transactions, a mechanism is to be implemented for m-payments. Two key issues need to be addressed in this regard namely identity verification and transaction authorization. Mobile devices are small and can be easily stolen or misplaced. Before processing any mobile payment request, the identity of the user needs to be verified. Once the identity is verified, a code or a security mechanism is needed to authorize the payment.

Location-Aware Applications

Some information is only intended for citizens within a specific geographical area or location. Using the Global Positioning System (GPS) will enable the service provider to send customized information to specific users within a specific area. Weather forecast, storm warnings, school closure, emergency situations, scheduled power or other services outages are only few examples of such applications (Unni & Harmon, 2003).

Content-Display Management

The mobile devices are still having limitations when it comes to storage, speed, and display when compared to the traditional wired internet computers or laptops. Display area size, keyboard, browsers, graphics and color support, memory, bandwidth capacity and transmission rate are few limitations to mention. Different mobile devices manufacturers develop different hardware and software standards for the different devices. This resulted in an additional burden on the side of the governments or the service providers. They need to design their application in a way that it can deal with the so many different hardware and software standards (Donegan, 2000).

CASE STUDY: "SAHER" TRAFFIC SYSTEM

Background

On April 2009, the Saudi ministry of interior announced that traffic cameras will begin to make their appearance on Kingdom's roads and highways. This decision was welcomed by most of the citizens and residents of Saudi Arabia due to the fact that this will certainly contribute to the overwhelming number of deaths and property damage that regularly take place here. It is estimated that a traffic death occurs in Saudi Arabia every 90 minutes.

The ministry started its six-month campaign to educate drivers about the new "SAHER" (Arabic word for awake all the time) system so that once traffic citations start to arrive in the mail, there will not be any confusion as to what has exactly happened. To ensure that the system improves road safety, it is imperative that the system be applied to all drivers equally. SAHER is an automated system for control and management of traffic that uses digital cameras network technology linked to the Information Center at the Ministry of Interior.

The system will be installed in several stages inside and outside the cities. On highways, cameras will be installed at fixed locations as well as on the vehicles of the Highway Security patrols.

At the next step, authorities must ensure that everyone pay their fines, no matter who they are. There is no room for delays or manipulations in a safety program. Drivers regularly ignore traffic citations now. In fact, there are a number of drivers on Kingdom's roads who drive without a license.

The government has an obligation to protect the lives of its citizens when circumstances that can be controlled are present. The roads are public property openly available for use to all who are licensed to use them. No one has a right, legal or moral, to put another person's life in danger, yet it is done constantly by those who appear to have no sense that the vehicles they are driving are lethal weapons.

The new "SAHER" system will be put into effect in a number of cities upon the completion of a six-month campaign to make motorists aware of the workings of the system. SAHER will use a network of digital cameras linked up to the National Information Center (NIC) which will provide personal information on the motorist in question and then issue violations related to speeding and ignoring traffic lights. Cameras will capture the vehicle's registration plate and send an image to the Traffic Violations Center to check the veracity of the infraction.

When it has been decided that a violation has indeed occurred, the NIC will be asked for the vehicle owner's personal details and a traffic violation form will be issued to his address as recorded on the information database. In Saudi Arabia, they mainly depend of mobile phone number and e-mail addresses as means of communication rather than physical address.

Fixed sensory cameras, detecting any jumping of lights, will be located at traffic lights on main and side roads, capturing images of the motorist and his vehicle's front and rear sides. Mobile cameras will cover other arteries. The cameras, which are equipped with flashes and will function at all hours, are capable of capturing detailed images of vehicles traveling at high speeds. The SAHER system is part of moves to clamp down on the nine million traffic infractions registered per year with traffic police, resulting in death, injury, and material losses of approximately USD 3.5 billion.

"Every 90 minutes a death is recorded due to motor accidents," said Fahd Bin Sa'oud Al-Bashar, head of the General Traffic Administration. "Someone is injured or left permanently disabled every fifteen minutes." Al-Bashar added that the new system would raise safety standards on the Kingdom's roads by improving the monitoring of traffic circulation, speeding up the response to incidents, and addressing traffic violations and swiftly informing those responsible via their e-mail addresses or mobile phones (SMS) registered at the interior ministry's NIC. Traffic fines will be payable through the usual system of payment. Motorists can make inquiries concerning any violations using the interactive voice system, through the ministry of interior site, or by sending a SMS to a designated number followed by the National Identification Number (NIN).

Element of the Project

The Saher system consists of five subsystems (TMS, AVL, LPR, VMS, CCTV) and the main command and control center.

Systems of the project:

- Traffic Management System (TMS)
- Auto Vehicle Location (AVL)
- License Plate Recognition system (LPR)
- Variable Message Sings (VMS)
- Closed Circuit TV (CCTV)
- Law Enforcement System (LES)

All these systems will be linked with the command and control centers located in eight cities Kingdom wide.

Command and control centers: SAHER system project includes the establishment of Command and Control centers through which all systems to be linked and operated.

Main Functions of the System

Traffic Management System (TMS): Highly sophisticated electronic system designed to improve movement of traffic automatically through automated control of traffic lights based on monitoring of traffic movement in all directions in each intersection, which called Green Wave.

Auto Vehicle Location system (AVL): An electronic system designed to track the location of Traffic police vehicles to direct them to deal quickly with certain traffic cases as well as to manage all field patrols.

License Plate Recognition system (LPR): An electronic system installed at the entrances and exits of cities in order to identify vehicles for statistical purposes, as well as for traffic wanted and stolen vehicles through license plates of these vehicles.

Variable Messaging Sings system (VMS): Network of electronic guidance signs for live broadcast designed to guide motorists to avoid traffic congestion on the roads.

Closed Circuit TV systems (CCTV): Electronic system designed to monitor live traffic movement on the main roads.

Law Enforcement system (LES): Network of cameras, fixed and mobile radars to automatically, without human intervention, monitor and control traffic violations, as well as issue traffic violation tickets and notifies violators.

For a violation to be ticketed, it goes through the following cycle:

- The violated vehicle automatically monitored by cameras
- Photo of the violated vehicle license plate broadcasted (over speeding, running a red light and other traffic violations)

- The violation received at the Violation Processing Center
- Information about be owner of the vehicle obtained from the National Database at the National Information Center
- Violation ticket issued
- The violation ticket issued and mailed to the violator to his mailing address registered at the National Information Center at Ministry of Interior.
- Settlement of traffic tickets may be made by Sadad[1] payment system through ATM.

When implemented properly, the traffic authorities hope to achieve the following objectives:

- To improve level of traffic safety
- To utilize the latest and most advanced technology in the field of intelligent transportation (ITS) in order to create a safe traffic environment.
- To upgrading the existing road network.
- To enhance the public security by using the latest surveillance systems.
- To ensure strict, accurate and constant implementation of traffic regulations.

The Saher system has some unique features that distinguish this system from the regular manual traffic control. Among those features:

- Live monitor of traffic (24/7).
- Better management of traffic.
- Quick handling of traffic cases.
- Increase the efficiency of traffic patrols.
- Live monitor of traffic situations and accidents.
- Automated control of traffic violations.

STUDY FINDINGS

The SAHER system has been proven to be effective in controlling reckless driving and reducing the number of vital accidents in countries like, Australia, Singapore, parts of Europe, and the United States. In Melbourne (Australia), during the first three years of implementation, the system reduced the number of annual car crash's deaths from 1350 to only 400.

When trying to adopt the same system in Saudi Arabia several factors need to be taken into consideration. Some of these factors are related to pre-implementation stages and others have to do with verification of information and violation notification. Compared to the European and the American systems, mail in Saudi Arabia is not being delivered to your home address (i.e. your physical location). This due to the fact that the street and houses are not numbered or named in Saudi Arabia. Either you pay a fee to have your own mail box at the mail center or they will simply call you to pick your mail from the mail center at designated hours. As a result, violations from the SAHER system will never get to the violator or simply will not arrive in a timely manner. Consequently, the violation charges will be pushed to its maximum limit due not paying on time.

Alternatively, mobile technology can be utilized to deliver notifications using SMS. In 2008, it has been reported that Saudi Arabia has more than 36 million mobile phone lines. With such a high mobile penetration ratio and the absence of a good mail delivery services, SMS is the most suitable delivery candidate for the notifications. Though this solution is promising and handy, it raises concerns about updating users' personal information. It is quite normal that users change their cell phone number without updating it at the National Information Center (NIC). One could look into the possibility of linking the mobile phone company's subscribers' database with the database at the NIC (real time update).

Other social or cultural factors could be present in particular societies but not in others. In Saudi Arabia, it is quite normal to drive your father's, brother's, uncle's, or cousin's car. In other words, you are driving a car registered under someone else name. In that case, they will be receiving tickets for violations you have committed yourself.

On the technical side, the infrastructure in the big cities can easily support the newly proposed system but this is not the case for small or remote cities. Mobile media technologies could be utilized to transmit the data to control and processing centers. The same or similar mobile technology could be used to pass the message back to the driver that you have been ticketed for over speeding or crossing the traffic light in that particular location.

CONCLUSION

The transformation from the usual face-to-face interaction to the electronic media in delivering government services to residents and citizens opened new horizons to deliver the services in a more efficient and effective manner. Though e-services were more convenient than the traditional face-to-face transaction, they were limited in many ways. They usually require an internet connection which as a result requires an access to a computer and a considerable technical knowledge. On the other hand, mobile services were successful in reaching to the customers in their locations rather than bringing them in.

The case under study demonstrates the increase in the range and the level of application when adopting the m-business model. It also supported the close relevance between the different m-business model success factors. As such, technology is not the only inhibiting factor.

On the other hand, most if not all mobile devices are characterized by small display areas, limited memory and processing power, low-speed data transmission, short-life batteries, limited coverage areas, and most importantly the questionable security. In light of the advances in mobile technology, most if not all of these limitations will vanish over time. Upon overcoming these timely limitations with more secured applications, m-application is undoubtly the future technology for providing business and government services putting in mind: the ease of use, real added value, and the price.

ACKNOWLEDGMENT

The author wishes to acknowledge King Fahd University of Petroleum and Minerals (KFUPM) Saudi Arabia and Hafr Al-Batin Community College for their support in providing the various facilities utilized in the process of producing this chapter and the book in general. This work was supported by the Deanship of Scientific Research (DSR) program of King Fahd University of Petroleum and Minerals (KFUPM), under Project Number: **# IN101001.**

REFERENCES

Banister, F., & Remenyi, D. (2000). Acts of faith: instinct, value and IT investments. *Journal of Information Technology, 15*(3), 231–241. doi:10.1080/02683960050153183

Banister, F., & Remenyi, D. (2004). Value Perception in IT Investment Decisions. Retrieved May 7, 2005 from http://ejise.com/volume-2/volume 2-issue2/issue2-art1.htm

Banister, F., & Remenyi, D. (2005). The Social Value of ICT: First Steps towards an Evaluation Framework. Retrieved May 27, 2006 from http://www.ejise.com/volume6-issue2 /issue2-art21.htm

Benjamin, R. J., & Blunt, J. (1992). Critical IT issues: The next ten years. *Sloan Management Review, 33*(4), 7–19.

Bias, R. G., & Mayhew, D. J. (Eds.). (1994). *Cost-Justifying Usability.* Boston, MA: Academic Press.

Chang, Ai-Mei, & Kannan, P.K. (2002). *Preparing for Wireless and Mobile Technologies in Government.* IBM Center for the Business of Government.

Devadoss, P. R., Pan, S. L., & Huang, J. C. (2002). Structural analysis of e-government initiatives: a case study of SCO. *Decision Support Systems, 34,* 253–269. doi:10.1016/S0167-9236(02)00120-3

Donegan, M. (2000). The m-commerce challenge. *Telecommunications, 34*(1), 58.

Dumas, J. S., & Redish, J. C. (1994). *A Practical Guide to Usability Testing.* Norwood, NJ: Ablex.

Easton, J. (2002). *Going Wireless: transform your business with wireless mobile technology.* USA: HarperCollins.

Ehrlich, K., & Rohn, J. (1994). Cost-justification of usability engineering: A vendor's perspective. In Bias, R. G., & Mayhew, D. J. (Eds.), *Cost-Justifying Usability.* Boston, MA: Academic Press.

ESCWA. (2005). *Regional profile of the information society in western Asia.* New York: United Nations.

Gandon, F., & Sadeh, N. (2004). Semantic Web Technologies to Reconcile Privacy and Context Awareness, Proceedings of the 1st French-Speaking Conference on Mobility and Ubiquity Computing, CD-Format, New York, USA.

Ghyasi, A., & Kushchu, I. (2004). Uses of Mobile Government in Developing Countries. Retrieved June 18, 2005 from mGovLab, http://www.mgovlab.org

Goldstuck, A. (2004). *Government Unplugged: Mobile and wireless technologies in the public service.* Center for public services innovation, South Africa.

Gould, J. D., & Lewis, C. (1985). Designing for usability: Key principles and what designers think. *Communications of the ACM, 28*(3), 300–311. doi:10.1145/3166.3170

Head, M., & Yuan, Y. (2001). Privacy Protection in Electronic Commerce – a Theoretical Framework. *Human Systems Management, 20,* 149–160.

Heeks, R. (2003). Causes of e-government success and failure. Retrieved October 12, 2004 from http://www.e-devexchange.org /eGov/ causefactor.htm

Heeks, R., & Lallana, E. C. (2004). M-Government Benefits and Challenges. Retrieved May 15, 2005 from http://www.e-devexchange.org/ eGov/ mgovprocom.

Ives, B., & Learmonth, G. P. (1984). The Information System as a Competitive Weapon. *Communications of the ACM, 27*(12), 1193–1201. doi:10.1145/2135.2137

Kakihara, M., & Sorensen, C. (2002). Mobility: An Extended Perspective. 35th Hawaii International Conference on System Sciences, Hawaii, USA.

Keen, P. G. W. (1981). Information systems and organizational change. *Communications of the ACM, 24*(1), 24–33. doi:10.1145/358527.358543

Kristoffersen, S., & Ljungberg, F. (1999). Mobile use of IT. In the proceedings of IRIS22, Jyvaskyla, Finland.

Kushchu, I., & Kuscu, H. (2003). From e-government to m-government: Facing the Inevitable? In the proceeding of European Conference on e-government (ECEG 2003), Trinity College, Dublin.

Layne, K., & Lee, J. (2001). Developing fully functional e-government: A four stage model. *Government Information Quarterly, 18,* 122–136. doi:10.1016/S0740-624X(01)00066-1

Lewis, J. R. (1991a). An after-scenario questionnaire for usability studies: psychometric evaluation over three trials. *SIGCHI Bulletin, 23,* 79. doi:10.1145/126729.1056077

Lewis, J. R. (1991b). Psychometric evaluation of an after-scenario questionnaire for computer usability studies: The ASQ. *SIGCHI Bulletin, 23,* 78–81. doi:10.1145/122672.122692

Lewis, J. R. (1991c). *User satisfaction questionnaires for usability studies: 1991 manual of directions for the ASQ and PSSUQ* (Tech. Report 54.609). Boca Raton, FL: International Business Machines Corporation.

Lewis, J. R. (1992a). *Psychometric evaluation of the computer system usability questionnaire: The CSUQ* (Tech. Report 54.723), Boca Raton, FL: International Business Machines Corporation.

Lewis, J. R. (1992b). Psychometric evaluation of the post-study system usability questionnaire: The PSSUQ. In *Proceedings of the Human Factors Society 36th Annual Meeting* (pp. 1259-1263). Santa Monica, CA: Human Factors Society.

Lucas, H. C. Jr. (1975). *Why Information Systems Fail.* New York, London: Columbia University Press.

Markus, M. L. (1983). Power, politics, and MIS implementation. *Communications of the ACM, 26*(6), 430–444. doi:10.1145/358141.358148

Markus, M. L., & Benjamin, R. J. (1996). Change agentry – the next information systems frontier. *Management Information Systems Quarterly, 20*(4), 385–407. doi:10.2307/249561

May, P. (2001). *Mobile commerce: opportunities, applications, and technologies of wireless business.* New York: Cambridge University Press. doi:10.1017/CBO9780511583919

Muller, M. J., Wildman, D. M., & White, E. A. (1993). Equal opportunity PD using PICTIVE. *Communications of the ACM, 36*(4), 64–66. doi:10.1145/153571.214818

Nichols, R. K., & Lekkas, P. C. (2002). *Wireless Security Models, Threats, and Solutions.* New York, NY: McGraw-Hill.

Nielsen, J. (1993). *Usability Engineering.* Boston, MA: Academic Press.

Nielsen, J. (1994). Heuristic evaluation. In Nielsen, J., & Mack, R. L. (Eds.), *Usability Inspection Methods* (pp. 25–64). New York, NY: John Wiley & Sons.

Nielsen, J., & Landauer, T. K. (1993). A mathematical model of the finding of usability problems, *Proceedings of the ACM INTERCHI'93 Conference,* Amsterdam, the Netherlands, 206-213.

O'Hara, K., & Stevens, D. (2006). Democracy, Ideology and Process Re-Engineering: Realising the Benefits of e-Government in Singapore. In Proceedings of Workshop on e-Government: Barriers and Opportunities, WWW06 (in press), Edinburgh. Huai, J., Shen, V. and Tan, C. J., Eds

Odedra, M. (1991). Information technology transfer to developing countries: is really taking place? In J. Berleur & J. Drumm (Eds.) *The 4th IFIF.TC9 International Conference on Human Choice and Computers*, North Holland, Amsterdam, Netherlands, HCC 4 held jointly with the CEC FAST Program.

Roggenkamp, K. (2004). Development Modules to Unleash the Potential of Mobile Government: Developing mobile government applications from a user perspective. In the proceedings of the 4th European Conference on e-Government, Dublin, Ireland.

Sadeh, N. (2002). *M-Commerce: Technologies, services, and business models.* Hershey, PA: Wiley Computer Publishing.

Schwiderski-Grosche, S., & Knospe, H. (2002). Secure mobile commerce. *Electronics and Communication Engineering Journal, 14*(5), 228–238. doi:10.1049/ecej:20020506

Senn, J. A. (2000). The emergence of m-commerce. *IEEE Computer Magazine, 33*(12), 148–150.

Shackel, B. (1971). Human factors in the P.L.A. meat handling automation scheme. A case study and some conclusions. *International Journal of Production Research, 9*(1), 95–121. doi:10.1080/00207547108929864

Siau, K., & Shen, Z. (2003). Mobile communications and mobile services. *International Journal of Mobile Communications, 1*(1-2), 3–14. doi:10.1504/IJMC.2003.002457

Smith, M. D., Bailey, J., & Brynjolfsson, E. (2000). Understanding Digital Markets: Review and Assessment. In Brynjolfsson, E., & Kahin, B. (Eds.), *Understanding the Digital Economy.* Cambridge, MA: MIT Press.

Tachikawa, K. (2003). A perspective on the evolution of mobile communications. *IEEE Communications Magazine, 41*(10), 66–73. doi:10.1109/MCOM.2003.1235597

Tanenbaum, A. S., & Van Steen, M. (2002). *Distributed Systems: Principles and Paradigms.* Upper Saddle River, N.J.: Prentice-Hall.

Turban, E., King, D., Lee, J., & Viehland, D. (2004). *Electronic Commerce 2004: a Managerial Perspective.* Englewood Cliffs, NJ: Pearson/Prentice-Hall.

Unni, R., & Harmon, R. (2003). Location-based services: models for strategy development in m-commerce. *In proceedings of IEEE International Conference on Management of Engineering Technology,* pp. 416-424, Portland, USA.

Varshney, U. (2002). Mobile commerce: framework, applications and networking support. *Mobile Networks and Applications, 7*(3), 185–198. doi:10.1023/A:1014570512129

Varshney, U., & Vetter, R. (2000). Emerging mobile and wireless networks (Technology information). *Communications of the ACM, 43*(6), 73–81. doi:10.1145/336460.336478

Voydock, V. L., & Kent, S. T. (1983). Security Mechanisms in High-level Network protocols. *ACM Computing Surveys, 15*(2), 35–71. doi:10.1145/356909.356913

Wasserman, A. S. (1989). Redesigning Xerox: A design strategy based on operability. In Klemmer, E. T. (Ed.), *Ergonomics: Harness the Power of Human Factors in Your Business* (pp. 7–44). Norwood, NJ: Ablex.

West, D. (2002). *Global E-Government.* Providence, Rhode Island: Brown University.

Yuan, Y., & Zhang, J. J. (2003). Towards an appropriate business model for m-commerce. *International Journal of Mobile Communications, 1*(1-2), 35–56. doi:10.1504/IJMC.2003.002459

Zalesak, M. (2003). *Overview and opportunities of mobile government.* Retrieved June 21, 2005 from http://www.developmentgateway.or g/download/218309/mGov.doc

ENDNOTE

[1]   Automated payment system in Saudi Arabia.

Chapter 7
Processing Change Instigated by Immersed New Media Usage and its Implications for School-Based and Informal Learning

Ġorġ Mallia
University of Malta, Malta

EXECUTIVE SUMMARY

This case presented in this chapter[1] revolves around the hypothesis that information processing has changed from a linear format, within a chronological progression, to a partially controlled chaotic format, with tracking achieved primarily through hypertextual nodes which goes against the enforced linearity of most institutionally imposed hierarchical learning. Suggestions are given as to how basic schooling methodologies may need to be modified to conform to new learning practices. The possibility of the informal learning option more amenable to hypertextual processing is also explored. Online whimsical searches and acquisition of information through social software interaction and other new media technology immersion has changed the breadth of informal learning, particularly self-directed and incidental learning. In a study of University of Malta students that requested self-perceptive descriptions of learning preferences (formal study/independent acquisition). 70% opted for formal study, explainable by their traditional academic context. 30% preferred flexibility and the intrinsic motivation stimulated by self-direction; a significant number given that a decision about a life choice was requested.

BACKGROUND

Internet usage in more technologically advanced continents has grown massively as shown in Table 1. There has been a huge usage growth since 2000, and there is a 50.1% penetration in Europe, 60.1% in Oceania/Australia, and a massive 73.9% in North America. At least in Europe, quoting slightly older statistics, 73% of young people aged 16 to 24 use the Internet at least once a week (Eurostat News Release, 2006). There can be no doubt that this has grown exponentially.

In the main the majority of researchers agree that the Web permits, among many other intrinsic and extrinsic gains, "learning through frequent interaction and feedback" (Donnerstein, 2002, p.

DOI: 10.4018/978-1-60960-015-0.ch007

320). The same applies to video games, which are multi-layered problem-solving experiences in which, for example, identities are assumed that promote intrinsic learning (Gee, 2003, Shaffer, 2006). More formally, learning can even be digital game-based, all about "the coming together of two seemingly diametrically opposed worlds: *serious learning* in schools and in businesses, and *interactive entertainment* – computer games, video games..." (Prensky, 2007, p.15)

Some research results are not so positive, indicating the possibility of Internet addiction. For example McKay, Thurlow and Tommey Zimmerman (2005) treat optimistic research about motivation resulting from immersed internet usage with caution and wonder as to whether young users are becoming little more than "techno slaves." This goes as far back as Greenfield's 1999 reference to "netheads [and] cyberfreaks." Internet addiction seems to be a well-analysed social fear (Chou, Condron, & Belland, 2005). The same applies to video games, with research indicating that immersed users' scholastic grades suffer (Anand, 2007) while at the same time admitting that determining whether this is because of time management disruption caused by dependence or because of other, collateral factors is difficult. Time loss through video gaming was considered to have both negative and positive outcomes in

research by Wood, Griffiths, and Parke (2007), though the contexts of this research are predominantly social. Teaming up video gaming with the internet in the form of Massive Multi-user Online Role-Playing Games (MMORPGs) is often considered lethal and addiction almost a natural and accepted side-effect (Young, 2009).

The focus in this chapter is on processing changes caused by New Media immersion that are more intimately related to cognitive acquisition which have recently begun to be explored (Salonius-Pasternak & Gelfond, 2005), rather than to Internet-affected social interaction. The negative effects of Internet and other New Media usage may be exaggerated and sensationalized and may blind researchers to other intrinsic changes that are happening because of the usage. I am not negating that addiction is a distinct possibility, given the affective strength of the media in question, but my arguments are that if the literature were to concentrate entirely on that aspect, the side to New Media immersion that invokes, provokes and consolidates processing changes, and that needs understanding, can easily lag behind.

As a result of this immersion, informal learning — that "vast reservoir of learning possibilities" (Tuschling & Engemann, 2006[2]) — is gaining an advantage over more formalized, school-based learning. This chapter also deals with the growing

Table 1. Internet usage and world population dtatistics for June 30, 2009

World Regions	Population (2009 Est.)	Internet Users Latest Data	Penetrati on (% Population)	Growth 2000-2009	Internet users by World Region
Africa	999,002,342	65,903,900	6.7%	1,359.9%	3.9%
Asia	3,808,070,503	704,213,930	18.5%	516.1%	42.2%
Europe	803,850,858	402,380,474	50.1%	282.9%	24.2%
Middle East	202,687,005	47,964,146	23.7%	1,360.2%	2.9%
North America	340,831,831	251,735,500	73.9%	132.9%	15.1%
Latin America/Caribbean	586,662,468	175,834,439	30.0%	873.1%	10.5%
Oceania/Australia	34,700,201	20,838,019	60.1%	173.4%	1.2%
World Total	6,767,805,208	1,668,870,408	24.7%	362.3%	100.0%

Source: www.Internetworldstats.com. © 2001-2009, Miniwatts Marketing Group

preference for informal learning, presenting a brief review of relevant literature and limited research that indicates how inroads are being made into formally structured, traditional tertiary contexts.

Immersion also leads to deeper change, going beyond content influence and intrusive persuasive manipulation — most likely it is affecting the very structure of information processing, defined by Perry (2003) within a cognitive science, problem-solving context as encoded information which is acted on and transformed in the resolution of a goal held by a cognitive entity.

These new informal venues of knowledge acquisition also have a new structure embedded into their architectures — a semi-structured architecture of semantic links that connect related knowledge with immediate access. Experts with these structures may have a fundamentally different approach to information processing.

The architecture of New Media languages has a pervasive effect on the cognitive perceptions and usages particularly of young immersed users of the media.

SETTING THE STAGE

The change that has been brought about by New Media immersion is more than societal. It is deep rooted and has affected cognition in ways that might determine the nature of teaching and learning for decades to come.

There are a number of ways in which this change has come about. New Media immersion can take many forms and is as wide-ranging as are the definitions of New Media itself. The term is old, and goes as far back as the 1980's, but interpretations are new and renew themselves regularly.

This chapter intends to look generally at New Media and how habitual usage has brought about a perceptual mutation that has led to a clash with societal norms, particularly when it comes to methodological practices in educational institutions.

If one were to think of New Media in terms of:

a. Computer-based technologies
b. Web 2.0 interactivity and Social Software usage
c. Interactive gaming (both personal and online)
d. Mobile technologies

It would be quite obvious that there are very few digital natives (Prensky, 2001) who are not in some way affected by the massive influx of these media.

There is an ongoing debate as to whether these young people are so massively influenced as to go through a disaffection with the norms of education and all other non-digital aspects of society in general (Bennett, Maton, & Kervin, 2008), but there can be little doubt that some sort of affective and cognitive change is taking place because of immersion in these media.

Highly representative of the research being carried out about digital natives is this statement from Marsh et al. (2005):

Young children are immersed in practices relating to popular culture, media and new technologies from birth. They are growing up in a digital world and develop a wide range of skills, knowledge and understanding of this world from birth. (p. 75)

Some of the learning in these new environments is as adventitious and haphazard as learning in the real world, with unexpected challenges and feedback. Some of it is more structured and controlled, as in the interlinked networks of a wiki. These environments may take advantage of the learning skills honed in the real world, and they may challenge the structured modes of institutional learning as uninteresting and stultified.

The earliest literature on video games has indicated that they have affected cognition, particularly in iconic or analog representation (Greenfield, deWinstanley, Kilpatrick, & Kaye, 1994). Extended immersion provides extensive indications that there is an ongoing transformation of cyber users' cognitive processing capabilities. The result is a change that permits ease of navigation, problematisation of situation and circumstance, and decision-making in environments that have moved architecturally away from the incremental, step-by-step demands made in traditional educational environments.

The essential base providing change is hypertextual in nature. Hypertext itself was deemed to be the fundamental element in the constructivist "textbook of the future" as far back as 1993 (Cunningham, Duffy, & Knuth, 1993).

There is an extensive literature examining Hypertext Assisted Learning (Niederhauser & Shapiro, 2003; Shapiro & Niederhauser, 2004), with its singling out of the main features of hypertext, primarily its non-linear structure, its flexibility of information access, its bite-sized approach to structuring knowledge, and its greater degree of learner control. Like the real world, it brings distantly related events and constructs into juxtaposition. Like the real world, it lets learners question their own understanding of the events and select aspects to ponder. Unlike the real world, it lets learners explore those connections they find interesting and personally meaningful, and provides a consistent interface and structured avenues for that exploration.

The early literature too found strong differences among learners in the way they used hypertext links. The distinction is made between "self-regulated readers" and "cue-dependent readers" (Balcytiene, 1999), with the second scoring better on content acquisition than the first, but with the first being more independent and exploratory in the way hypertext is read.

A number of theories have explored the need for learners to adjust their cognitive processes in the face of hypertextuality and conceptual complexity and irregularity in knowledge domains, predominantly Cognitive Flexibility Theory (Spiro, Feltovich, Jacobson, & Coulson, 1991).

As in that theory, what is being proposed in this chapter also demands adaptability to an ir-regular stimulus. The metacognitive processes involved put the learner firmly in the centre of the learning in a cyclical process, the medium feeding the learner's own conscious approaches to the usage and the subsequent learning, with that same usage modifying the mechanisms of perception and application, and reflecting on the actual medium. This is particularly true in the contexts of independently-used, flexible learning environments (IUFLEs) in which the learning itself provides motivational impetus.

The social reality surrounding technology-heavy environments in which immersed users thrive is that informal, independent, flexible learning is much more in line with the new random processing. Research shows social software's effectiveness in this regard, both as reinforcement of existing learning and as a motivational instigator of learning all by itself (see, for example, Milheim, 2007; Selwyn, Gorard, & Furlong, 2006).

It is almost a superfluity to state that the spread of personal computing and mobile technologies, together with, static and mobile gaming consoles, has revolutionised the dissemination of information on demand. This information includes ephemeral, transient facts that might be useful only to (say) the game being played, or it might include more detailed, fully-fledged online searches. In all cases, the change is persistent and though more common in the younger digital natives, it reaches quite far into society since cyberculture has permeated all generations at present, with some more amenable to integration with the culture than others, since a formidable adherence to formal modes of information acquisition is also evident in some contexts.

Cross- and inter-active Web 2.0 applications such as Weblogs and wikis and such user-addictive phenomena as YouTube and peer-to-peer audio sharing, social networks, as well as online fora and chat environments, are proving a ready source of byte-sized, non-hierarchically scaled items of information. These resources cumulatively build into a library attuned to this new kind of

HTP learning, but it does not necessarily have an institutionally accepted focus. Mobile technology also contributes directly to "learning-on-the-go" — creating a perpetual chain of information through technology. All of this is beginning to be used tentatively in schools (Sang Hyun, Holmes, & Mims, 2005).

Immersed internet users, and heavy users of social software, as well as many forms of video gaming, live in an environment in which knowledge acquisition is at their fingertips, and the processes they have mastered to interact with the software also gives them the rudimentary skills needed to navigate, absorb and integrate the learning into a cohesive, if chaotically absorbed, body of learning. In this sense, the acquisition is both substantive and procedural – the content of the learning, teamed with the navigational process (for the internet) and manipulative skills (for gaming) that utilises that content in tiered, sometimes hierarchical, at others random, ways.

"The structure sought here is integrative, a self-reflective technique of self performance ideally centered in the individual. It seeks to make learning independent from setting, from personal and financial effort. Informal learning can take place regardless of circumstances" (Tuschling & Engemann, 2006, pp. 456-457), and it can take place any time and anywhere, given that New Media technologies are both desktop and mobile.

A lot has also been written about how the blog has created an invaluable vehicle for vociferous self-expression. Can the blog itself be a means to producing feedback from independent learning? "Could blogging be the needle that sews together what is now a lot of learning in isolation with no real connection among the disciplines?" (Richardson, 2004). Certainly the use of blogging and beyond - the immersion into the interactive multiverse that links together so many different users/feeders of knowledge and opinion, is providing an enormous amount of learning 'on the run'. The "e is for everything" concept spearheaded by Katzand Oblinger (2000) and interpreted by Wheeler

(2007) as "extended learning," "enhanced learning," and "everywhere learning," emphasizes the all-encompassing presence of the learning source, and the persistent, erratic, but ubiquitous learning that is totally learner directed and informal.

Informal (or non-formal, as described by Eraut, 2000) learning is a persistent happening that we often find difficult even to conceptualise as actual learning. It is incidental in the main, and can take the form of anything from reading instructions in a recipe booklet to reaching out for an encyclopedia to look for a reference.

A more formal definition is given by Livingstone (2001), "Informal learning is any activity involving the pursuit of understanding, knowledge or skill which occurs without the presence of externally imposed curricular criteria." (p.4). Meaning that there is no help offered to the person acquiring the learning, and no structured studies programme to follow. This also means that no institutional learning of any type is a part of it, nor is any type of online instruction, or learning that is organized in any way, directly or indirectly.

The three forms that informal learning usual takes are (1) Self-Directed Learning, (2) Incidental Learning, and (3) Socialization (Schugurensky, 2000).

To define the individual forms: *Self-Directed Learning*: or that learning that is taking on as a "project" by the individual. A lot of informal learning that happens online is of this type. *Incidental Learning*: non-intended learning that happens on the side of an activity, or even as an indirect result of self-directed learning. In informal learning online this can happen, for e.g., through hypertextual meanderings beyond the web-pages sought consciously by the person browsing. *Socialization (tacit learning)*: "refers to the internalization of values, attitudes, behaviors, skills, etc. that occur during everyday life. Not only we have no a priori intention of acquiring them, but we are not aware that we learned something." (Schugurensky, 2000, p.4).

Informal, on-a-whim searches for information have, by necessity, redimensioned the concept of informal learning, with volume often (though never totally) compensating for a lack of learning organisation.

Efforts have been made to find ways of integrating informal learning into a more structured, formal design. One form this takes is the recognition of prior learning (RPL), "a process whereby people are provided with an opportunity to have the skills and knowledge they have developed outside the formal education system assessed and valued against qualifications frameworks" (Hargreaves, 2006, p.1), often surfacing in the field of Adult Education, and taking the form of the acceptance of assessible competence, possibly accrued through experience and the other venues of informal learning (for e.g. in Sweden, Andersson & Fejes, 2005; in France, Pouget & Osborne, 2004; and in Australian Universities, Pitman, 2009).

In the case of on-a-whim searches, though there is no denying the massive infusion of informal learning that happens on a daily, purely personal basis, there is no cumulative objective to the learning, nor is it built against an assessable framework, in most cases making accreditation very difficult.

As is the case with a reformatted school-based learning, the issue of motivation is essential in this type of learning. In this case motivation is hardly ever extrinsic, as it often is in schooling, but intrinsic. It is the impulsive need-to-know about some aspect of a personally appreciated topic. In the case of young people this takes the form of searches related to music, gaming, films, etc., and is often a side-task during social-software interaction.

Because of the transient nature of the information searching, and the questionable qualifications of many of the websites consulted – Wikipedia being forefront in this, with academics split on its use by students (Eijkman, 2009) – it is contended that the process defies integration within a formalised

academic setting, though attempts at self-paced project work that demands web-searching have often been made at both secondary and tertiary levels of education. But in these, the all-important motivational elements that infuse the process are almost always missing since it is only the vehicle that is integrated within the formalised learning, and not the essential need-to-know motivational drive that normally fuels the use of independently-used, flexible learning environments. This is also the case with online learning systems, or, indeed, a lot of forms of e-learning, in which motivation is more difficult to stoke than in face-to-face teaching and learning, to the point where it needs to be singled out for interventional consdieration (ChanLin, 2009).

But IUFLEs are inscrutable in many ways. Not only are they very difficult to define, given the diversity of source and the whimsical nature of usage, they are also prone to negative effect by factors as divergent as national scholastic inclinations, academic and social traditions, and individual drive.

IUFLEs more often than not defy accreditation. While "assessment should be a vehicle for educational improvement", and "lecturers may need to provide different but equivalent assessment activities "(Cummings, 2003), the main problem with the new independence and flexibility in learning is not acceptance, it is that no formalized way of accrediting information is gained through Web interaction or direct individual research, in spite of some National Qualification Frameworks' statement to the opposite (Young, 2007). The problems for the formalization of what is essentially the most informal of all ways of accessing information are legion, and very few fit in with the quantifiable assessment practices in use today in most universities. This is particularly true of the more traditional universities, and in spite of the fact that "wider inclusion in a learning society may come more easily from greater recognition of tacit knowledge than from more participation" (Gorard, Fevere, & Rees, 1999, p. 451).

Other Considerations

Learner control depends extensively on how individuals who use the hypertext use the baggage of prior knowledge they bring with them to the usage and how this affects whether learner control predominates. The indications from the literature (for example, Gail & Hannafin, 1994) are that those with high levels of prior knowledge are more in control than those with low levels of prior knowledge, who prefer more structured program-controlled hypertexts. However, hierarchically-structured texts, so often touted in research on learning from traditional text, are not necessarily indispensable when used by novices using hypertext. Surface information seems to be acquired regardless of structure (Shapiro, 1998), though deeper meaning does benefit from a structured approach. Hierarchies can be built even in unstructured hypertext links, providing they have cues to meaning (Shapiro, 1999).

Interestingly, eye-tracking research about novices learning how to use computer games indicates the preference of a trial-and-error strategy, with little time given to actual teaching hints as they learnt how to use the game (Alkan & Cagiltay, 2007). Documentation was not easily available in the experiment, but none of the participants complained about this, as they immediately began overcoming the obstacles and independently figured their way around the gameplay, the learning of which they deemed to be easy.

Among many learners, strong, independent problem solving seems to be prevalent in self-regulated users' navigation of these media, with metacognitive processes at work creating a schema-driven means of procedural acquisition.

The hypothesis that is being presented in this chapter is that the process goes beyond this, and the cognition of the structures reflects the navigational processes in the media. The result is an intrinsic, cognitive and affective move from predominantly linear processing to a more lateral one. In many cases this takes the form of hypertextual leaping.

This moves the onus from the singular focus to a more diversified, multi-focus, superficial in content but quite wide in spread, taking advantage of the freedom associated with hypertext that is evident even in the early literature on its use (e.g., Rouet & Levonen, 1996; and George Landow's seminal volume on the topic, now updated, Landow, 2006), and in direct structural links with, for example, the cinema (Mancini, 2005) and literature (Schneider, 2005), and more broadly perhaps with real world exploration.

This is a cognitive strategy that has also already found mirroring on such popular stations as MTV with its multi-focal-point announcer presentations and erratic camera movement in sequential narrative, and its use of the fragmented, juxtaposed editing of visuals that interacts with and responds to the rhythm and lyric of the sounds of the music (Williams, 2003).[3] Indeed, traces of hypertext-induced influence have been evident for a while in a lot of postmodern works of fiction, film and the visual arts (Gaggi, 1997).

There is a byte-sized communications revolution. This includes the abbreviated mobile phone instant text message, the short burst message on social networks Twitter and Facebook, as well as the language used in internet chat rooms. They are by themselves changing the nature of language – creating nu-speak (Herther, 2009). This is further corroborated by the quick-flip style of editing in television advertising, not to mention the minutes long television serial sequences in between frequent advertising breaks, and even the short sentence, short chapter mode of novel writing, exemplified by several bestseller *novels*, all contribute directly to corroborate the context and effects of hypertextuality.

Speculatively, the result of persistent immersion is Hypertextual Processing (HTP) which organizes perceived information into an erratic, loosely grouped number of simultaneous focal points resulting in coherent, if sporadic, information gain (Mallia, 2007). This provides a change from a linear format within a chronological progression to a partially-controlled chaotic format, with tracking achieved primarily through hypertextual nodes. One such unit, taken out of a typically hap-hazard set for the sake of analysis, would contain a large number of random information/'instructional clusters, strung together by means of an arbitrary lattice-work of hypertextual points (or nodes), themseles independent of each other, though at times periferally linked through wide-ranging topic or keyword relationship.

In turn, this conflicts with the perceived linear (if stratified) organization of thought processes on which presumption most traditional school-based pedagogies and training programmes are built. The conflict makes for a very limited attention span and a resultant lack of follow through.

Nor does the move towards HTP appear to be limited to certain age groups, though the vulnerability of the young does single them out for particular influence. Digital natives are by far more susceptible to this than digital immigrants – though it seems that it is the volume of media immersion creates the processing diversity rather than the age itself. Though I am unaware of any laboratory testing for this particular presumed change specifically, it would be interesting to conduct a diachronic study of similar IQ subjects diversified in media exposure (perhaps on the basis of their past experiences and preferences) – linear/chronological (books, certain tv programmes, radio) and non-linear/saltatory (the Internet and multimedia, including game console software). To date, many of the links posited in the literature between video games and education are quite ephemeral, concentrating more on how gaming can be accepted by teachers and how it can be utilized in a format that integrates with ongoing classroom methodologies (see, for example, Hutchinson, 2007).

HTP affects to varying degrees and is dependent on a number of variables, not least of which are varying cognitive styles (Riding & Rayner, 1998). As well, the individual learning strategies of the immersed user can determine how and in

which way hypertextual architecture is perceived and handled (Graff, 2005).

Another important variable is cognitive load (Sweller, van Merrienboer, & Pass, 1998), for which each user has a particular threshold, and for which individual solutions need to be found, including users adopting varying cognitive tools that also determine mind-set and cognitive change (Ozcelik & Yildirim, 2005).

CASE DESCRIPTION

Most of the assumptions presented here have been derived from an analysis of primrarily qualitative data gathered in the main from the following:

- Qualitative observation of *in situ* subjects — intensive observation of young people aged 13 to 18 playing platform and role-playing games in a self-regulating manner noting timing in the decision-making process, eye-hand coordination speeds and variations, browsing style and ease, hyper-linking frequency and patterns, and navigation through stratification. Each subject showed an evolving grasp of navigation and goal-oriented problem solving. There was a progressive mastery of content, so both substantive and procedural gains were noted.

- Focus groups with young people about media immersion and resultant effects — the ages of participants varied from 18 to 22, in the main University of Malta students. All were New Media users to varying degrees. All participated in online chat (from under 1 to 6 hours a day), all used mobile phones extensively, particularly to send SMS's, and around a third were gamers (from casual to fully immersed). Effects of lengthy immersion in both gaming and online browsing varied, but lack of focus, alienation, and an inability or preference not to follow linear conversations and follow uni-directional lectures were particularly noted.

- Semi-structured interviews with school teachers who recognise a rising lack of rapport between traditional methodologies and student interest — the interviews were for another area of research, but a number of questions were about student interest and motivation, the result of which brought out what they believed to be the collocation between technological immersion and diminishing attention span, corroborated by the noting of increased motivation and focusing when HTP was used as a back up to top-down, class-based teaching.
- One directed and one open-ended question on preference between formal and informal tertiary-level learning, as part of a longer questionnaire in the process of analysis. Information about this part of the research is given further below in this chapter.

This last research point needs to be gone into in detail because of the implications it has on the effect that HTP has on formal education.

The question that needs to be asked, and which underscores the case, is: Are we on the brink of the inception of informal "universities" owned by immersed cyber users? How credible will the product be of these populist non-institutions that bring together non-registered learners who browse and surf and get their problem-solving skills from RPG (online or on games consoles) and strategy gameware? How will formal institutions take on board such learning, which, arguably, is motivationally and stylistically more suited to lateral processing than what can be accredited by both traditional and online universities and schools, even if they take on board the suggestions for methodological rerouting to be found in the present work?

In order to determine just how many would actually opt for a life-choice of informal acquisi-tion as opposed to institutionalized learning, the following limited research was undertaken.

The research in this regard has been carried out on the Mediterranean island republic of Malta, an EU member state, and with 413,609 crammed into a total area of 316 km^2, one of the most densely populated countries in the world (information taken from Wikipedia).

Internet access in Malta in 2008 stood at 59.0% (NSO, 2008), just below the 60% average of the EU27 according to Eurostat (Lööf, 2008). Eurostat also indicates that across the EU27, by far the greatest users are between the ages of 16 and 24, and educational background only creates a minor disparity in this age bracket.

Only undergraduate research has been carried out on the internet usage habits of the University students in Malta, so a study in this regard, albeit with a slant in favor of discovering browsing behavior, was in order.

A questionnaire on internet usage was sent to 6000+ University of Malta students by internal mail. 1,600 valid questionnaires were returned to the researcher. All respondents had an internet connection, either at home, or at University, or both. The questionnaire was multi-faceted in content, and sought information about student habits regarding their use of the internet, with particular regard to individual, non-directed use. Information was sought on which sites were most visited by the students for independent search, and which were used mostly for academic searches. Other areas tested were multi-tasking, multi-focusing, hypertextual processing, self-perceptive distinc-tion between directed and non-directed searching, as well as online communication and socialisa-tion habits.

As this chapter is being written, the question-naire is in the process of analysis, but, for the purpose of getting at least an idea with regards to formal/informal learning preference of Uni-versity Students, most of whom can lay claim to being digital natives, a number of offshoots us-ing random samplings from the instrument have yielded a telling glimpse into Maltese student learning format preferences. One open-ended question in particular was intended to provide insight into student preference regarding specifically formal/informal learning. It is true that this relies entirely on respondent perception, and there is no validating exercise to corroborate this take on the question, but perceptions are also useful and indicative.

The question was: "Given a life choice between formal, directed study (for e.g. a university degree course) and independent, non-directed acquisition of information (for e.g. non-accredited, internet based, incidental learning), which would you choose?" In the next field, participants were asked to give an explanation for their choice in as much detail as possible. A random 300 replies (across faculties and roughly 50-50 by gender) were chosen from among the submitted questionnaires, and the explanations were in the main analyzed qualitatively.

Apart from the move to independent, flexible learning, a number of residual permutations and implications of the possible change to HTP exist. For example, limited qualitative research in a school for lower-achieving students (mostly all illiterates) but who are quite well versed in the use of games consoles has led to experiments regarding how the visual dimension can act as a replacement to symbolic literacy (Mallia, 2003). The link with HTP manifested itself in a mapping of their use of a digital editing suite, in which their sequencing proved quite non-linear, but very intuitively effective. A number of variables may explain this away, but the narrative in each case was relatively clear and complete, with only the intrinsic linearity of sequencing often missing.

Findings

70% of the random sampling ticked the *Formal Study* field, whereas 30% ticked the *Independent Acquisition* field. This is interesting on many levels, not least in its profiling of the learning

methodology preferences of University of Malta students. The University of Malta is a traditional, teaching University, which has embraced technology in its many facets (uses SITS campus wide for all registration, marks posting, etc.; has a progressing, fully integrated website; uses one-password access for all services), but is still to have formally accredited e-learning, though a VLE was officially chosen recently, and, in all fairness, Moodle had been used randomly by individual academics to varying degrees for years prior to its sanctioned embracing by the University itself. However, in the main, courses are delivered face-to-face and the lecturing system is predominantly top-down.

The indications are that this influenced students in their choice of formal study. The inverse could actually be true, and that their presence at the university might indicate their need for supervised learning. Unfortunately this cannot be corroborated, since the University of Malta is the only university on the island, so there is no room for informed student choice in this regard.

This chapter is considering only that informal learning that comes from self-directed online searches and any incidental learning that comes from it. Socialization as defined can have a very important online dimension, particularly through social networks, as well as VOIP usage – a large percentage of all those who submitted the questionnaire listed as participating actively in one or more social networks, and very few did not make use of communications networks and VOIP. However, for many of those who chose the formal study field, socialization factors were reasons to do so. What was often described as "real" socialization played an important part in making many respondents opt for formal study. Malta's size could also be a significant factor in this.

Also confirming the predominant style of teaching and learning of their *alma mater*, the need for guidance and the fear of redundancy in their online searches figured quite extensively. This was corroborated by an airing of insecurities about individual abilities, with "wouldn't know what to look for", and "deadlines help get the job done", along with an adulation (inversely mirrored in the other field) of professional academics who pass on their knowledge and experience.

The third and final most important factor was accreditation. The qualifications needed to get a job, that one respondent described as "something which I think is the main engine driving students to learn, and not intrinsically for the sake of learning". Whereas in some EU countries there is a tentative move to accredit informal learning within a formal context (Colardyn & Bjornavold, 2004), there are few indications of this in Malta to date, so the reasoning is understandable.

On the other hand, most of those who opted for Independent Acquisition had a number of varied arguments, to make their point, for e.g. flexibility in subject change to avoid boredom; personal interest promoting concentration; not learning under pressure; enjoyment because of personal preference; relevance to the person's lifestyle; self-pacing permitting deeper delving; a more relaxed exercise; vaster choice of topics (i.e. not restricted to the curricular); no imposition. As one respondent put it, "nourishing yourself with knowledge".

There were those who believed that this fostered independent thinking and creative decision making, as opposed to working within the envelope of structured, formal learning. One respondent said that his browsing helped him get a "leg-up" when working in a team of people who preferred formal study. But all in all, the main motivation was "a mixture of personal interest, curiosity and wanting to learn."

Only one participant from the 300 said that "I prefer books, to be honest".

Given the limitation of the sampling, there is no more than an indication of preferences here, placed against an academic and social backdrop that seems to influence quite extensively the choice made by students as they interact with and are immersed in New Media technologies. The indications are, however, that there are those, so far in the minority, who opt for informal acquisition. The fact that this 30% exists at all, given that a "life-choice" was asked for, is an indication of flux in learning format preference. Informal learning as an option seems to be finding a place even among those studying in a formal institution.

The above deals with the highest level of institutionalized education, the University. But the implications of HTP and its effects reach back to all levels of education. For example, one potential direct effect of HTP is the clear pointing out of the lack of most schools' preparedness for coping with students who do not process linearly, as per the traditional approach to hierarchically-structured teaching and text-based resources (Collins & Halverson, 2009).

And it might even go further than that. The majority of teachers interviewed by the author, who have been in post for over ten years, stated that students are finding focusing progressively more difficult. This is predominantly the case in non-technologically aided traditional instruction, but some who supplement their face-to-face teaching with limited e-learning support have indicated that this is also true in formal online learning programmes that lack flexibility and are time constrained. So the indications are that HTP does not affect just formal class-based learning, but also many structured teaching methodological approaches, conveyed through whichever medium permits quantification for accreditation purposes, since that seems to be the intended aim of most institutional teaching and learning.

This brings forth a number of dilemmas within the context of schooling as it stands in a many countries. Often the changes caused as a direct or indirect result of HTP create a huge differentiation in learner approaches within the same learning community. This continues to load difficulty on the demands of inclusive learning environments. Also, currently many teachers come from the generations of either digital semi-literates or digital immigrants, meaning that there is little or no natural affinity with HTP students. This necessitates acquiring a mind set that discerns heightened individual differences and moving to a hyperpedagogy in which "learning can become an endless process of democratic inquiry wherein essences emerge to fit the purposes of individual students and communities" (Dwight & Garrison, 2003, p. 718).

An understanding of the architecture of HTP change is a necessary base on which to build approaches to methodologies that can be effective with those who will otherwise be incompatible with traditional schooling, and be added to the existing long list of those who are deemed as "unteachables."

The following elaborations break down what can be deemed to be the cause, effects and possible modifications needed for change. The change can only be implemented if, first of all, some sort of acceptance of the reality of HTP occurs. Once that acceptance is in place, then the change needs to happen in order for learning within a formal environment to conform to HTP. The suggestions presented here are based on my research in schools, exploring the contrast between set methodologies and student reaction; my experience as a teacher within the educational system; and on interviews with teachers, with bases for the submissions corroborated by the observations and focus group data.

SOLUTIONS AND RECOMMENDATIONS

It is the hypothesis of this chapter that Hypertextual Processing affects attention, focusing, and cognitive processing. A look at the inferred cause and effect on each of these, and their effect in turn on pedagogical practice in school-based learning, can suggest ways in which that practice can change to accommodate the mutated processing.

Attention Span

Internet users are used to short, quickly accessed information instances that can easily be diversified and are often multi-media based; video-gaming often demands speed of sudden decision making and multiple switching; often instantaneous. Multimedia products also give information in small chunks, interlinked and cohesive, but individually compact. As a result of this, long readings and/or long dedicated explanations become daunting, and attention is lost after the first few paragraphs and/or sentences. Unless there are short, multiple media treatments, there is little to draw attention back to the task at hand. Concentrating for longer than an instant on any task defies the need for quick switching between (possibly inter-related) tasks, so often the chance of schematic mapping of the longer process is not possible, and the possibility of understanding is quickly lost. This is a perspective Ben Shneiderman championed throughout his career (Shneiderman & Kiersley, 1989).

If one were to take present pedagogical practice within a traditional teaching environment – a generalised top-down, teacher-student relationship – one can say that lessons are based on pre-planned chunking, each chunk hierarchically or independently listed within a lesson duration scheme of work. Chunks may vary in length, but each covers a topic or activity, and might last as long as a whole lesson.

In order to take on board the effect of HTP, it can be suggested that schemes of work should be based on seemingly random short activities, each of which links to the next at different moments, so there can be independent divergence by individual students. An overarching framework can be determined by the teacher, so that all possible outcomes of each activity should cohere to meet the overall pedagogical objectives for the lesson or sequence of lessons.

Multifocusing

Many uni- and vari- focal actions occur simultaneously during the playing of videogames. This is also prevalent on some Web pages, with flash adverts and pop-ups vying for (and usually getting) instantaneous attention. This has also found itself in the styles of many short streaming video clips, the brevity demanding a large number of cuts. This multifocal activity can also be seen in some young people's television programming. Depth of specific information is sacrificed for spread of stimuli and variety. The predominant effect of this persistent multi-focal reading is a resultant ability to spread focus on a network of equally attracting focal points. Most often the data input from the spread is relatively superficial, so the multifocusing, as opposed to persistent single focusing, is at the price of input depth.

What is most frequently being done in schools at the moment (also presuming a generalised norm) is the focusing on a single pedagogical objective, plumbing its depths and exploring its every aspect before moving on to another point to focus. This practice demands constant and dedicated attention by the students, forsaking even less focused distractions. Many of the summative exams held in the middle and at the end of scholastic years emphasise depth of knowledge as opposed to spread, although spread and depth are also demanded in the more exclusive schools. What can be done to counteract this and be more compliant with HTP is to break down of whole individual activities into short, flexibly accessed actions, researched and discovered by the students themselves, both individually and collectively. Actions that need to be taken might be simultaneous, or separate over a short period of time. The teacher can find ways to interlink the activities carried out over a period of time into a cohesive and coherent whole that further interlinks with other lessons learnt in this way.

Lateral Processing

On the Internet, as well as in multimedia and video game playing, there is a constant directionally chaotic navigation which has no linear, chronological progression as, for example, exists in the case of books. Hyperlinks can be found anywhere on a page, and hypertextual leaping from one page to another, or one element of the page to another, or even across pages and Websites (in the case of the Internet) is constant. A result of the use of hyperlinks on Internet sites and in multimedia products and the making of lateral, interlinked strategic movements in video game playing is a move away from linear processing, which is replaced by lateral and/or multi-directional processing. This makes concentrated uni-directional thinking difficult to achieve, and it is often replaced by seemingly chaotic instances of thought, that, however, might be tracked through thematic, stylistic or contextual nodes.

In most schools, teaching is chronologically directed, and this is particularly the case whenever textual resources (such as books) are used. The progression of lessons is hierarchical and the schemas that are scripted are mostly repetitive and formulaic. The result of the learning is usually summative and often tested primarily for cognitive recall in formal exams.

A suggested pedagogical practice in this case would be the instigation of flexible classroom learning in which computer and other media aided teaching can be used in individual projects determined by the students themselves against a backdrop of loose curricular structuring. Work should be self- or *ad hoc* group-paced and planned to link to flexible classroom teaching through hypertextual modules that can link at any step in the development of each project or module.

What is being suggested here is not the adoption of actual resources, such as specially authored didactic games or the inclusion of, for example, blogging within a formal, quantifiable instructional design. While social software coming to the attention of instructional designers is laudable (e.g., Beldarrain, 2006), many of the focus group participants said that they find very difficult engaging with anything that subverts for didactic ends what they normally use purely for entertainment or non-directed informal knowledge gathering.

What is suggested here is the adoption of techniques that duplicate to some extent the pacing and syntax of main sources of HTP stimulation used as a base for a total restructuring of classroom and other learning routines.

CONCLUSION

Immersed usage of the Internet, with its predominantly hypertextual architecture, along with heavy usage of New Media technologies such as video gaming consoles, within a context of curt, swiftly shifting communications environments, has brought about a variable but quite evident information processing change that demands we rethink the paradigms of individual learning differences for educational purposes if schooling is to be considered. An understanding of the move towards informal, independent acquisition, given that a limited, but significant number seem to be moving in that direction, is also desirable if one is to fully understand the change in learning mentalities that have been instigated by New Media immersion.

Within schooling, teaching and learning methodologies that simulate cyber-technological environments may help bridge the gap between institutionally accepted instructional processes and more hypertextual processing-friendly approaches to educational acquisition.

However, the slow, but apparently logical move towards informal, independent learning, using the very vehicles of change themselves (the Internet, particularly Web 2.0 applications, and other New Media) seems to be the commonsensical way to go, with heavy users of New Media technologies finding a motivational setting away from institu-

tions that are finding difficult discovering ways of formalizing for accreditation purposes the informal body of both substantive and procedural knowledge that is acquired by New Media users.

It can even be speculated that the non-linear, or hypertextual, processing which leads to informal, independent and flexible learning, has brought about a potential new route to Transfer of Learning, so elusive within rigid curricular face-to-face and online teaching environments. Speculatively, the diffusion and multi-focusing that are at the base of HTP, and the personalization, diversification and acquisition of general knowledge that infuse independent, flexible learning can create an amenable setting for the generalization and abstraction needed for effective transfer (Mallia, 2009). But more research is needed in this area to clarify variables and test the practice.

A number of ways forward exist. One way that can help young HTP learners is for formal institutions to adopt variants of the methodological styles suggested in this chapter, which might help reroute to institutional formats traits that would otherwise exclude the subverted learner from benefiting from a institution-based education. But the change goes beyond the classroom and is inherent to varying degrees in the affective and cognitive character-set of immersed New Media and social software users, which makes informal, independent routes to learning much more motivationally attractive to them and their mindset. This leads to a social, educational dilemma and for these informal learners not to be marginalized within an industrial system that often demands formal certification of learning, will require a roots-up institutional changes once the acknowledgment of the processing transformations is in place.

This chapter proposes that fundamental changes are underway in the preferred modes of learning by a whole generation.

The literature seems to be in two minds about whether to work towards integrating digital natives within already-existing structures, possibly sidelining the changes that have been instigated by immersion, or to understand better what the changes are and change the methodological base of schooling. Another possibility is to embrace informal, incidental learning, and as is happening in certain areas of industry, accept that this can be a preferred way of skill, information and learning acquisition.

How institutions will eventually adapt to take advantage of these transformations, or whether they will do so, is unclear. A few modest proposals towards a better understand of the situation, and a possible adjustment of norms in order to embrace the change within learners, are offered here. However, the fundamental proposal is that more research needs to be carried out to help us understand better the nature and the extent of the change that is actually happening.

More discussion of future alternatives also needs to be conducted in thoughtful research-based and speculative fora, and more broadly within academic institutions themselves, as they begin to change to adapt to this new future.

REFERENCES

Alkan, S., & Cagiltay, K. (2007). Studying computer game learning experience through eye tracking. *British Journal of Educational Technology, 38*(3), 538–542. doi:10.1111/j.1467-8535.2007.00721.x

Anand, V. (2007). A study of time management: The correlation between video game usage and academic performance markers. *Cyberpsychology & Behavior, 10*(4), 552–559. doi:10.1089/cpb.2007.9991

Andersson, P., & Fejes, A. (2005). Recognition Of Prior Learning As A Technique For Fabricating The Adult Learner: A genealogical analysis on Swedish adult education policy. *Journal of Education Policy, 20*(5), 595–613. doi:10.1080/02680930500222436

Balcytiene, A. (1999). Exploring individual processes of knowledge construction with hypertext. *Instructional Science, 27,* 303–328. doi:10.1007/BF00897324

Beldarrain, Y. (2006). Distance education trends: Integrating new technologies to foster student interaction and collaboration. *Distance Education, 27*(2), 139–153. doi:10.1080/01587910600789498

Bennett, S., Maton, K., & Kervin, L. (2008). The 'digital natives' debate: A critical review of the evidence. *British Journal of Educational Technology, 39*(5), 775–786. doi:10.1111/j.1467-8535.2007.00793.x

ChanLin, L-J. (2009). Applying Motivational Analysis in a Web-based Course. *Innovations in Education and Teaching International, 46*(1), 91–103. doi:10.1080/14703290802646123

Chou, C., Condron, L., & Belland, J. C. (2005). A review of the research on Internet addiction. *Educational Psychology Review, 17*(4), 363–388. doi:10.1007/s10648-005-8138-1

Colardyn, D., & Bjornavold, J. (2004). Validation of Formal, Non-Formal and Informal Learning: Policy and practices in EU Member States. *European Journal of Education, 39*(1), 69–89. doi:10.1111/j.0141-8211.2004.00167.x

Collins, A., & Halverson, R. (2009). *Rethinking Education in the Age of Technology*. New York: Teachers College Press.

Cummings, R. (2003). *Equivalent assessment: Achievable reality or pipedream*. Paper presented at ATN Education and Assessment Conference. Retrieved May 11, 2008, as Word Document from http://www.unisa.edu.au/.

Cunningham, D. J., Duffy, T. M., & Knuth, R. A. (1993). The textbook of the future. In McKnight, C., Dillon, A., & Richardson, J. (Eds.), *Hypertext: A psychological perspective* (pp. 19–49). New York: Ellis Horwood.

Donnerstein, E. (2002). The Internet. In Strasburger, V. C., & Wilson, B. J. (Eds.), *Children, adolescents & the media* (pp. 301–321). Thousand Oaks, CA: Sage.

Dwight, J., & Garrison, J. (2003). A manifesto for instructional technology: Hyperpedagogy. *Teachers College Record, 105*(5), 699–728. doi:10.1111/1467-9620.00265

Eijkman, H. (2009). The Epistemology War: Wikipedia, Web 2.0, The Academy, And The Battle Over The Nature And Authority Of Knowledge. Ken Fernstrom (Ed.), *Readings in Technology and Education: Proceedings of ICICTE 2009* (pp. 516-529). Abbotsford B.C., Canada: UCFV Press.

Eraut, M. (2000). Non-Formal Learning, Implicit Learning and Tacit Knowledge in Professional Work. In Coffield, F. (Ed.), *The Necessity of Informal Learning* (pp. 12–31). Bristol, UK: Policy Press.

Eurostat News Release 146/2006, 1-3. Nearly half of individuals in the EU25 used the internet at least once a week in 2006. Luxembourg: Eurostat Press Office.

Gaggi, S. (1997). *From text to hypertext: Decentering the subject in fiction, film, the visual arts, and electronic media*. Philadelphia, PA: University of Pennsylvania Press.

Gail, J., & Hannafin, M. (1994). A framework for the study of hypertext. *Instructional Science, 22*(3), 207–232. doi:10.1007/BF00892243

Gee, J. P. (2003). *What video games have to teach us about learning and literacy*. New York: Palgrave Macmillan.

Gorard, S., Fevre, R., & Rees, G. (1999). The apparent decline of informal learning. *Oxford Review of Education, 15*(4), 437–454. doi:10.1080/030549899103919

Graff, G. (2005). Differences in concept mapping, hypertext architecture, and the analyst–intuition dimension of cognitive style. *Educational Psychology, 25*(4), 409–422. doi:10.1080/01443410500041813

Greenfield, D. N. (1999). *Virtual addiction: Help for netheads, cyberfreaks, and those who love them*. Oakland, CA: New Harbinger Publications.

Greenfield, P. M., de Winstanley, P., Kilpatrick, H., & Kaye, D. (1994). Action video games and informal education: Effects on strategies for dividing visual attention. *Journal of Applied Developmental Psychology, 15*, 105–123. doi:10.1016/0193-3973(94)90008-6

Hargreaves, J. (2006). *Recognition of Prior Learning: At a glance*. Adelaide, Australia: National Centre for Vocational Education Research.

Herther, N. K. (2009). The Changing Language of Search Part 1. Nu Speak. *Searcher, 17*(1), 36–41.

Hutchinson, D. (2007). Video games and the pedagogy of place. *Social Studies, 98*(1), 35–40. doi:10.3200/TSSS.98.1.35-40

Katz, R., & Oblinger, D. (Eds.). (2000). *The "e" is for everything: Ecommerce, e-business, and e-learning in the future of higher education*. San Francisco, CA: Jossey-Bass.

Landow, G. P. (2006). *Hypertext 3.0: Critical theory and new media in an era of globalization*. Baltimore, MD: Johns Hopkins University Press.

Livingstone, D. W. (2001). *Adults' Informal Learning: Definitions, Findings, Gaps and Future Research*. NALL Working Paper 21. Toronto, Canada: Centre for the Study of Education and Work.

Lööf, A. (2008). *Eurostat: Data in focus 46/2008*.

Mallia, G. (2003). Pushing media democracy: Giving marginalized illiterates a new literacy. In K. Fernstrom (Ed.), *4th ICICTE Proceedings* (pp. 387–392). Athens: National and Kapodistrian University of Athens.

Mallia, G. (2007). A Tolling Bell for Institutions? Speculations on student information processing and effects on accredited learning. In *Readings in Technology in Education* (pp. 24–32). Abbotsford, BC, Canada: UCFV Press.

Mallia, G. (2009). Transfer through Learning Flexibility and Hypertextuality. In Wheeler, S. (Ed.), *Connected Minds, Emerging Cultures: Cybercultures in Online Learning* (pp. 185–208). Charlotte, N.C.: Information Age Publishing.

Mancini, C. (2005). *Cinematic hypertext: Investigating a new paradigm*. Amsterdam: IOS Press.

Marsh, J., Brooks, G., Hughes, J., Ritchie, L., Roberts, S., & Wright, K. (2005). *Digital beginnings: Young children's use of popular culture, media and new technologies*. Sheffield: University of Sheffield. doi:10.4324/9780203420324

McKay, S., Thurlow, C., & Toomey Zimmerman, H. (2005). Wired whizzes or techno slaves? Teens and their emergent communication technologies. In Williams, A., & Thurlow, C. (Eds.), *Talking adolescence: Perspectives on communication in the teenage years* (pp. 185–203). New York: Peter Lang.

Milheim, K. L. (2007). Influence of technology on informal learning. *Adult Basic Education and Literacy Journal, 1*(1), 21–26.

Niederhauser, D. S., & Shapiro, A. (2003, April). Learner Variables Associated with Reading and Learning in a Hypertext Environment. Paper presented at the meeting of the *American Educational Research Association*, Chicago, IL.

NSO. (2008). *Nso News Release. December 15, 2008*. Malta: National Statistics Office.

Ozcelik, E., & Yildirim, S. (2005). Factors influencing the use of cognitive tools in Web-based learning environments: A case study. *The Quarterly Review of Distance Education, 6*(4), 295–308.

Perry, M. (2003). Distributed cognition. In Carroll, J. M. (Ed.), *HCI models, theories, and frameworks: Toward a multidisciplinary science* (pp. 193–222). San Francisco, CA: Martin Kaufmann. doi:10.1016/B978-155860808-5/50008-3

Pitman, T. (2009). Recognition of Prior Learning: The accelerated rate of change in Australian universities. *Higher Education Research & Development, 28*(2), 227–240. doi:10.1080/07294360902725082

Pouget, M., & Osborne, M. (2004). Accreditation or *Validation* of Prior Experiential Learning: Knowledge and *savoirs* in France – a different perspective? *Studies in Continuing Education, 26*(1), 45–66. doi:10.1080/158037042000199452

Prensky, M. (2001). Digital Natives, Digital Immigrants. *Horizon, 9*(5), 1–6. doi:10.1108/10748120110424816

Prensky, M. (2007). *Digital Game-Based Learning*. New York: McGraw-Hill.

Richardson, W. (2004). Personal mail to Stephen Downes, quoted in Educational Blogging. *EDUCAUSE Review, 39*(5), 14–26.

Riding, R., & Rayner, S. (1998). *Cognitive styles and learning strategies: Understanding Style differences in learning and behaviour*. London: David Fulton Publishers.

Rouet, J. F., & Levonen, J. J. (1996). Studying and learning with hypertext: Empirical studies and their implications. In Rouet, J.-F. (Eds.), *Hypertext and cognition* (pp. 9–24). Mahwah, NJ: Lawrence Erlbaum Associates.

Salonius-Pasternak, D. E., & Gelfond, H. S. (2005). The next level of research on electronic play: Potential benefits and contextual influences for children and adolescents. *Human Technology, 1*, 5–22.

Sang Hyun, K., Holmes, K., & Mims, C. (2005). Opening a dialogue on the new technologies in education. *TechTrends: Linking Research & Practice to Improve Learning, 49*(3), 54–89.

Schneider, R. (2005). Hypertext narrative and the reader: A view from cognitive theory. *European Journal of English Studies, 9*(2), 197–208. doi:10.1080/13825570500172067

Schugurensky, D. (2000). *The Forms of Informal Learning: Towards a Conceptualization of the Field.* NALL Working Paper 19. Toronto, Canada: Centre for the Study of Education and Work.

Selwyn, N., Gorard, S., & Furlong, J. (2006). Adults' use of computers and the Internet for self-education. *Studies in the Education of Adults, 38*(2), 141–159.

Shaffer, D. W. (2006). *How Computer Games Help Children Learn.* New York: Palgrave Macmillan. doi:10.1057/9780230601994

Shapiro, A., & Niederhauser, D. (2004). Learning from hypertext: Research issues and findings. In Jonassen, D. (Ed.), *Handbook of research for educational communications and technology* (2nd ed., pp. 605–620). Mahwah, NJ: Lawrence Erlbaum Associates.

Shapiro, A. M. (1998). Promoting active learning: The role of system structure in learning from hypertext. *Human-Computer Interaction, 13*(1), 1–35. doi:10.1207/s15327051hci1301_1

Shapiro, A. M. (1999). The relevance of hierarchies to learning biology from hypertext. *Journal of the Learning Sciences, 8*(2), 215–243. doi:10.1207/s15327809jls0802_2

Shneiderman, B., & Kiersley, G. (1989). *Hypertext hands on!* New York: Addison-Wesley.

Spiro, R. J., Feltovich, P. J., Jacobson, M. J., & Coulson, R. L. (1991). Cognitive flexibility, constructivism, and hypertext: Random access instruction for advanced knowledge acquisition in ill-structured domains. *Educational Technology, 5*, 24–33.

Sweller, J., van Merrienboer, J. G., & Paas, F. G. (1998). Cognitive architecture and instructional design. *Educational Psychology Review, 10*(3), 251–296. doi:10.1023/A:1022193728205

Tuschling, A., & Engemann, C. (2006). From education to lifelong learning: The emerging regime of learning in the European Union. *Educational Philosophy and Theory, 38*(4), 451–469. doi:10.1111/j.1469-5812.2006.00204.x

Wheeler, S. (2007). Learning with "e"s: Defining technology supported e-learning within a knowledge economy. In Fernstrom, K. (Ed.), *Readings in Technology in Education* (pp. 306–312). Abbotsford, BC: UCFV Press.

Williams, K. (2003). *Why I (still) want my MTV: Music video and aesthetic communication.* Cresskill, NJ: Hampton Press.

Wood, R. T. A., Griffiths, M. D., & Parke, A. (2007). Experiences of time loss among videogame players: An empirical study. *Cyberpsychology & Behavior, 10*(1), 38–44. doi:10.1089/cpb.2006.9994

Young, K. (2009). Understanding Online Gaming Addiction and Treatment Issues for Adolescents. *The American Journal of Family Therapy, 37*(5), 355–372. doi:10.1080/01926180902942191

Young, M. (2007). Qualifications frameworks: Some conceptual issues. *European Journal of Education, 42*(4), 445–457. doi:10.1111/j.1465-3435.2007.00323.x

KEY TERMS AND DEFINITIONS

Information Processing: The psychological process whereby information is coded, processed, memorized, retrieved and utilized.

Institutionalized Education: School-based education, ranging from early schools to University teaching and learning. The offshoot of institutionalized Education is often summative and based on an accreditation system.

New Media Technologies: Communication technologies that are more often than not computer based, using the world wide web as a means of communicating information. Mobile technologies and interactive gaming also form part of what can be referred to as New Media Technologies.

Immersed Technology Usage: Refers to those that dedicate a large percentage of waking time to the use of technology. There is often, though not necessarily, an addiction to the use, and change in processing makeup and socialization practices often result from the immersion.

Hypertextual Processing (HTP): The result of persistent New Media Technology immersion, and which organizes perceived information into an erratic, loosely grouped number of simultaneous focal points resulting in coherent, if sporadic, information gain.

Independently-Ued, Flexible Learning Environments (IUFLEs): Often as distinct from institution-based, formal educational environments, these environments are populated by on-a-whim searches for information and that provide for incidental learning.

Independent Learning: Learning of which the learner takes charge. It can be formal learning that is done independently by the learner, or informal learning determined and indulged in persistently or intermittently by the learner.

Flexible Learning: Self-paced learning the parameters of which are determined by the learner. The flexibility can be in the time when to learn and for how long, and in the content undertaken. If the flexible approach is from the teaching side, this could apply to instructional methodologies and resources, as well as in delivery.

Digital Natives: A phrase coined by Prensky in 2001 that refers to those for whom digital technologies already existed before they were born. This is counterbalanced by the phrase (also coined by Prensky) Digital Immigrants, that refers to those who came into digital technologies later in life.

ENDNOTES

[1]   Parts of this chapter are based on a paper published in the electronic journal UFV Research Review. Other parts are based on a paper presented at the CELDA 2009 Rome Conference.

[2]   Quoting the Commission of the European Union, 2000.

[3]   Text used here comes from a review of the book by K. Brittain McKee (2004) in *Journalism and Mass Communication Quarterly, 81*(3), 718-720.

Section 3
Information Technology Outsourcing

Chapter 8
Information Technology Outsourcing Cost and Policy in Developing Countries:
A Case Study of Malaysia

Abdul Jaleel Kehinde Shittu
University Utara, Malaysia

Nafisat Afolake Adedokun-Shittu
International Islamic University, Malaysia

EXECUTIVE SUMMARY

Information Technology Outsourcing (ITO) practices in developing countries have come with numerous problems ranging from organisational setup, absence of mutual trust between IT suppliers and clients, inconsistent policies and lack of deployable ITO model and several others. These and other problems are well pronounced among the developing countries who are tapping from the global outsourcing resource market. Malaysia being one of the leading ITO destinations is not an exception in these problems. Therefore, in this chapter, we took an in-depth look into various challenges facing Malaysia's ITO industry especially from suppliers' perspectives. We looked at problems facing ITO practices in the light of government policy and ITO model in this chapter. We also used qualitative research method with special reference to interpretive and exploratory approach for the analysis of relevant issues in the chapter.

INTRODUCTION

In the late 70s and early 80s, outsourcing was referred to as 'bureaux'. This shows that outsourcing itself is not a new concept (White, 2002: 15). Outsourcing fell from favour at the beginning for several reasons which are still relevant in the outsourcing environment today. The IT industry has added mystique to describe outsourcing by establishing its own vernacular, though these vernaculars are sometimes controversial (Cullen & Willcocks, 2005). Phrases such as; strategic partnering, strategic alliances, co-sourcing, value-added outsourcing, have been coined to suggest greater depth to the prospective relationship between client and ITO supplier. Kern et al. (2002) lamented thus:

DOI: 10.4018/978-1-60960-015-0.ch008

More recently, ITO has seen the somewhat false start of what it called netsourcing that is renting applications, services and infrastructure over a network. This idea is considered to have profound applicability in the medium term to 2010.

As more functions become candidate for outsourcing, a new language is spoken by a generation of globally savvy business executives. To these executives, outsourcing connotes strategic flexibility, a return to core competencies, focus, discipline, leverage, cost consciousness, nimbleness etc. In short, outsourcing to some of these business gurus means: progressiveness; modernity; open-mindedness and the likes. In contrast to old pejorative labels on outsourcing such as defeatism, laziness, or incompetence, where outsourcing was seen as an admission of limitations for small firms and as a sign of failure for large firms as commonly known in the 1950s, there is a paradigm shift in the reasons behind outsourcing (Anderson & Trinkle, 2005).

Nowadays, large and small firms outsource virtually anything. Large companies go to the extent of announcing their outsourcing moves with the hope that such news will lift their stock price, which according to Anderson and Trinkle (2005), it often does. The outsourcing revolution that took place in the late 1990s and continued into the new millennium has made the logistic options in corporate supply chains to easily make or mar a company's manufacturing and supply chain model (Cook, 2007). This millennium change has made outsourcing to become "*downright fashionable*" (Anderson & Trinkle, 2005). To this research, this phrase symbolizes a constant growth in ITO management, and at the same time, indicates some of the challenges that continue to arise in the face of client/supplier relationship and IT Outsourcing management.

During the last decade, outsourcing has emerged as a major strategic option in information technology management (Jae-Nam et al., 2008). Cobb (2005) noted the continued wave of billion dollars from outsourcing deals. Citing International Data Corp (IDC), the estimated worldwide outsourcing market size has increased from $100 billion in 1998 to $152 billion in 2000 to whooping increase of £1200 billion by 2005. Kern et al., (2002) projected $US190+ billion by 2006 as global market revenues on information technology outsourcing. Cobb (2005), while referring to IDC, observed that the U.S. outsourcing market will increase by 5.6 percent to $268.7 billion in 2005 and ultimately reach $355 billion by 2009. There is a sharp increase in the projection made by IDC in 1998 and 2005, which indicates that IT outsourcing market is growing tremendously from $152 billion to $268.7 billion.

Similarly in Malaysia, a report from *Price Water House*, a research market firm, indicates that Malaysia can attract at least RM11.4 billion out of RM1.9 trillion global outsourcing businesses by year 2008. Kearney (2007) index of the 50 most attractive offshoring locations also ranks Malaysia third in the world indicating that Malaysia is an appealing domain for outsourcing among the developing countries. Thus, this research has chosen Malaysia as a suitable site for putting into perspective the challenges of IT outsourcing with special reference to cost and policy implications.

STUDY POPULATION SAMPLE AND INTERPRETATION PROCEDURE

At the onset, we estimated 120 IT vendor companies in Malaysia that have attained MSC status and have been recognized and licensed by the Malaysian government to engage in IT/IS services. However, at end of the day, due to unforeseen obstacles lesser number of IT outsourcing vendors responded and granted the much-needed interview. Nevertheless, this research gained the required data with the adoption of the interpretive approach, which calls for less number but qualitative and in-depth interview. MAXQDA data analysis tool and constant comparative analysis (CCA) method were used to analyze the data on both:

1.   Effects of Government policies on IT outsourcing and
2.   High cost of IT outsourcing services.

Thematic approach is used in this chapter to analyze data collected from the interviewees. This makes this chapter to be very practical in addressing related problems of IT outsourcing in Malaysia. IT outsourcing vendors were grouped into five major categories called Case ranging from Case 1 to Case 5 to further ease our analysis.

Background

In the literal sense, outsourcing can be defined as a process in which a company delegates some of its in-house operations/processes to a third party. Although this definition is not complete in the full sense and seems very much close to contracting, contracting and outsourcing are in no way related. Grossman and Helpman (2005) simply said that *"we live in an age of outsourcing"*. Outsourcing is an accepted business strategy. The current interest of many companies in making outsourcing a key component of their overall strategy and their approach to supply chain management represents a big departure from the way companies used to deal with their suppliers and vendors.

Outsourcing has variously been defined in the IS literature as a conscious decision to abandon or forgo attempts to perform certain activities internally and instead to farm them out to outside specialists and strategic allies (Thompson et al. 2008). Some have defined it as the organizational decision to turn over part or all of an organization's IS functions to external service provider(s) in order for an organization to be able to achieve its goals. Nowadays, each scenario in outsourcing carries its own unique flavours and nuances; therefore, outsourcing can no longer be defined straightaway as before.

In order to get a full-fledged definition of outsourcing, one has to take into consideration the issue of ownership or control. Grossman and Helpman (2005) claimed that generally in contracting, the ownership or control of the operation/process being contracted lies with the parent company, whereas in outsourcing the control of the process is with the third party and not with the parent company. Outsourcing is seen as an activity where the supplier provides for the delivery of goods and / or services that would previously have been offered in-house by the buyer organisation in a predetermined agreement. It equally appears as a phenomenon in which a company or organisation delegates a part of its in-house operations to a third party with the third party gaining full control over that operation/process.

Outsourcing can be described as the option of using external sources for the provision of services by an organisation as traditional outsourcing, where potentially any service may be bought rather than built. This involves transferring IT assets, leasing staff and management responsibility for delivery of services from internal IT functions to third-party vendors. This situation or cooperation between two parties can be temporary or designated for an agreed length of time and aided by existing policies in the transacting environment.

The culmination of these had been succinctly explained by Shittu, et al. (2009) who construed outsourcing as a practical step to allow an organisation to focus its resources on key areas of value-added capability, or core competencies, rather than spreading resources too thinly and overloading the capacity of the organisation. Meanwhile, we define IT outsourcing, for the purpose of this chapter, as the process of contracting out any information technology (IT) internal activity or function to a trusted IT (supplier/vendor) party that shares the same or similar policies with either the IT based or non IT-based (client) organisation. We realised that, this definition accommodates the range of outsourcing options while preserving the inside-to-outside transfer of IT functionality (Shittu, 2009).

IT Outsourcing: A Management Tool

Information technology outsourcing has outlived the five-year period typical of a management fad and is now regarded as a standard IT management tool (Cullen and Willcocks, 2005). The concept of outsourcing as a management tool has been popularized by a number of authors such as; Heeks (2002), Heywood (2001), Tho (2005), Burkholder, (2006), Bragg, (2006) among numerous others. We noticed that all these authors realized and analysed ITO as a tool in the management and business environments. This approach adopted by other authors spurred us in writing this chapter, though from a critic dimension. These critics come from our study focus which highlighted the impacts of policy and vendors service cost on ITO. We will further look into ITO success model from the policy integration and harmonized service cost consolidation. We will trace a brief developmental study on the trend of ITO in Malaysia in the next section.

Malaysia IT Outsourcing Environment

Kearney's 2007 index of the 50 most attractive offshoring locations ranks Malaysia third in the world, hot on the heels of India and China in the criteria of financial attractiveness and workforce skills/availability (Goolsby, 2007). She proclaimed Malaysia as *"the natural choice for offshore services"*. In the business environment criteria, Malaysia scored 2.0, higher than the 1.4 of India and China. In the same vein, Singh et al. (2007) in their study conducted under the *Gartner* rated Malaysia as 'good' for outsourcing based on ten criteria listed. In contrast to the above statements, the International Data Corporation (IDC) in 2007 favored several cities for IT outsourcing destination; neither Kuala Lumpur nor any city in Malaysia was included in its study.

Nevertheless, we discovered that an emerging country like Malaysia views IT outsourcing as a value-added service in generating more revenues and improving IT service and performance. A report from *Price Water House*, a research market firm, indicates that Malaysia can attract at least RM11.4 billion out of RM1.9 trillion global outsourcing businesses by year 2008. In the ninth Malaysia Plan (2006-2010) released by the former Prime Minister, a substantial allocation was provided for IT and telecommunications industries in the development of infrastructural plan and development of IT solutions for modernizing the country. An amount of RM5.7 billion has been allocated for various ICT projects. Therefore, a substantial amount will be further awarded to IT service providers. This could demonstrate that the future path for IT outsourcing growth in Malaysia is promising.

Malaysian government agencies and private sectors are continuously seeing a rising trend in engaging in IT outsourcing arrangements involving significant amount of deals. For instance, *Bank Negara* (Central Bank) Malaysia sparked these large outsourcing deals as an effort to soften the 1997 financial crisis in the Malaysia banking industry. Massive computation projects were outsourced in the early 1990s in an attempt to mobilize Malaysian government's large-scale systems integration projects. Implementation of Multimedia Super Corridor (MSC) flagship applications marks the beginning of ICT project in the public sector, which includes E-Government (EG) initiatives. Malaysia IT clients are ranging from those wanting minimal e-services solutions to those with mega IT needs.

In 2005 Budget, a sum of RM500 million was set aside for infrastructure outsourcing projects especially in the education and health sectors (Ahlan & Shittu, 2006). Outsourcing has been realized as a strategic means to accelerate IT projects in order to achieve the Vision 2020 envisaged by the Malaysia government. However, in 2009 budget, the former Malaysian Prime Minister advocated for greater utilisation of ICT as an essential tool for businesses to remain competitive. The budget emphasized that the use of ICT requires companies, especially SMEs, to incur large expenses to replace and upgrade ICT assets. The Government proposed an Accelerated Capital Allowance (ACA). In essence, Malaysia 2009 budget gave room for wider direct foreign investments (FDI), which is not limited to IT multinationals only. The Malaysian budget 2009 read thus:

To ensure Malaysia remains an attractive investment destination in the region, particularly among multinational companies, the tax framework has to be transparent and business friendly. To enhance certainty on pricing issues for inter-company trades within a group, the Government proposes to introduce an Advanced Pricing Arrangement mechanism.

This mechanism is believed to be widely practiced in developed countries and has succeeded in resolving issues relating to transfer pricing. Lesser interest has been shown in the study of IT outsourcing from the vendor's window, especially in reference to government policy and high cost IT service for the developing world in general and in Malaysia specifically.

Identifying Outsourcing Problems

Outsourcing originated and became popular as a cost-saving strategy during a recessionary period and environment. This had made the world's largest organizations to call into question the efficacy of outsourcing in today's economy. Companies offshore are mainly to seek cost efficiencies by exploiting wage differentials. Pfannenstein and Tsai (2004) pointed out information technology (IT) hourly rates for workers in Asia and other emerging markets are reported to be anywhere from 30% to 75% lower than what is obtainable for the IT professionals in the United States. This could generate close to 50% savings for offshoring an activity outside United State.

In contrast, the rising cost of outsourcing services, coupled with the enterprises' incapability of information technology and systems has made IT outsourcing a nightmare. Small scale enterprises (SMEs) were the most affected by this phenomenon. This development had led several SMEs to fold up, due to their inability to compete even within their local environments (Hashim, 2007). Another study conducted by DiRomualdo (2005) also presents a mixed picture of outsourcing experiences, where the number of buyers that have "abnormally terminated" an outsourcing relationship soared to 51 percent from 21 percent last year. The primary reasons for those mass terminations were poor provider performance (36%), a change in strategic direction of the buyer (16%), decision to move the function in-house (11%), and not achieving cost savings (7%).

With the rapid evolution of information technologies, to many enterprises, the importance of IT has been unceasingly increasing; more and more is getting into the main business of an enterprise in depth, and IT eventually becomes a vital part of the enterprise's core competence, which definitely has a great influence on the decision-making and the development strategies of an enterprise in the long run. However, most IT suppliers in Asia are relatively inexperienced with the management of IT outsourcing relationships. Not only the IT suppliers are inexperienced, the outsourcing companies do not have a track record in the management of IT-outsourcing relationships. Even though outsourcing is an effective way to help the enterprises manage their IT system management, it is not an easy job, if it is not properly handled. Outsourcing may result in a nightmare instead of the expected benefit (Tan & Sia, 2006). This occurs when there is no standard IT outsourcing management system in place. Absence of a perfect IT outsourcing management system is borne out of inadequate government policy and arbitrary cost of IT service.

IT Outsourcing Service Cost

Many of the world's largest organizations that were quick to participate in IT and business process outsourcing (BPO) are bringing operations back in-house and exploring alternatives. According to a new study released by Deloitte Consulting (April, 2005), dissatisfaction in areas that traditional outsourcing was expected to improve, such as costs and complexity, was found to be the primary reason behind participants' negative responses.

The study, *Calling a Change in the Outsourcing Market*, revealed that 70% of participants have had significant negative experiences with outsourcing projects and are now exercising greater caution in approaching outsourcing. The study revealed that one in four (25%) participants have brought functions back in-house after realizing that they could be addressed more successfully and/or at a lower cost internally, while 44% did not see cost savings materializing as a result of outsourcing (Deloitte, 2005). Moreover, 57% of participants in this study absorbed costs for services they believed were included in the contracts with vendors. Nearly half of the study participants identified hidden costs as the most common problem when managing IT outsourcing projects.

There are fundamental differences between product outsourcing and the outsourcing of service functions. These differences were earlier overlooked but have now come to the fore. We highlighted certain IT services expected from an IT outsourcing vendor in aiding our differential analysis. At the end of the day, we realized that IT outsourcing vendors and companies may have conflicting objectives, which might put at risk clients' desire for innovation, cost savings, and quality.

The structural advantages envisioned do not always translate into cheaper, better, or faster services. As a result, larger companies are scrutinizing new outsourcing deals more closely, re-negotiating existing agreements, and bringing functions back in-house with increasing frequency.

In an earlier study, Shittu (2007) realized that participants (IT clients) originally engaged in outsourcing activities for a variety of reasons such as: cost savings, ease of execution, flexibility, and lack of in-house capability. However, instead of simplifying operations, the company under study then had found that outsourcing activities can introduce unexpected complexity, add cost and friction into the value chain, and require more senior management attention and deeper management skills than anticipated, especially when the outsourcing deal is done with a total stranger.

IT Outsourcing Government Policy

The pervasiveness of information and communication technology (ICT) in society, and the perception that it can form the basis of a national competitive advantage has led to a flurry of national policies geared towards strengthening the society's capacity to adopt and skillfully adapt ICTs (Chini, 2008). Proactive institutional intervention from the government has been a legitimate step to take. The appreciation of ICT as source of provision for a distinct competitive advantage has prompted the involvement of regional and international authorities in joining the ICT policy field, as the issue was deemed to be too important to allow uncoordinated action or inaction to stifle the economic potentials of the state. Such organizations include state-based organisations such as Multimedia Super Corridor (MSC) in Malaysia, The National Information Technology Development Agency (NITDA) in Nigeria, Communication and Information Technology Commission (CITC) under Saudi Communications Commission, National Information Development Authority (NiDA) of Cambodia, *Sistem Informasi Nassional* (SISFONAS) of Indonesia, Information Technology Authority (ITA) Sultanate of Oman etc. Also there are regional authorities such as the European Union; supranational organisations, such as the Organisation for Economic Cooperation and Development (OECD); and international organisations, such as ITU and the World Bank. These organizations have all stepped forward to create their own ICT visions, backed by policies and programmes of action. In the year 2000, ASEAN as a body entered into the e-ASEAN framework agreement to facilitate the establishment of the ASEAN Information Infrastructure and collectively promote the growth of e-services and e-commerce in business (Kotler, Kartajaya & Huan, 2007). Gulf Cooperation Council (GCC), an official body for the Cooperation Council for the Arab States of the Gulf, followed suit by formulating GCC eGovernment where information technology initiatives such as e-business, e-payment, e-commerce, e-retailing, e-banking, among others are formulated and encouraged.

The impetus for e-ASEAN is due to the explosive growth of ICT worldwide and the speed of growth, which had inadvertently made it harder for less developed countries to catch up with rapid changes. We equally believed that this agreement is out of shared belief that technology is a key growth driver with ability to accelerate production and innovation, which in turn speeds up economic progress. We acknowledge that the expansion of markets is most visible in today's convergence in information and communication technologies (ICT). Consequently, ICT convergence has led to myriad possibilities for innovative applications and immense opportunities for bridging the digital divide between the haves and have-nots. This convergence has equally brought about new directions in the business and economic reality under ICT, by adopting outsourcing as a tool in developing a country's economy.

As applicable in several countries, information technology outsourcing, shared services and outsourcing in general play an important role in Malaysia because they contribute to economic growth and development in numerous ways. IT outsourcing directly contributes to economic growth. ICT-enhanced sectors developed the economy faster than envisaged, thereby catapulting Malaysian position in the global outsourcing scenario. Several benefits and incentives introduced by the Malaysian government to enhance her competitiveness in the arena of ITO are discussed in details later under MSC.

Among other developing countries, the Indian government is the first to realize that Information Technology outsourcing has the potentials to influence extensive economic development in the country. ITO is now one of the top priorities of the Indian government and favorable policies are being formulated to extract maximum benefits from the industry. Here, we are highlighting some of the government policies which have proved very beneficial in the growth of IT/BPO industry. These favorable government policies have gone a long way in making India a BPO/IT hub (Cronin & Motluk, 2007). We used India ITO policy as a benchmark for ITO success in terms of policy formation and implementation. For instance, India has reduced licensing requirements and made foreign technology accessible. Also the Indian government is actively promoting FDI and investments from NRIs (Non-Resident Indians). Among the celebrated ITO policies in India is formulation and implementation of more transparent and investment policies.

In India, the Ministry of Communications and Information Technology is overseeing the Indian electronic and IT industry which includes software industry and Indian BPO industry among others. The National Association of Software and Services Companies (NASSCOM), the premier trade body and 'voice' of the Indian IT-BPO industry functions like Multimedia Super Corridor (MSC) in Malaysia. It has been playing a crucial role in helping the IT industry achieve the IT and ITES vision and make India far ahead of other players in the field of IT and BPO. It has helped the government to implement almost all the original recommendations of the last NASSCOM-

McKinsey Report concerning the capital markets, venture capitalists, SEBI and the Companies Act.

ITO Questions: Policy and Service Cost

In the light of the issues stated above and the information technology outsourcing trend in Malaysia, this chapter addresses, how developing countries respond to the increasing cost of outsourcing services and inconsistent government policy. The emphasis of this chapter is on the IT supplier which is also called IT vendor. Furthermore, in this chapter, two factors are identified as major contributors to the success of information technology outsourcing and they are:

a. The cost of ITO suppliers' services (*Analyze and evaluate government policies that are affecting IT outsourcing services especially on the suppliers' side in Malaysia*).
b. Effect of government policy on ITO practices in Malaysia (*Analyze and evaluate the extent to which the global IT outsourcing market price is affecting outsourcing services in Malaysia*).

Effects of Government Policies on ITO

Under this thematic heading, seven questions emerged during the interview sessions with identified organisations. The questions relate to ITO incentives from government, types of government policy, need for government to hands-off ITO, need for government stake in ITO, effectiveness of government policy, obstacles emanating from government policy, and government requirements for ITO. These set of questions were fashioned in line with the in-depth and explanatory nature of this research. Though the major responses came from government organisations, most of the respondent organisations declined to give detailed responses, which was one of the earlier limitations of this research. However, to overcome this challenge, the researchers were impelled to redirect certain set of questions to the government officers interviewed. There is a unanimous opinion on the fact that the government policies on ITO are affecting the ITO suppliers. However, most of the interviewees/Cases were reluctant to give any further elaboration.

ITO Incentives from Government

There are several motivating factors behind multiplication of multinational IT companies establishing their regional headquarters, global center, outlet, etc. in Malaysia. This study finds out that this is not unconnected with incentives being provided by the Malaysia government. Beside a ten year tax-free policy, ownership right and ease movement of capital among others are part of superlative incentives provided by Malaysia. The interviewees made these researchers believe that incentives provided by MDeC are second-to-none and irresistible to investors. An interviewee pointed out that Multimedia Development Corporation (MDeC) one-stop service agency has made it easy for any MSC status organisation to complete his or her needs at one place, without unnecessary delay.

(Figure 1) represents interviewees' responses on information technology outsourcing incentives from government.

Types of Government Policy

Government policies are mainly to protect and promote certain interests; it may be economic, social or political. In the case of ITO, at macro level, the policies guiding it are mainly to improve and protect economic interests of the nation. However, due to current level of ITO in Malaysia, most policies are leaning towards micro interest, or attempt to make use of the policies to promote and reposition Malaysia ITO global participation. These diverse perceptions are shown in below

Figure 1. Types of government policy (Shittu, 2009)

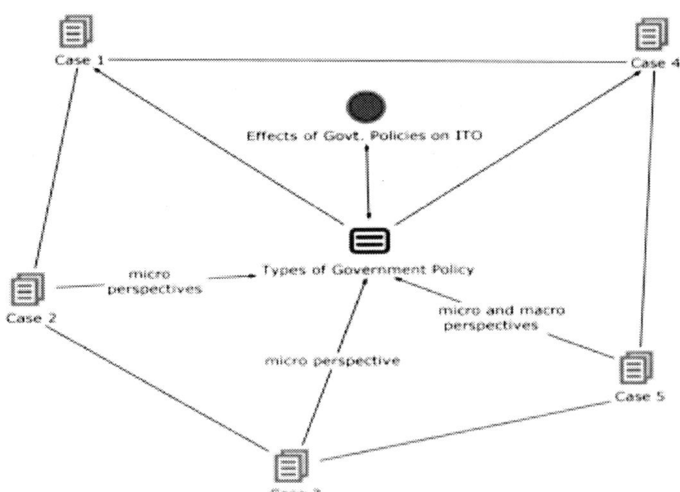

Figure 1, relationships where some respondents view government policies from micro perspectives only and others see the policies from both micro and macro outlooks, probably because these later interviewees were directly involved in formulating government policies on outsourcing.

However, most interviewees did not give any comment probably due to lack of awareness of ITO policies put in place by the government. At this juncture, we discovered that the level of awareness of ITO policies in the IT industry is very low; only the top and middle managers were concerned about such policies. This also affects the research culture in the Malaysia IT community, as every organisation tries to hide under non-disclosure of data. This development is taking toll on quality of research and at the same time affecting the research students and organisation' research and development move.

Need for Government's Hands-Off over ITO Industry

There were discord from some quarters on the need for the government to hands-off the day-to-day control of information technology outsourcing in Malaysia, though ulterior motive for such calls could be deciphered from one of the interviewees' statement when he said: "*Too much of government helping, I think the Malaysia government should step back. Everybody depends on the government, every single time; every little problem they want the government to help*". He elaborated his statement that inability of the local ITO suppliers to be independent of government has been a major obstacle in creating a viable ITO industry in Malaysia. What we can infer from the above statement is that the inability of some local IT vendors to operate without unnecessary dependence on the government is one of the major reasons why ITO industry has not been flourishing in Malaysia because this might lead to fear of the unknown for these kinds of vendors when they need to venture into unprotected global environment.

In contrast to the above call, we found that some interviewees believe that there is still need for the government to exercise its control over the ITO industry for reasons such as market control and economic interest. Besides these two groups, other interviewees considered this question to be political in nature and avoided giving any specific answer to it. This development is one of the reasons why Multimedia Development Commission (MDeC) was included in this research.

This government corporation maintained that: *"... the government should be more involved not less involved"*. MDeC believe that such government involvement will increase the number of participating organisations and help Malaysia to promote IT outsourcing through the power of number of organisations in the industry. We however suggested that the involvement of government agency in IT policy should be supervisory in order to create a viable competitive environment for IT development.

Need for Government Stake in ITO

This section focuses on the need for government stake in ITO in general. There is a unanimous support for government to maintain its stake in the ITO industry. Some see it as a measure to control unnecessary monopoly that might arise and a way for the government to protect the economic interest of the state which encompasses the GDP. An interviewee said, *"...if you release it freely, people can actually abuse it and start monopolizing the market, giving the government hard time"*. Some equate outsourcing to economic development; therefore, they emphasized on the need for government to tap from the economic benefits that come with outsourcing. While agreeing with this, a respondent submitted thus; *"because outsourcing is equivalent to economic growth nowadays, therefore government should rather look into how to benefit more from outsourcing"*. In the same vein, another interviewee supported the economic stance that:

...but you cannot expect the Government also to fold its arms on ITO because it's related to the economy. You know that the Malaysian outsourcing income for 2007 only was worth US$ 300 million and is growing at CAGR of 30% year on year

He further asserted:

We are working towards making IT outsourcing to generate 10% of Malaysia's GDP by 2012. You can now understand why government is having stake in ITO.

In another dimension, the stake was looked at from the perspective of contribution being made by government to develop the ITO industry, starting from budget to allocation and training, etc. This stake is conceived in terms of financial support, specialised training programs and guarantee on infrastructures like electricity and telecommunication by government agencies. Interestingly, some others only see the need for government involvement in ITO only when it comes to protecting some sensitive information. These arguments were considered vital to this research, firstly, because global ITO participation might not be achieved if there are lapses in information security, and no organisation would compromise its information security. Secondly, the economic situation of a country is scrutinized before it is considered as an outsourcing destination. The figure depicts the diversities of the interviewees/Cases on the need for government to have stake in Malaysia ITO industry. Some ITO vendors believe that government is protecting its interest in the IT industry. While some IT vendors view this protection of interest from economic perspectives others interpret it from long and short term interests dichotomy.

Effectiveness of Government Policy

One of the essences of this research is to evaluate how effective is the government policy on ITO. In doing this, the assessment will be solely on the interviewees, though their responses might not be appropriate for the purpose of generalization as the case of interpretive approach is. However, their responses should be considered as valid for the sake of ITO development in Malaysia. Because most of the interviewees considered such a question not only sensitive but also political, thereby, turning down the questions, only few of these individuals braced up to voice their opinions on this. This research assumes that it is most likely to come to the same conclusion if same question is repeated among other ITO vendors in Malaysia either in similar or different situations.

Respondents are categorized into three. The first category consists of some local employees who found it difficult to criticize any activity championed by government even if it is a constructive criticism. The second category comprises some foreign workers who see their future in this country and want to create an enabling environment for the ITO progress. They believe that an improved government policy would at least help them secure their job for a longer time and at the same time favour economic future of this country. The third category consists of ITO consultants working under government own corporations; they do not only see any wrong thing in the policies but actually promote the existing ones. For instance, an interviewee said *"in principle we ensure no censorship of Internet"* whereas in reality internet censorship is still going on (Gartner, 2007). These mixed responses would, instead of helping government to formulate or enhance its existing policies, create more confusion which might end up derailing the government. Figure 2 represents interviewees' responses on effectiveness of government policy.

Obstacles Emanated from Government Policy on ITO

There is no policy that is not confronted with certain level of obstacles, although some of the hindrances may emanate either from internal or external influences or effect of the policy. Most of the interviewed organisations declined to point out any obstacle instead they outlined some problems facing ITO policy vis-à-vis that of the organisation but not as government policy. Some industries expressed their frustration on IT outsourcing starting from manpower, labour law, industrial law, local laws, etc. Salary scale policies and the working

environment were also seen as problems related to IT outsourcing. In actual sense, some of these identified policy-related problems are directly related to the government though these organisations tried to present the problems in a general outlook instead of government-policy-related-problems. One IT vendor related these problems to situation of ITO industry where learning culture has been absent thus; *"I don't think there is anything else the government can do without the change in the situation of industry. It is the industry that has to go and learn what the problem is, which they don't do".*

Government Requirements for ITO

It was revealed to us during some of the interview sessions that some of the IT vendor organisations in Malaysia are not willing to share any information related to government with third party. This notion was apparent from responses got from some organisations who considered question on government's requirement as political. They failed to realize that the success of IT policies, though gazetted by the government, depends on the implementation outcome.

Some organisations gave an inward look at the government requirements for ITO. They assumed that the basic ITO requirements revolved around level of security and standard of facilities provided by IT outsourcing vendors. However, the government requirements as enumerated by MDeC are similar to India IT development provision which this study used to benchmark Malaysia IT provisions.

High Cost of ITO Services

Under this theme issues such as high service cost, big organisations vs. SMEs, duration of contract, methods of charging, steps to reduce ITO cost and local service cost were questioned and raised during interview sessions. The set of questions asked and generated in the course of several interview

Figure 2. Effectiveness of government policy (Shittu, 2009)

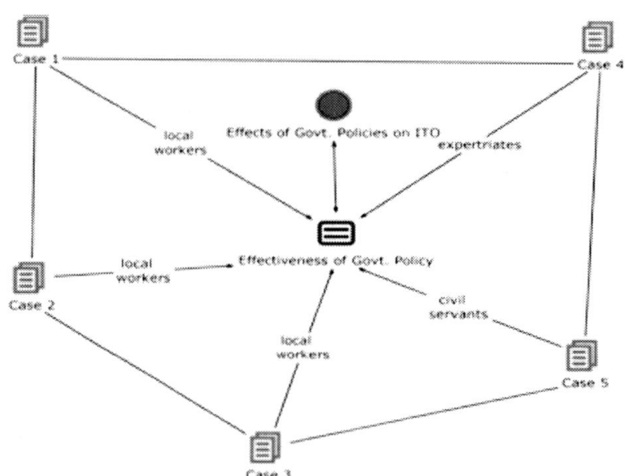

sessions were towards identifying the reasons and rationale behind high cost of ITO services and at the same time understanding the perception of ITO vendors.

These questions addressed under this theme are meant to provide possible answer(s) to one of the problems identified by this research which is on high cost of ITO service in Malaysia, as one of the challenges of ITO service. Figure 3 shows that all the interviewees/Cases in the study agreed in principle that the cost of ITO service is relatively high but not too enormous. Though there are diverse opinions regarding this claim, this theme will be addressing high cost of ITO services in detail.

High Service Cost

Most vendors' organisations interviewed agreed with the fact the cost of ITO is not too enormous, however, they claimed that only small scale enterprises (SMEs) thought that the ITO vendors' charges are too expensive. Some attributed this 'misconception' to lack of awareness, misplacement of priority and education on the side of SMEs as major factors that led to outrageous cost concept. An ITO vendor believed that SMEs do not have the requisite knowledge, which is the reason why they say IT service charges are expensive. This vendor went further to accuse SMEs that information technology facilities are always the least priority when setting an organisation.

Actually, those who understand the dot of IT will not make this kind of acquisition because outsourcing services business drivers are: lower cost, ride on talents and proven processes. This indicates long term and immediate benefits to be derived from outsourcing IT functions. However, only futuristic organisations would look beyond money and realize the abundant benefits of outsourcing information technology. This can be done by patronizing small but reliable IT vendors instead of big names that go with big money. Clearer insight could be inferred from below statement:

Basically, a big IT vendor is concerned about securing big contract. So the smaller companies who cannot afford to pay that much, there are many smaller IT outsourcing companies that can render their services depending on the fees paid, how much they can afford. So, get more concern with big money they don't really care much for small businesses.

Another possible step to assist local organisations and SMEs is by sourcing their potential

Figure 3. High cost of ITO services (Shittu, 2009)

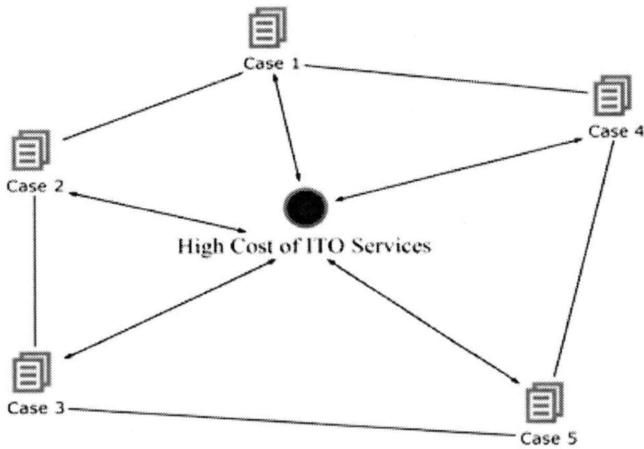

clients through a local organisation called Outsourcing Malaysia. Definitely, the service cost might not be easy to control however, what we can do is to help some stakeholders such as *Outsourcing Malaysia*. Though, in organisations such as this clients can source for local Outsourcing companies in order to reduce costs. This measure creates access to all local IT organisations that provide the service needed by clients. Besides this, it would also give room for a healthy competitive environment. The Figure 4 gives a diagrammatic representation of interviewees/Cases opinions on high service cost of ITO.

Big vs. SMEs

Certain characteristics of big and small non-IT organisations were explored in this section based on the interview conducted in our research. Most interviewees believe that it is only the SMEs that could complain about the price of ITO services due to the fact that majority of SMEs are not aware of IT services tailored for them by several IT vendors. This might be due to poor consultation and/or lack of basic knowledge on importance of information technology services.

Figure 4. High service cost (Shittu, 2009)

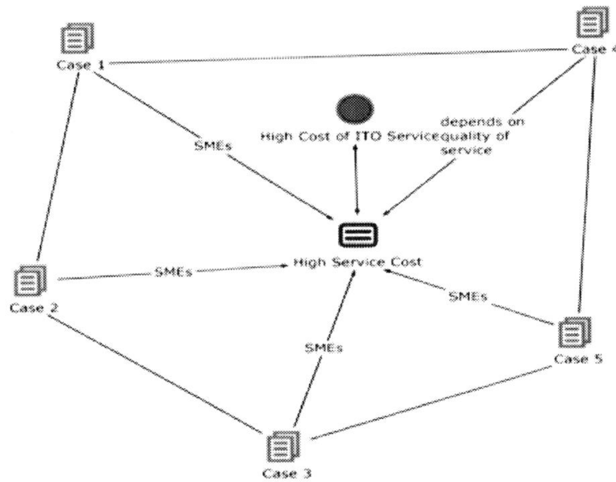

Another characteristic pointed out by the interviewees is lack of quality awareness among SMEs compared to big organisations. This factor was identified from the rate at which big ITO vendor organisations were struggling to achieve world standards and global ISO certifications. Some big ITO vendors refer to their dealings with small organisations as *out-tasking* instead of outsourcing, because outsourcing, according to them, has to do with passing over the entire IT infrastructure to an IT vendor, thereby making their clients focused on their core business. To these big IT vendor organisations, this arrangement can also be called partnership. The Figure 5 gave graphical representation of interviewees' opinions on how ITO vendors relate with big organisations and small and medium-scale enterprises.

Duration of Contracts

Contract duration varies from one organisation to other; however, most ITO vendors agreed upon the minimum of one year duration for a project. One of the interviewees observed:

...any contract less than a year is not an effective contract. It means you are not ready to assist your clients and your organisation as well. SLA assessment is quarterly-based; it will be difficult to measure development if the period is less than a year

Although some of ITO vendor organisations pointed out that one year is not enough for most outsourcing contracts since they (the ITO vendors) consider outsourcing as part of organisation strategies, some believe that the duration of any IT outsourcing contract should be determined by the complexities entailed in such a contract and that a big scale contract should be at least up to five years while the small scale project should be at least one year.

Methods of Charging

Organisations differ in their charging approaches based on the type of services rendered. Internet service providers mostly based their service charges on three pivots; space, bandwidth and response time [1-1], with different levels of flexibility. Apart from the standard service cost, some organisations purposefully give their clients access to bigger bandwidth size, beside what was initially agreed upon. The reasons for such extra

Figure 5. Big vs. SMEs (Shittu, 2009)

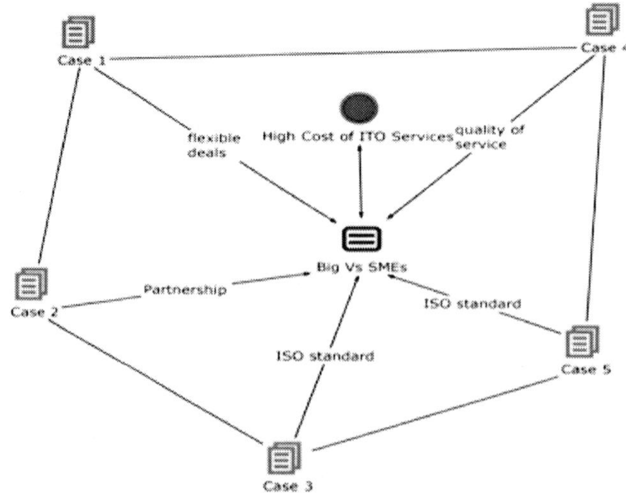

bandwidth size are: Firstly, to establish client's loyalty to the service or application provider, and secondly, to create a sense of belonging for the clients, though such clients would be informed of the extra bandwidth usage and appropriately advised to increase to bigger size. Any client that wants higher level of service should be ready to bear higher service cost.

There are standards, for example, if you pay certain amount you will get this kind of response [within] four hour... but if you want to have less than one hour you should pay extra. These are the variables ...

Another interviewee said that:

We charge based on SLA. We have some identified measures that we agreed upon, though we have our standard to maintain. Duration of contract period is also a factor in charging clients, because we have discount method or some kind of flexibility mode of charging. For data centre, it has to do with space per cubic, plus associated charges.

In the case of application service providers, most of their service charges are based on service level agreement (SLA) as agreed with the clients in the contract. This research noticed that some individuals in some organisations do not possess adequate knowledge of ITO processes related to their organisations. For instance, a senior manager claimed ignorance of module charging clients by claiming that that was not his area of specialisation. He submitted that "*I am not in the right position to answer that, I am in a very specialized area. I wouldn't know what is actually going on in the finance and promotions unit*".

This development in organisations might not augur well for the proper development of organisation in particular and ITO in general. This is because organisation's openness on the contracts is one of the criteria to assess organisation's readiness to partake in the ITO global economic market. In that case, Malaysia's aspiration to compete evenly with other global ITO players might be jeopardized if this trend continues.

Figure 6. Duration of contracts

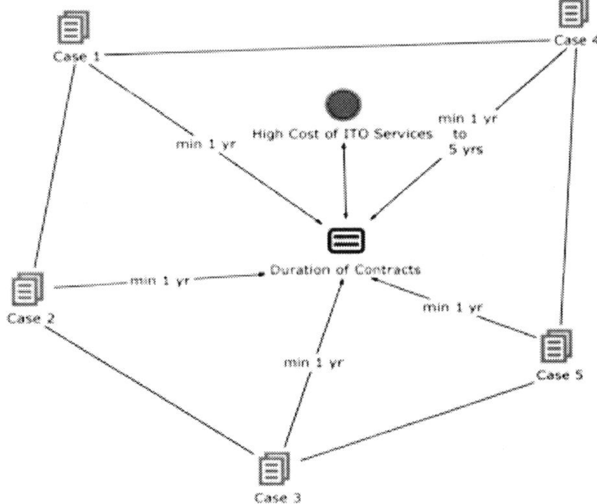

Steps to Reduce ITO Cost

In light of the study on "*Method of Charging*", we argued that there should be a pragmatic approach to reduce service cost being charged by ITO vendors. This vision led to the questions that relate to measures and possible steps towards reducing the service costs which happened to be one of the aims of this research. The Figure gives some organizational view and response to this motion. Some organisations believe that this can be done only by identifying the goal of vendors' organisations, whether the IT vendor is after volume or value. An opinion was expressed thus:

... [either] you want volume or you want value. If you want value you charge high and you go for premium clients; if you want volume, then you can just spread your cost. This means we have to set some infrastructure. It is what we call value vs. volume.

He also expressed the possibility of having *demarcated services*, which according to him is a combination of both volume and value. Some vendors believe that the steps to reduce ITO cost had been taken into consideration while mapping out strategies for their organisations. This concept made them to operate *global model* which allows them to provide low budget website design and web based application solutions in a very efficient and quality manner. Consequently, this flexibility enabled several SMEs (ITO clients) to go online fast and at reduced costs.

However, some vendors might see this flexibility as counter-productive and that it could affect their standard practice and possibly put the reputation of the organisation at stake. These vendors advised that instead of small IT clients (SMEs) patronizing big vendors, the SMEs could execute their IT outsourcing deals with small IT vendors rather than enshrined themselves with big budget IT vendors. Despite these two dissenting opinions, the two groups, that is, big ITO vendors and Medium scale ITO vendors could create a leeway for cost reduced services especially for SMEs. One interviewee advised further:

Most ITO vendors should build leverage on cost over a few customers. They will also leverage on the skills already developed to deliver the services. That's how vendors make their margin and at the same time should offer lower cost to their customers. But if the clients are looking at innovation and re-engineering of their business processes, then there is value for the vendor to

Figure 7. Steps to reduce ITO cost

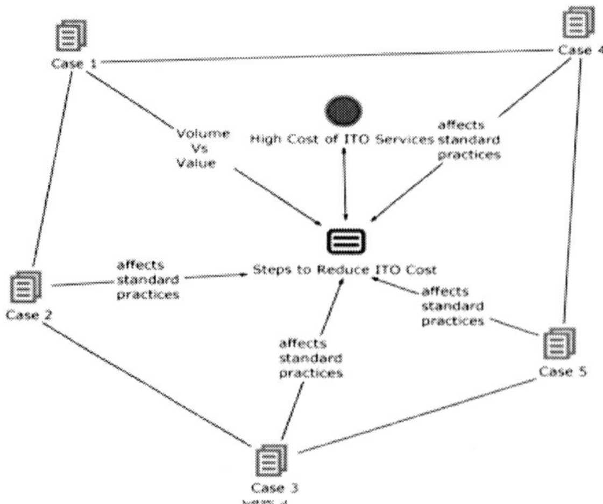

charge more. In any case, the additional cost should be cheaper and innovation can be achieved at much quicker time. But please bear in mind that not all outsourcing projects take cost cutting as the main criteria.

Another interviewee realized that in order to build a formidable ITO in Malaysia, SMEs need to be carried along. That is, if we really want to improve the ITO practices in Malaysia we would have to consider the SMEs along.

Local Service Cost

In an attempt to reduce ITO service costs, this study took into consideration the ranges of local factors that might assist or hinder the actualization of cost reduction agenda. It started from government policy/policies such as budget, to some local and foreign organisations available in Malaysia. The first factor that is contributing to the scheme of vendors' charges is culture. For instance the global culture in outsourcing practices had made it possible for several multinational organisations to practice in Malaysia without any hitch. Most of these foreign organisations are not actually meant for the Malaysian markets; therefore, the practices have been towards their global outreach. In con-

trast, most local ITO vendors used local factors as the basis of their operations. This made them to benchmark their services with local economic reality not with global practices compared to the multinational ITO vendors domiciled in Malaysia. And this had helped them in creating a niche market for not only Malaysia but the region as well.

A lot of outsourcing companies talk about call centers, for example, DELL has an outsource call center; we don't do that. DELL has foreign subsidiary companies. They open up an Internet Data Center here offering services, but our value is always there because we are local to local; so we understand culture, so we go on that strength.

Some of these local ITO vendors claimed that they deliver services at reasonably low cost. In fact, they believe that their organisations deliver high quality web-based solutions and IT enabled services at low and reasonable costs. This belief is borne out of certain comparative analysis done with some global ITO vendors. It was also easy for local ITO vendors to input some personal touch for their clients. This may also create a competitive edge for local ITO vendors.

Figure 8. Local service cost (Shittu, 2009)

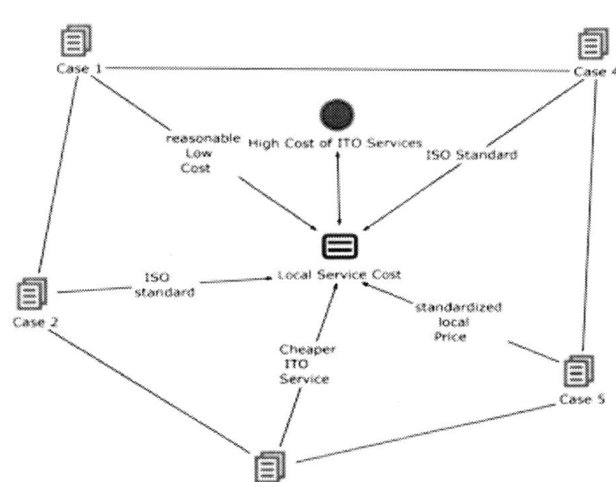

You know client like to have personal touch; that is the keyword. For example, Case 1 we do offer personal services because our clients are all long time clients, they can call us anytime, so the main reason why they want to be with you is because of personalized services offered rather than customized.

Language also gave local vendors another edge over foreign vendors. These advantages over foreign vendors should make ITO services become cheaper considering some local factors that give local ITO some competitive edge, such as language. However, going by the reality on ground, it shows that patronage from local organisations is very minimal probably because of inadequate awareness and lack of standardized prices. In the light of this, some have suggested that if local companies in Malaysia have standardized pricing policies, they would probably have more competitive pricing than the multinational companies.

CONCLUSION

The aim of this chapter is to identify and understand how IT outsourcing being practiced in a developing country such as Malaysia can contribute effectively to the country's economic development and maximise global opportunity rendered by IT outsourcing practices. In order to realise this aim, this chapter looked into two out of numerous problems facing ITO vendors. We looked at policy-related problems and IT service costs. We conclude that in order to have a successful IT outsourcing model, these two elements must be incorporated into either the existing ITO models or a new model that can be easily adapted into the systems of developing countries. In essence, this chapter has attempted to identify challenges posed by lack of standard cost practice and policies to govern ITO in developing countries.

REFERENCES

Ahlan, A. R., & Shittu, A. J. K. (2006). Issues in Information Technology Outsourcing: Case study of PETRONAS Bhd. In *Proceeding ICT4M 2006*. Kuala Lumpur. Malaysia.

Anderson, E., & Trinkle, Bob. (2005). *Outsourcing Sales Function: The Cost of Field Sales*. Thomson, OH.

Annesley, C. (2005). *Outsourcing works better when based on trust*. Retrieved June 17, 2008 from. http://www.computerweekly.com/Articles/2005/11/24/213137/outsourcing-works-better-when-based- on-trust-survey.htm

Barrar, P., & Gervais, R. (2006). *Global Outsourcing Strategies: An International Reference on Effective Outsourcing Relationships*. Gower Publishing.

Beaver, G., & Prince, C. (2004). Management, strategy, and policy in the UK small business sector: a critical review. *Journal of Small Business and Enterprise Development, 11*(1), 34–49. doi:10.1108/14626000410519083

Beulen, E., & Ribbers, P. (2002). *"Lessons learned: Managing an IT-partnership in Asia:* Theme Study: The relationship between a global outsourcing company and their suppliers." In *Proceedings of Hawaii International Conference on Systems Sciences.*

Chini, I. (2008). ICT Policy as A Governable Domain: The Theme of Greece and the European Commission. in IFIP International Federation for Information Processing: *Vol. 282. Social Dimensions of Information and Communication Technology Policy; Chrisanthi Avgerou, Matthew L. Smith, Peter van den Besselaar* (pp. 45–62). New York: Springer.

Cook, T. A. (2007). *Global Sourcing Logistics: How to Manage Risk and Gain Competitive Advantage in a Worldwide Marketplace. American Management Association.* New York: AMACOM.

Cronin, F. J., & Motluk, S. A. (2007). Flawed Competition Policies: Designing 'Markets' with Biased Costs and Efficiency Benchmarks Published online: 24 August 2007. New York: Springer Science+Business Media, LLC 2007.

Cullen, S., & Willcocks, P. (2005). *Intelligent IT Outsourcing: Eight Building Blocks to Success.* Oxford, UK: Elsevier Butterworth-Heinemann.

Dibbern, J., Goles, T., Hirschheim, R., & Jayatilaka, B. (2004). Information systems outsourcing: A survey and analysis of the literature. *The Data Base for Advances in Information Systems, 35*(4), 6–102.

Grossman, G. M., & Helpman, E. (2005). Outsourcing in a Global Economy. *The Review of Economic Studies, 72*(1), 135. doi:10.1111/0034-6527.00327

Hashim, M. K. (2007). *SMEs in Malaysia: A Brief Handbook.* Petaling Jaya, Malaysia: August Publishing Sdn. Bhd.

Heeks, R. (2002). *Reinventing Government in the Information Age: international practice in IT-enabled Public Sector Reform, Routledge, Research in Information Technology and Society.* London: Routledge.

Hirschheim, R., & Lacity, M. (2006). Four stories of information systems insourcing. In Hirschheim, R. Heinzl A. & Dibbern J. (Ed.), *Information Systems Outsourcing: Enduring Themes, New Perspectives and Global Challenges.* Berlin, Germany: Springer-Verlag (pp. 303-346).

Hongxun, J. et al. (2006). Research on IT Outsourcing based on IT Systems Management. ICEC 06, Fredericton, Canada, *Journal of ACM 1-59593-392-1.* 533-537.

Jae-Nam, L., Huynh, M. Q., & Hirschheim, R. (2008). An integrative model of trust on IT outsourcing: Examining a bilateral perspective. *Information Systems Frontiers, 10,* 145–163. doi:10.1007/s10796-008-9066-7

Shittu, A. J. K. (2009). Information Technology Outsourcing in Developing Countries- an Exploratory, Interpretive Case study of Malaysia Suppliers' Perspective. Unpublished doctoral dissertation, University Technology PETRONAS, Malaysia.

Shittu, A. J. K., Mahmood, A. K.. & Ahlan, A. R (2009). Information Security and Mutual Trust as Determining Factors for Information Technology Outsourcing Success. *International Journal of Computer Science and Information Security IJCSIS* – July 2009.

Tan, C., & Sia, S. (2006). Managing flexibility in outsourcing. *Journal of the Association for Information Systems, 7*(4), 179–206.

White, T. (2002). *Reinventing the IT Department.* Oxford, UK: Butterworth-Heinemann.

Willcocks, K. T., & Heck, E. (2002). The Winner's Curse in IT Outsourcing: Strategies for Avoiding Relational Trauma-. *California Management Review, 44*(2), 47–69.

Chapter 9
Key Health Information Systems Outsourcing Issues from Six Hospital Cases

Chad Lin
Curtin University, Australia

Yu-An Huang
National Chi Nan University, Taiwan

Chien-Fa Li
Puli Veterans Hospital, Taiwan

Geoffrey Jalleh
Curtin University, Australia

EXECUTIVE SUMMARY

Traditionally, little attention has been paid by hospitals to the key issues in the health information systems (HIS) outsourcing decision-making process. This is important given that the HIS outsourcing can play a key role in assisting hospitals in achieving its business objectives. However, the decision-making process of HIS outsourcing in hospitals is under-studied, especially in the management of their HIS outsourcing contracts. Therefore, the main objectives of this book chapter are to: (1) examine key issues surrounding the management and implementation of HIS outsourcing in Taiwanese hospitals; and (2) identify issues that are crucial in managing and implementing HIS outsourcing in hospitals. Four key issues and problems were identified in the HIS outsourcing process: lack of implementation in IS investment evaluation process, problems in managing HIS outsourcing contracts, lack of user involvement and participation in HIS outsourcing process, and failure to retain critical HIS contract management skills and project management capabilities in-house. Solutions and recommendations are provided to deal with key issues that are critical in the management and implementation of HIS outsourcing in hospitals.

DOI: 10.4018/978-1-60960-015-0.ch009

INTRODUCTION

Health Information Systems (HIS) outsourcing is to partially or completely contracting out HIS functions to external service contractors. These include: setup and maintenance of the required functions, manipulation of systems, management of networks and communication, end-user computing support, systems planning and management, and procurement of application software (Young, 2003). Outsourcing in IS – since the Kodak's 1989 milestone decision, the transferring of internal IS assets, hiring and lending of assets, employees and management responsibilities to a third party service contractor has become a popular trend. Ever since this milestone decision, the process of transferring of internal IT functions to a third party service contractor to deliver required services has become a popular trend (Shinkman, 2000). In recent years, both public and private organizations worldwide have outsourced their major IS functions to external contractors (Lin et al., 2007).

Some of the main reasons for these organizations to outsource their IS functions are to: save costs, concentrate on other activities or core activities, improve services and productivity, and contract out the maintenance of existing systems. The setup (and maintenance) of a HIS/IS function is usually an expensive exercise. Outsourcing contractors have the advantage of economies of scale due to their large client bases (Menachemi et al., 2007a; Young, 2003). This is not something that a single organization can afford to do it. Therefore, cost saving is one of the reasons for IS outsourcing (Diana, 2009; Hsaio et al., 2009; Marek et al., 1999). Another reason for IS outsourcing is to increase efficiency (Liu et al., 2008; Moschuris and Kondylis, 2006; Roberts, 2001). Outsourcing contractors are able to keep up the trend and provide necessary leading edge software and systems to their clients. Moreover, IS outsourcing contractors have usually possessed more technical know-hows and skilled person-

nel to solve their clients' problems than a single organization (Beaver, 2003; Lorence and Spink, 2004; Ondo and Smith, 2006).

Hence, management of IS outsourcing contracts has become one of the top key management issues for IS executives in recent years (Luftman et al., 2006). Although a plethora of IT outsourcing studies have been published in the literature in the past, HIS outsourcing in the hospital setting, however, is still under-studied. Very few studies have examined how the hospitals manage their HIS/IS outsourcing contracts as well as how they consider key issues and problems in making HIS outsourcing decisions (Diana, 2009; Lorence and Spink, 2004). This may be due to the fact that only 20% of healthcare organizations' budgets are spent on outsourcing compared with 33% for other industries such as manufacturing, banking, insurance, and finance as healthcare organizations tend to have less experience in managing external relationships such as IS outsourcing (Shinkman, 2000). Not surprisingly, it is not unusual for hospitals and other healthcare organizations to make mistakes in developing and managing their HIS outsourcing process (Guy and Hill, 2007). Indeed, understanding key HIS outsourcing decision-making issues will help hospitals to better manage and select appropriate outsourcing arrangements. This will also help hospital managers to decide about when to consider outsourcing as an option. Therefore, the main objectives of this study are to: (1) examine issues surrounding the management and implementation of HIS outsourcing in Taiwanese hospitals; and (2) identify issues that are crucial in managing and implementing HIS outsourcing in hospitals. One contribution of the study is the recommendations provided to deal with issues that are critical in the management and implementation of HIS outsourcing in hospitals. Most of the key issues identified have not been discussed in the relevant HIS outsourcing literature in the hospital context.

THEORETICAL BACKGROUND

Total spending on IS outsourcing worldwide has been predicted to be about $441 billion in 2008, an increase of 8.1% from 2007 (Gartner, 2008). It has become a worldwide phenomenon with no signs of a slowdown in its use (Barthelemy and Geyer, 2004; Computer Economics, 2006; Gartner, 2009). According to Frost and Sullivan (2006), HIS outsourcing in the European market is likely to reach approximately US$700 million in 2010. Many outsourcing experts believe that extensive outsourcing by healthcare organizations assist in creating an outsourcing market and culture that other healthcare organizations can tap into in meeting their requirements as well as in developing industry-wide standards and protocols among outsourcing contractors (Burmahl, 2001; Lorence and Spink, 2004).

Motivation and Benefits for IS Outsourcing

IS outsourcing in healthcare tends to generate strong emotions among the senior executives and external outsourcing contractors. There are many motivation and benefits contributing to the growth of the outsourcing in the healthcare industry. Some of the reasons for outsourcing are:

- *Gain access to requisite skills:* Outsourcing allows healthcare organizations to improve the skill level of their internal IT personnel. Hospitals often utilize outsourcing to leverage resources and knowledge outside of their domains for issues such as assisting with a system development or to resolve a technical problem (Beaver, 2003; Lorence and Spink, 2004; Ondo and Smith, 2006);
- *Improve services and operations of the healthcare organization's systems:* Many IT functions have become stable commodities that can be turned over to external outsourcing contractors for more effi-

cient processing and management (Liu et al., 2008; Moschuris and Kondylis, 2006; Roberts, 2001);

- *Reduce costs and capital outlay:* There is tremendous downsizing and cost-reduction pressures on many healthcare organizations. This is often the number one reason for IT outsourcing (Diana, 2009; Hsaio et al., 2009; Marek et al., 1999);
- *Increase customer satisfaction:* It is extremely important for hospitals to attract new customers and retain their existing customers by improving patient care and services (Moschuris and Kondylis, 2006; Roberts, 2001; Shinkman, 2000);
- *Focus on core competencies:* Outsourcing of important but non-core HIS functions has become an effective business strategy for healthcare organizations. By focusing on its core competencies and strengths, healthcare organizations are more able to provide better quality of medical care (Beaver, 2003; Menachemi et al., 2007a; Wholey et al., 2001);
- *Resolve high IT staff turnover/shortage problem:* Outsourcing of HIS functions might assist healthcare organizations experiencing high staff turnover to obtain the required IT personnel and skills from external outsourcing contractors. It can also be used to retain IT personnel for the core competencies and outsource non-core competency workforce (Diana, 2009; Hsiao et al., 2009; Young, 2003);
- *Reduce the problem of managing industrial relations:* Outsourcing can be used to increase the power of top management and reduce the power of trade unions (Young, 2005);
- *Align with government policy and regulations:* Decision makers of public sector agencies including hospitals sometimes are motivated by a desire for power and see this being fulfilled by acting in the interests

of the government. Outsourcing can also be forced upon hospitals by numerous government regulations that govern all aspects of hospital IS operations (e.g. electronic patient records). In some instances, it can also be used to get around government regulations in limited full-time-equivalent staff ratio (Hsiao et al., 2009; Shinkman, 2000);

- *Keep up with competitors:* Sometimes decision to outsourcing can be influenced by the action of competitors of healthcare organizations (Lorence and Spink, 2004);
- *Increase flexibility*: It allows hospitals or healthcare organizations to acquired skills and support from external outsourcing contractors to quickly implement or build a HIS with little or not capital outlays (Haley, 2004); and
- *Economies of scale:* Outsourcing can provide economies of scale for smaller and rural hospitals as they are more likely to outsource than bigger hospitals (Menachemi et al., 2007a; Young, 2003).

Moreover, IS outsourcing can vary according to organizational needs, structure and changing technology. According to Menachemi et al. (2007a), smaller and rural hospitals are more likely than bigger hospitals to outsource. In addition, the number of branch hospitals and clinics with dissimilar HIS systems and platforms owned by a healthcare organization can also force healthcare organizations to rethink their outsourcing strategies (Lorence & Spink, 2004).

Risks and Disadvantages of IS Outsourcing

However, despite the promised savings from the IS outsourcing contracts, there have been risks and disadvantages for healthcare organizations to undertake IS outsourcing. Some of the major IS outsourcing problems in the healthcare industry include:

- *Inexperienced employees:* There is a risk that external outsourcing contractors might not have the right staff to meet outsourcing hospital's needs (Ondo and Smith, 2006);
- *Employee resistance:* It is possible that some employees might resist the transition from hospital-run HIS to the outsourced HIS. They can see outsourcing as a threat to their job security (Boardman and Hewitt, 2004; Hsiao et al., 2009; Meyers, 2004);
- *Inability to manage outsourcing contracts:* In addition to problems and issues with the contracts between the hospitals and external outsourcing contractors, it is difficult to know whether hospital IS managers will be any better at managing an external outsourcing contractor (Ondo and Smith, 2006; Roberts, 2001);
- *Poor strategic similarity between healthcare organizations and external contractors:* There is no guarantee that both outsourcing hospitals and external contractors have similar objectives and visions for the outsourcing projects (Ondo and Smith, 2006);
- *Poor quality:* Something can always go wrong in HIS outsourcing and external outsourcing contractors may fail to provide good quality services and products (Boardman and Hewitt, 2004);
- *Dependency:* If external outsourcing contractors cease contract suddenly, hospitals might not have the required skills and knowledge to operate the outsourced HIS. This dependency problem shifts power to the external outsourcing contracts and weakens the bargaining power of the outsourcing hospitals (Hsiao et al., 2009);

- *Hidden costs:* Lower outsourcing bids may not translate into additional savings for the outsourcing healthcare organizations as there are still many hidden costs and service issues that have not been written into the contracts. These costs may be due to ambiguities in the contract (Gonzalez et al., 2004). Learning curves, management cost, contractor search, technological discontinuities should be weighted against the promise of early cash-flow and long-term cost savings (Aubert et al., 1998; Barthelemy, 2003; Hsiao et al., 2009); and
- *Government regulations:* Public sector organizations including public hospitals need to conduct the tendering process to select external outsourcing contractors every few years, making it difficult to outsourcing contractors to consistently provide quality services and products (Hsiao et al., 2009).

Strategies for IS Outsourcing

According to Sinton (1994), IS outsourcing can vary according to organizational needs, structure and changing technology. For example, there is an option to have long or short term contracts with external contractors. In situations of high business uncertainty and/or rapid technological change shorter term contracts are more appropriate (Willcocks & Lester, 1997). Currie (1998) and Willcocks and Lester (1997) have found that selective rather than total outsourcing (80% or more of IS budget spent on outsourcing) tended to be the lower risk and the more successful option to take. Moreover, organizations that invite both internal and external bids tend to have higher success rates than organizations that merely compare external bids with current IS costs (Lacity & Willcocks, 1998). Furthermore, senior executives and IS managers who make decision together have higher success rates than either stakeholder group acting alone (Lacity & Willcocks, 1998).

RESEARCH METHODOLOGY AND CASE DESCRIPTION

Case studies were carried out in six Taiwanese hospitals involved in major HIS outsourcing projects. The six cases were deliberately chosen in order to focus efforts on theoretically useful cases (following the theoretical, non-random sampling strategy by Eisenhardt (1989)). The hospitals in Taiwan are accredited by Department of Health into three levels: medical centers (Level 3), regional teaching (Level 2) hospitals, and district (Level 1) hospitals. Hospitals which are classified as "medial centers" generally have more than 800 beds and are affiliated with a medical school. District hospitals are usually the smallest hospitals while the size of regional teaching hospitals are usually somewhere between Level 3 and Level 1 hospitals. The first hospital (hereafter referred to as Hospital A) was a private Regional Teaching hospital with five smaller branch hospitals in other parts of Taiwan. The second hospital (hereafter referred to as Hospital B) was a public District hospital with one small external clinic. The third hospital (hereafter referred to as Hospital C) was a private regional hospital with three external branch clinics. The fourth hospital (hereafter referred to as Hospital D) was a public-owned medical center whereas the fifth hospital (hereafter referred to as Hospital E) was a private regional teaching hospital with one external branch hospital in another city. The sixth hospital (hereafter referred to as Hospital F) interviewed was one of the biggest medical centers in Taiwan with six different branch hospitals across the country. In total, two of the interviewed hospitals were medical centers, three were regional teaching hospitals, and one was a district hospital.

The data collection at these six cases continued until a point of theoretical saturation, which is when the value of an additional interview was considered to be negligible (Eisenhardt, 1989). In total, 14 participants were interviewed (a mixture of CIOs, IS/IT managers, senior contract managers, and senior project managers). The interviews focused on these six hospitals' HIS outsourcing contracts, the contractual relationship between the hospitals and their external outsourcing contractors, IS investment evaluation process, HIS outsourcing tendering process, HIS outsourcing management, and user involvement in the HIS outsourcing process. Each interview lasted between 1 to 2 hours. Other data collected included some of the actual contract documents, planning documents and some minutes of relevant meetings. Qualitative content analysis was used to analyze the data from the case studies (Miles and Huberman, 1994). Finally, the analysis of the case study materials was also conducted in a cyclical manner and the issues identified were double-checked by the researchers and other experts.

CURRENT CHALLENGES FACING THE CASES

A number of issues and problems emerged from the analysis of the text data and some of the key issues surrounding the HIS outsourcing contracts are presented below in some detail.

Lack of Implementation in IS Investment Evaluation Process

Relevant literature has stressed the need for proper IS investment evaluation on outsourcing contracts and projects (Willcocks et al., 1999). However, a review of relevant documents obtained from interview participants and hospital website as well as closer examination of the interview responses reveal only two out of the six hospitals interviewed had a proper internal IS investment evaluation process for their HIS outsourcing contracts. In most cases, hospitals started the tendering and contract negotiation processes before any IS investment evaluation process was carried out. This is despite the fact that almost all of the hospitals had claimed that evaluation of HIS outsourcing contracts or

projects had been conducted by the hospital itself (for private hospitals) or by the relevant government department (for public hospitals).

The two public hospitals (Hospitals D and F) that had an IS investment evaluation process are among the biggest hospitals in the country and have been classified as level 3 (medical center) hospitals. Although the government has a final say on the HIS outsourcing contracts or projects for all public hospitals, level 3 hospitals have more resources than other types of public hospitals (level 1/district hospitals or level 2/regional hospitals) in their HIS outsourcing processes. Level 3 hospitals are among the biggest hospitals in the country whereas Level 1 hospitals are usually the smallest. Level 3 public hospitals are also required by government regulations to put in place proper processes and procedures for dealing with all IS procurement and outsourcing needs. The other public hospital (Hospital B) had no internal IS investment evaluation process on its HIS outsourcing contracts but an evaluation process was conducted by the government beforehand. For the three private hospitals (Hospitals A, C, and E), the decisions to outsource were made by the top management without the use of IS investment evaluation process or methodology.

Most of the case studies participants also showed the lack of understanding of the IS investment evaluation process by indicating that a formal methodology was used. No formal IS investment evaluation methodology was mentioned by any of the participants (but two hospitals had an IS investment evaluation process). Many participants either mistakenly thought terms and conditions specified within the service level agreement constituted their formal IS investment evaluation process or methodology; or that evaluation had been carried out by the government (for public hospitals) or top management (for private hospitals). For example, IT manager of Hospital B stated that proper IS investment evaluation of their outsourcing contracts or projects had been conducted by the government and that *"the gov-*

ernment was responsible for conducting IS investment evaluation on HIS outsourcing contracts or projects ……and the decision as to whether to go ahead with it rested with the relevant government department."

Problems in Managing HIS Outsourcing Contracts

One key ingredient of achieving stated outsourcing objectives is the ability of outsourcing organization to manage them (Graham & Scarborough, 1997; Lin et al., 2007). Results from the case study revealed that the ability to manage HIS outsourcing contracts had something to do with the complexity of the hospitals' HIS systems as well as the number of IT centers a hospital possessed. Hospitals D and F had admitted that their ability to manage large-scale HIS outsourcing contracts were limited as they possessed more complicated and larger IT and HIS systems than most other hospitals in the country. Some of their HIS outsourcing projects failed in the end and they had to develop and build their own IT and medical systems internally with some external assistance. Similar, Hospitals A and F had the same problem as each of them had owned several subsidiary hospitals and had problems in managing certain HIS outsourcing contracts and projects across different subsidiary hospitals. They struggled to manage their outsourcing contracts because of different IT needs among different IT centers. For example, IT manager of Hospital A stated that: *"We are a regional teaching hospital……We have five different branch hospitals…… They all have different IT needs and it was difficult to manage and implement HIS outsourcing contracts across these subsidiaries."*

By contrast, Hospitals B, C, and E were more able to manage their HIS outsourcing projects as most of their outsourced HIS systems were less complicated than those of Hospitals A, D, and F. In addition, Hospitals B and E had either no or only 1 subsidiary hospital and the size of their

IT centers were relatively smaller than those in Hospitals A, D, and F.

Lack of User Involvement and Participation in HIS Outsourcing Process

IS literature has stressed that there is a direct relationship between user involvement and success of any information systems (e.g. Davidson, 2002; Lin & Shao, 2000). The case study results showed that private hospitals (Hospitals A, C, and E) and the smaller public hospital (Hospital B) had failed to involved their key users and stakeholders their HIS outsourcing processes. Decisions to undertake HIS outsourcing in the private hospitals were generally made by either the top management or the head superintendent of the hospitals alone. No other key users or stakeholders were invited to participate in the processes. For example, IT manager of Hospital E stated that: *"……the HIS outsourcing decisions were entirely made by either the head superintendent or board of directors of the hospital."* The decisions to outsource for the smaller public hospital (i.e. Hospital B) were made by the government without any input from the hospital itself. In both cases, the use of these outsourced HIS systems were then forced upon the users. However, for the larger public hospitals (i.e. Hospitals D and E) the decisions to undertake HIS outsourcing were often made in a two-step process with both government (as the primary sponsor and decision-maker for outsourcing) and the hospitals (which had certain power to make recommendations and negotiate with the government on HIS outsourcing) having major inputs in the process. In both Hospitals D and F, key users and stakeholders were consulted and involved in the outsourcing process.

Lack of user involvement often resulted in distrust between the affected key users and stakeholders, the top management, external outsourcing vendors/suppliers, and the government (for public hospitals). These key users and stakeholders often felt that their requirements were not solicited before the commencement of the HIS projects. After all, it was difficult for the hospital as a whole to react positively to the HIS outsourcing decision if the overall goals of the decision were not communicated to the key users and stakeholders. However, this was not the case for bigger public hospitals (Hospitals D and F) in which their users and stakeholders were fully consulted and involved in the HIS outsourcing processes.

Failure to Retain Critical HIS Contract Management Skills and Project Management Capabilities In-House

Retention of appropriate information systems contract management skills and project management capabilities in-house is crucial for organizations undertaking outsourcing (Lacity and Willcocks, 1997). This would allow organizations to ensure that their outsourcing projects as well as their relationship with outsourcing contractors would be managed effectively and appropriately (Huang et al., 2005). All interview participants had indicated that they knew the importance of keeping all critical HIS contract management and planning skills in-house in order to manage the outsourcing contracts. However, this was only possible for larger hospitals (Hospitals D and F) where they had more resources and had selectively outsourced some of their HIS functions. They were able to retain and recruit skilled IT personnel to manage their HIS outsourcing projects and were more capable to manage and deal with any project issues with outsourcing contractors more quickly and effectively. For example, IT manager of Hospital F stated that: *"We outsourced mostly non-strategic HIS to external outsourcing contractors…… We have the required contract and project management skills and capabilities in-house to deal with any issues with external outsourcing contractors quickly and effectively."*

This was not the case for the smaller hospitals which did not have large IT budgets or required IT skills to proper manage HIS outsourcing contracts. The IT department within these smaller hospitals did not have good project management capabilities to deal with issues arising from the outsourcing contracts. As a result, they often had to reduce the number of HIS functions to be outsourced or had to rely on external outsourcing contractors to resolve these issues on their behalf.

SOLUTIONS AND RECOMMENDATIONS

The above-mentioned research findings indicate that HIS outsourcing is not a panacea and careful attention and evaluation are needed to ensure organizational success. Based on the literature review and the results from the case studies, there are several important factors that govern successful and less successful HIS outsourcing decisions. These are as follows:

Allocate Resources to Undertake IS Investment Evaluation Process

There are many potential pitfalls of outsourcing wrong HIS functions or choosing inappropriate external HIS outsourcing contractors. The adoption of an appropriate IS investment evaluation process by hospitals would ensure them to thoroughly evaluate external HIS outsourcing contractors on their contextual understanding of your outsourcing requirements. The IS investment evaluation process can assist hospitals in ranking the contractors based on certain pre-defined criteria and this can also this can also minimize the subjective influence on the selection. The adoption of IS investment evaluation process is also crucial for hospitals to measure the contribution of their investments in HIS to business performance. However, as noted in the literature most organizations fail to properly evaluate their IS outsourcing projects (Willcocks

& Lester, 1997). Indeed, most organizations do not have formal process to evaluate their IS outsourcing decision and, instead, relied on limited cost analysis associated with the outsourcing decision (McIvor, 2000) and as such the adoption of an IS investment evaluation process would ensure that hospitals not only measure and manage their tangible costs and benefits but also intangible costs and benefits such as customer satisfaction, access to flexible, scalable, and easy to maintain systems, leeway to focus on core strategic functions, and access to required technical skills.

Organizations that make extensive use of IS investment evaluation processes have higher perceived payoffs from IS (Tallon et al., 2000). It can also assist hospitals in managing their HIS outsourcing contracts more successfully as they have a better way of measuring, managing, and monitoring the costs and benefits of the projects. According to Misra (2004), this can: (a) lead to the desired behavior by both outsourcers and external outsourcing contractors; (b) be easily measured by both the outsourcers and external outsourcing contractors; and (c) can be aligned with business objectives. Failure to allocate appropriate resources by hospitals' top management to undertake IS investment evaluation process can result in letting politics cloud decision, letting external outsourcing contractors to take control of the process, and failure to understand the actual outsourcing requirements. Lack of the adoption of IS investment evaluation by hospitals can eventually result in HIS outsourcing failure.

Assess the Outsourcing Requirements Carefully

Hospitals need to first assess their in-house capability and needs before undertaking HIS outsourcing. There is no incentive for an organization to outsource its IS function when its in-house capability is equivalent to or better than that available in the external market (Willcocks & Lester, 1997). Pre-project justification and assessment processes must be carried out by hospitals to determine if in-sourcing is feasible and whether HIS outsourcing will negatively or positively impact on their performance and core business. One important consideration should also be the cultural fit or compatibility between the hospitals and the external outsourcing contractors. Contractor assessment also needs to be conducted. It is important to find an external outsourcing contractor that has similar work ethics, objectives, visions, and ways of doing things. Hence, it is better not outsource a HIS function when an appropriate outsourcing contractor with compatible cultural fit cannot be found. The other important factor to consider relates to hospitals' security and privacy concerns. This needs to be addressed before and during the selection of external outsourcing contractors.

Once the decision has been made to either outsourcing or in-sourcing, an IS benefits realization methodology (e.g. Cranfield Process Model of Benefits Management) should also be adopted immediately in order to manage, evaluate, and realize the expected benefits arising from the pre-project justification and assessment processes. Lacity and Willcocks (1997) found that the threat of the external outsourcing contractor bid actually galvanized in-house staff into identifying new ways of improving on IS performance, and into maintaining the improvement through putting in place, and acting on the output from, enhanced evaluation criteria and measures. This would also help hospitals to decide which HIS functions should be outsourced and whether there are any security and privacy concerns by outsourcing these functions. These would ensure that these hospitals will have a positive outsourcing experience.

Build an Appropriate Knowledge Retention Initiative

HIS outsourcing can often lead to a loss of crucial skills and corporate memory (Kakabadse & Kakabadse, 2000). Loss of key personnel with critical skills and knowledge can adversely affected outsourcing hospitals' ability to manage outsourcing contracts. Hence, possession of appropriate knowledge and understanding of the hospitals' HIS functions being managed are critical in a successful outsourcing contract arrangement. Corporate memory is often developed from previous business experiences, successes, and failures. Outsourcing hospitals need to retain key personnel with appropriate corporate memory and knowledge to effectively manage, monitor, and plan their HIS outsourcing contracts and projects. In order to manage contracts effectively, outsourcing organizations should develop a robust and practical mechanism for the capture, sharing and application of corporate memory. Hospitals possessing adequate corporate memory would also be more capable of managing more complicated and large HIS outsourcing contracts than those without much corporate memory. Moreover, possession of adequate corporate memory would also assist the hospitals in determining the appropriate strategy for undertaking HIS outsourcing (e.g. selective outsourcing or in-sourcing). For example, recognizing that they had more complicated and bigger HIS systems than the other hospitals and hence would pose a problem in their ability to manage their HIS outsourcing contracts or projects, Hospitals A, D, and F had tried to minimize the number of IT outsourcing projects. In-house or more selective outsourcing should be recommended for those hospitals with complicated IT and medical systems and those with several subsidiary hospitals.

Involve Users in the Outsourcing Process

Lack of user involvement in the outsourcing process can potentially result in systems that are not responsive to user requirements and hence the success of outsourcing projects (Sakhtevil, 2007). If key users and stakeholders are involved and updated during the outsourcing process, they may not view the outsourced systems as their own

systems (Nakatsu and Iacovou, 2009). Hence, user involvement is a key factor in delivering results in an outsourcing contract and this can assist hospitals in, for example, communicating, sharing, and clarifying organizational and business objectives as well as in resolving issues (e.g. job loss and resistance to change) arising from HIS outsourcing contracts and projects. This is particularly important in private hospitals and smaller public hospitals where either the top management or the government generally did not involve users in their outsourcing decision-making processes.

CONCLUSION

The findings suggest that the management of both public sector and private sector hospitals may not consider a range of issues that are important in making HIS (health information systems) outsourcing decision. This is consistent with findings by Lorence and Spink (2004) and Wholey et al. (2001) in which they found the impact of organizational management and outsourcing issues may affect the general level of comfort for outsourcing across healthcare organizations. In summary, hospitals have to be more realistic in their HIS outsourcing expectations. For an organization to achieve a big jump in savings, it would have to have been operating very inefficiently in the past. Outsourcing healthcare organizations need to carefully implement changes and assess their in-house capabilities. There is no guarantee that the IS outsourcing will be perceived as achieving its stated objectives due to the very different expectations held by the various stakeholders. Allocate appropriate resources to undertake IS investment evaluation process, assess the outsourcing requirements carefully, involve users in the outsourcing process, and the retention of corporate memory are crucial for the success of HIS outsourcing for hospitals. Hospital management will also need to assess external outsourcing contractors for existing capabilities. Hospitals can make use of assessment committees consisting different stakeholders or seek external assistance in selecting a suitable outsourcing contractors and in developing outsourcing implementation plans.

FUTURE TRENDS

HIS outsourcing spending will continue to rise in the future. The rising price of resources will put increasing pressure on healthcare organizations to both utilize technology and outsource to remain competitive. Despite the recent debates in the US and other western countries about outsourcing of skilled IS jobs to other low-cost countries such as India and China, and about organizations' obligations to the broader stakeholder community, offshore IS outsourcing has often been employed by most large organizations to reduce the cost of future IS investments and to improve the cash flow of the organizations (Burns, 2006; Hollands, 2004; Rottman & Lacity, 2004). Hospital IS executives from the six hospitals interviewed indicated that user satisfaction with external outsourcing contractors will greatly influence their future outsourcing decisions. All other things being equal, most of these hospital IS executives predicted a moderate or substantial increase of HIS outsourcing in the near future due to intense competitive environment and government regulations.

REFERENCES

Aubert, B. A., Patry, M., & Rivard, S. (1998). Assessing the Risk of IT Outsourcing, In *Proceedings of the 31st Annual Hawaii International Conference on System Science*, Hawaii, 685-692.

Barthelemy, J. (2003). The Hard and Soft Sides of IT Outsourcing Management. *European Management Journal, 21*(5), 539–548. doi:10.1016/S0263-2373(03)00103-8

Barthelemy, J., & Geyer, D. (2004). The Determinants of Total IT Outsourcing: An Empirical Investigation of French and German Firms. *Journal of Computer Information Systems, 44*(3), 91–97.

Beaver, K. (2003). *Healthcare Information Systems, Best Practices Series* (2nd ed.). Boca Raton, FL: CRC Presss, Auerbach Publications.

Boardman, A. E., & Hewitt, E. S. (2004). Problems With Contracting Out Government Services: Lessons From Orderly Services at SCGH. *Industrial and Corporate Change, 13*(6), 917–929. doi:10.1093/icc/dth034

Burmahl, B. (2001). Making the Choice: The Pros and Cons of Outsourcing. *Health Facilities Management, 14*(6), 16–22.

Burns, S. (2006). IT Industry Spends $66bn in Taiwan, VNU Business Publications, VNUNet.com.

Computer Economics. (2006). *IT Spending, Staffing, and Technology Trends 2006/2007 Study*. Computer Economics Inc.

Currie, W. L. (1998). Using Multiple Suppliers to Mitigate the Risk of IT Outsourcing at ICI and Wessex Water. *Journal of Information Technology, 13*, 169–180. doi:10.1080/026839698344819

Davidson, E. J. (2002). Technology Frames and Framing: A Social-cognitive Investigation of Requirements Determination. *Management Information Systems Quarterly, 26*(4), 329–358. doi:10.2307/4132312

Diana, M. L. (2009). (in press). Exploring Information Systems Outsourcing in US Hospital-based Health Care Delivery Systems. *Health Care Management Science*. doi:10.1007/s10729-009-9100-4

Eisenhardt, K. M. (1989). Building Theories From Case Study Research. *Academy of Management Review, 14*(4), 532–550. doi:10.2307/258557

Frost and Sullivan. (2006) Reports European Healthcare IT Outsourcing market to offer lucrative opportunities. *Hospital Business Week*, 37.

Graham, M., & Scarborough, H. (1997). Information Technology Outsourcing by State Governments in Australia. *Australian Journal of Public Administration*, *56*(3), 30–39. doi:10.1111/j.1467-8500.1997.tb01263.x

Guy, R. A., & Hill, J. R. (2007). 10 Outsourcing Myths That Raise Your Risk: Hospitals Should Be Wary Of Common Myths That Can Cause Them To Make Missteps In Developing Clinical Service Outsourcing Arrangements. *Healthcare Financial Management*, *61*(6), 66–72.

Haley, D. (2004). A Case for Outsourcing Medical Device Reprocessing. *AORN Journal*, *79*, 806–808. doi:10.1016/S0001-2092(06)60821-1

Hollands, M. (2004). *Status of Offshore Outsourcing in Australia: A Qualitative Study*. AIIA Report, Australian Information Industry Association.

Hsiao, C., Pai, J., & Chiu, H. (2009). The Study on the Outsourcing of Taiwan's Hospitals: A Questionnaire Survey Research. *BMC Health Services Research*, *9*, 78. doi:10.1186/1472-6963-9-78

Huang, Y., Lin, C., & Lin, H. (2005). Techno-economic Effect of R&D Outsourcing Strategy for Small and Medium-sized Enterprises: A Resource-Based Viewpoint. *International Journal of Innovation and Incubation*, *2*(1), 1–22.

Kakabadse, N., & Kakabadse, A. (2000). Critical Review – Outsourcing: A Paradigm Shift. *Journal of Management Development*, *19*(8), 670–728. doi:10.1108/02621710010377508

Lacity, M. C., & Willcocks, L. P. (1998). An Empirical Investigation of Information Technology Sourcing Practices: Lessons From Experience. *Management Information Systems Quarterly*, (September): 363–408. doi:10.2307/249670

Lee, J., & Kim, Y. (1999). Effect of Partnership Quality on IS Outsourcing Success: Conceptual Framework and Empirical Validation. *Journal of Management Information Systems*, *15*(4), 29–61.

Lin, C., Pervan, G., & Mcdermid, D. (2007). Issues and Recommendations in Evaluating and Managing the Benefits of Public Sector IT Outsourcing. *Information Technology & People*, *20*(2), 161–183. doi:10.1108/09593840710758068

Lin, W. T., & Shao, B. B. M. (2000). The Relationship Between User Participation and System Success: A Simultaneous Contingency Approach. *Information & Management*, *37*(6), 283–295. doi:10.1016/S0378-7206(99)00055-5

Liu, X., Hotchkiss, D. R., & Bose, S. (2008). The Effectiveness of Contracting out Primary Health Care Services in Developing Countries: A Review of the Evidence. *Health Policy and Planning*, *23*, 1–13. doi:10.1093/heapol/czm042

Lorence, D. P., & Spink, A. (2004). Healthcare Information Systems Outsourcing. *International Journal of Information Management*, *24*(2), 131–145. doi:10.1016/j.ijinfomgt.2003.12.011

Luftman, J., Kempaiah, R., & Nash, E. (2006). Key Issues for IT Executives 2005. *MIS Quarterly Executive*, *5*(2), 27–45.

Marek, T., Diallo, I., Ndiaye, B., & Rakotosalama, J. (1999). Successful Contracting of Prevention Services: Fighting Malnutrition in Senegal and Madagascar. *Health Policy and Planning*, *14*(4), 382–389. doi:10.1093/heapol/14.4.382

McIvor, R. (2000). A Practical Framework for Understanding the Outsourcing Process. *Supply Chain Management*, *5*(1), 22. doi:10.1108/13598540010312945

Menachemi, N., Burke, D., & Diana, M. (2007a). Characteristics of Hospitals that Outsource Information. System Functions. *Journal of Healthcare Information Management*, *19*(1), 63–69.

Menachemi, N., Burkhardt, J., Shewchuk, R., Burke, D., & Brooks, R. G. (2007b). To Outsource or not to Outsource: Examining the Effects of Outsourcing it Functions on Financial Performance in Hospitals. *Health Care Management Review, 32*(1), 46–54.

Meyers, S. (2004). ED Outsourcing: Is It Good for Patient Care? *Trustee, 57*, 12–14.

Miles, M. B., & Huberman, A. M. (1994). *Qualitative Data Analysis: An Expanded Sourcebook.* Sage Publications.

Misra, R. B. (2004). Global IT Outsourcing: Metrics for Success of All Parties. *Journal of Information Technology Cases and Applications, 6*(3), 21–34.

Moschuris, S. J., & Kondylis, M. N. (2006). Outsourcing in Public Hospitals: A Greek Perspective. *Journal of Health Organization and Management, 20*(1), 4–14. doi:10.1108/14777260610656534

Nakatsu, R. T., & Iacovou, C. L. (2009). A Comparative Study of Important Risk Factors Involved in Offshore and Domestic Outsourcing of Software Development Projects: A Two-Panel Delphi Study. *Information & Management, 46*, 57–68. doi:10.1016/j.im.2008.11.005

Ondo, K., & Smith, M. (2006). Outside IT the Case for Full IT Outsourcing: Study Findings Indicate Many Hospitals Are Turning to Full IT Outsourcing to Achieve IT Excellence. What's the Best Approach for Your Organization? *Healthcare Financial Management*, (February): 1–3.

Roberts, V. (2001). Managing Strategic Outsourcing in the Healthcare Industry. *Journal of Healthcare Management, 46*(4), 239–249.

Rottman, J. W., & Lacity, M. C. (2004). Twenty Practices for Offshore Sourcing. *MIS Quarterly Executive, 3*(3), 117–130.

Sakhtevil, S. (2007). Managing Risks in Offshore Systems Development. *Communications of the ACM, 50*(4), 69–75. doi:10.1145/1232743.1232750

Shinkman, R. (2000). Outsourcing on the Upswing. *Modern Healthcare, 30*(37), 46–54.

Sinton, J. (1994) *Outsourcing: Why Is It So? An Exploratory Study Into Factors That Contribute To Outsourcing Information Systems*, Research Report, Curtin University of Technology, Perth, November.

Tallon, P. P., Kraemer, K. L., & Gurbaxani, V. (2000). Executives' Perceptions of the Business Value of Information Technology: A Process-Oriented Approach. *Journal of Management Information Systems, 16*(4), 145–173.

Wholey, D. R., Padman, R., Hamer, R., & Schwartz, S. (2001). Determinants of Information Technology Outsourcing Among Health Maintenance Organizations. *Health Care Management Science, 4*(3), 229–239. doi:10.1023/A:1011401000445

Willcocks, L., & Lester, S. (1997). Assessing IT Productivity: Any Way Out of the Labyrinth? In Willcocks, L., Feeny, D. F., & Islei, G. (Eds.), *Managing IT as a Strategic Resource, Ch4* (pp. 64–93). London: The McGraw-Hill Company.

Willcocks, L. P., Lacity, M. C., & Kern, T. (1999). Risk Mitigation in IT Outsourcing Strategy Revisited: Longitudinal Case Research at LISA. *The Journal of Strategic Information Systems, 8*, 285–314. doi:10.1016/S0963-8687(00)00022-6

Young, S. (2005). Outsourcing in the Australian Health Sector: The interplay of Economics and Politics. *International Journal of Public Sector Management, 18*(1), 25–36. doi:10.1108/09513550510576134

Young, S. H. (2003). Outsourcing and Benchmarking in a Rural Public Hospital: Does Economic Theory Provide the Complete Answer? *Rural and Remote Health, 3*, 124–137.

KEY TERMS AND DEFINITIONS

Benefits: The tangible and intangible returns or payback expected to be obtained from a systems investment or implementation.

Healthcare Industry: The health profession industry which offers services in relation to the preservation of health by preventing or treating illness.

Health Information Systems (HIS): A data system which includes various health statistics from various sources, used to derive information about health reports, the delivery of services, costs, demographic, and health impact.

Information System (IS): It refers to the interactions between business processes, data, people, and technology. It includes a combination of hardware, software, infrastructure and people organized to assist in planning, monitoring, evaluation, and decision making.

IS Investment Evaluation: This is the weighing up process to rationally assess the value of any in-house IS assets and acquisition of software or hardware which are expected to improve business value of an organization's information systems.

IS Outsourcing: The practice of transferring IS assets, leases, staff, and management responsibility for delivery of services from internal IS functions to external contractors.

User Involvement: User participation. It is an act or a process for users to actively participate and/or or share their expertise, thoughts, and experience during a system development life cycle or project.

Section 4
Security Issues

Chapter 10
Graphs in Biometrics

Dakshina Ranjan Kisku
Dr. B. C. Roy Engineering College, India

Phalguni Gupta
Indian Institute of Technology Kanpur, India

Jamuna Kanta Sing
Jadavpur University, India

EXECUTIVE SUMMARY

Biometric systems are considered as human pattern recognition systems that can be used for individual identification and verification. The decision on the authenticity is done with the help of some specific measurable physiological or behavioral characteristics possessed by the individuals. Robust architecture of any biometric system provides very good performance of the system against rotation, translation, scaling effect and deformation of the image on the image plane. Further, there is a need of development of real-time biometric system. There exist many graph matching techniques used to design robust and real-time biometrics systems. This chapter discusses different types of graph matching techniques that have been successfully used in different biometric traits.

INTRODUCTION

Biometric systems (Jain, et. al., 2004; Jain, et. al., 2006) are considered as human pattern recognition systems. They can be used for individual identification and verification which is determined by some specific measurable physiological or behavioral characteristics (Jain, et. al., 2004; Jain, et. al. 2006; Jain, et. al., 2007). These characteristics can be obtained from fingerprint, face, iris, retina, hand geometry and palmprint, signature, ear, gait and voice, etc. which satisfy the properties like universality, invariance, measurability, singularity, acceptance, reducibility, tamper resistance, comparable and inimitable. There exist many computational intelligence techniques (Jain, et. al., 2007) applied to biometric systems for feature extraction (Jain, et. al., 2007), template updating (Jain, et. al., 2007), matching and classification (Jain, et. al., 2007). However, this type of systems seeks efficient and robust performance in real time environments. These robust systems often degrade their performance because of uncon-

DOI: 10.4018/978-1-60960-015-0.ch010

trolled environment and poor feature extraction, feature representation and pattern classification techniques.

There exist several graph matching techniques (Wiskott, et. al., 1997; Conte, et. al., 2003; Tarjoman, & Zarei, 2008; Fan, et. al., 1998; Mehrabian, & Heshemi-Tari, 2007; Abuhaiba, 2007) for identity verification of biometric samples which can solve problems like orientation, noise, non-invariant, etc that often occurred in fingerprint (Maltoni, et. al., 2003), face (Li, et. al., 2005), iris (Daugman, 1993), signature recognitions (Kisku, et. al., in press). Different graph topologies are successfully used for feature representations of these biometric cues (Jain, et. al., 2007). Graph algorithms (Conte, et. al., 2003; Gross, & Yellen, 2005) can be considered as a tool for matching two graphs obtained from feature sets extracted from two biometric cues (Jain, et. al., 2007). To describe the topological structure of biometric pattern, the locations at which the features are originated or extracted are used to define a graph. The small degree of distortions of features can easily be computed during matching of two graphs based on the position and distances between two nodes of the graph and also with the adjacency information of neighbor's features.

This chapter makes an attempt and explain the way a graph can be used in the designing an efficient biometric system. Next section discusses the use of graphs in fingerprint, face and iris recognition. In Section 3, a complete graph topology has been used in a SIFT-based face recognition system. Section 4 describes the method of using probabilistic graphs and fuse invariant SIFT features of a face. Next section deals with the problem of using wavelet decomposition and monotonic decreasing graph to fuse biometric characteristics. Experimental results are given in Section 6 which concluding remarks are in the last section.

USE OF GRAPHS IN BIOMETRICS

In Fingerprint Verification

Fingerprint verification (Maltoni, et. al., 2003) is method of verifying the identity of a user with the help of his fingerprint images. It requires several features of fingerprint impression, such as ridges and bifurcation information, minutiae features. A fingerprint pattern may contain arch, loop and whorl. The lines that flow in these patterns across fingerprints are called ridges and the spaces between two ridges are called valleys. An arch is a pattern where the ridges enter from one side of the finger and form an arch at the center and finally exit from the other side of the finger. The loop is a pattern where the ridges enter from one side of a finger, then form a curve and exit from the side they enter. In the whorl pattern, ridges form circular pattern around a center point on the finger. The method that most frequently used for fingerprint representation and matching is based on the distinguishable landmark points, called minutiae points. Minutiae points are of two types and they are terminating points of ridges, termed as ridge endings and are the points at which ridges are bifurcated, termed as ridge bifurcations. Thus, a minutiae is represented by three information – minutiae location (x, y), orientation (θ) and type of minutiae. In addition to minutiae, two other features that can be used for matching are core and delta. The core can be considered as the center of the fingerprint pattern while the delta is a singular point from which three patterns deviate.

In any minutiae based fingerprint system (Maltoni, et. al., 2003), matching between two fingerprints is done on the extracted minutiae points from the segmented, oriented and enhanced fingerprint images. Steps mentioned to extract minutiae are shown in Figure 1.

Apart from the minutiae based systems, there exist some robust graph based fingerprint systems (Tarjoman, & Zarei, 2008; Fan, et. al., 1998; Neuhaus, & Benke, 2005). A fingerprint verifica-

Figure 1. Steps for minutiae extraction

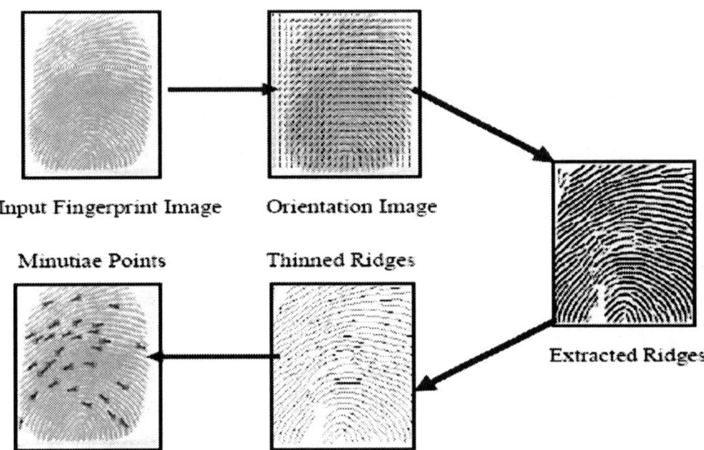

tion using relational graph proposed in (Tarjoman, & Zarei, 2008) has used directional image of fingerprint. The directional fingerprint image is segmented into a number of regions consisting of pixels with the identical direction as shown in Figure 2. On the segmented regions, relational graph is constructed as shown in Figure 3. The matching is performed with the model graph and the obtained graph using some predefined cost function. The accuracy of the proposed system can be increased by increasing the number of subclasses. The relational graph based fingerprint verification (Tarjoman, & Zarei, 2008) system can perform better when there is more number of subclasses.

In (Fan, et. al., 1998), a fingerprint based system has been discussed which uses fuzzy bipartite weighted graph for matching and verification. Initially a few preprocessing operations are applied on fingerprint image and it records the clusters consisting of feature points. Using fuzzy membership functions, 24 attributes are characterized for each feature point cluster. Verification is done by finding optimal matching graph between two feature point clusters of a query fingerprint and a database fingerprint which are the sets of left vertices and right vertices, respectively, in a bipartite weighted graph (Fan, et. al., 1998).

Even though there are several graph based fingerprint verification systems (Tarjoman, &

Figure 2. 4×4 blocks of segmented fingerprint images (Tarjoman, & Zarei, 2008)

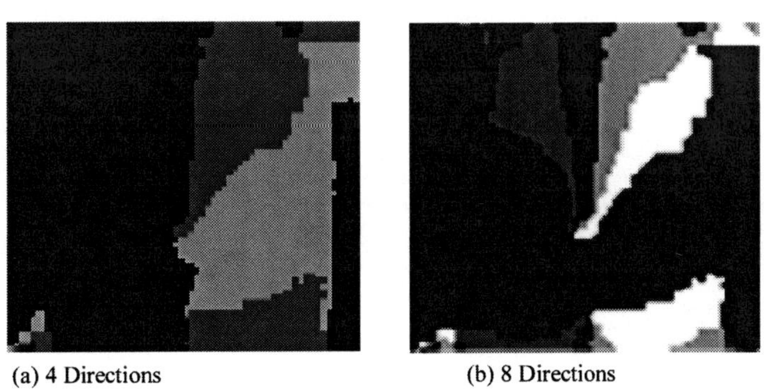

Figure 3. Relational graph for block directional fingerprint image (Tarjoman, & Zarei, 2008)

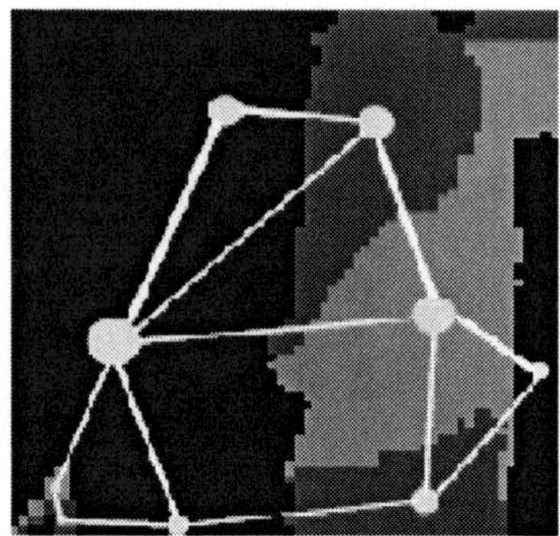

Zarei, 2008; Fan, et. al., 1998) but none of the fingerprint systems is tried to reduce its matching complexity for authentication. The graph based fingerprint system presented in (Neuhaus, & Benke, 2005) uses the concept of directional variance to extract regions of interest from fingerprint image relevant to classification based on Henry scheme (Maltoni, et. al., 2003). Finally, these regions of interest are then converted into attributed relational graphs. Identity verification of a query fingerprint is done by computing edit graph distance to a graph constructed on template fingerprint of a database image. This system is found to be very much useful to reduce matching cost. Figure 4 shows a fingerprint image with core and delta points and vertical orientation lines. It also shows the directional variance from core to

delta point which is used to extract the regions of interest for converting into attributed relational graphs. Figure 5 shows the modified directional variances.

Face Recognition using Graph Matching

Automated face recognition (Li, et. al., 2005) is used to verify the identity of personnel based on the face characteristics (Li, et. al., 2005). There are three approaches in face recognition – feature based approach (Li, et. al., 2005), appearance based approach (Li, et. al., 2005) and model based approach (Li, et. al., 2005). Different feature based graph representations have been successfully used in face recognitions. The computational costs of the graph matching techniques (Wiskott, et. al., 1997; Kisku, et. al., 2007; Kokiopoulou, & Frossard, 2009; Fazi-Ersi, et. al., 2007) are found to be compatible with those of the feature based and appearance based techniques. Graphs on face also have proved to provide robust feature representation for both controlled and non-controlled environments. Face recognition using graph matching (Wiskott, et. al., 1997; Fazi-Ersi, et. al., 2007) refers to a process in which graph is formed on detected fiducial points on face and it is used to match with the graph drawn on another face. The matching process of two graphs computes the matching probability of two corresponding users.

Figure 4. Left Loop Fingerprint Image with Core and Delta Points and Vertical Orientation Lines on Left Fingerprint (Neuhaus, & Benke, 2005). Directional Variance shown on the Right Image (Neuhaus, & Benke, 2005).

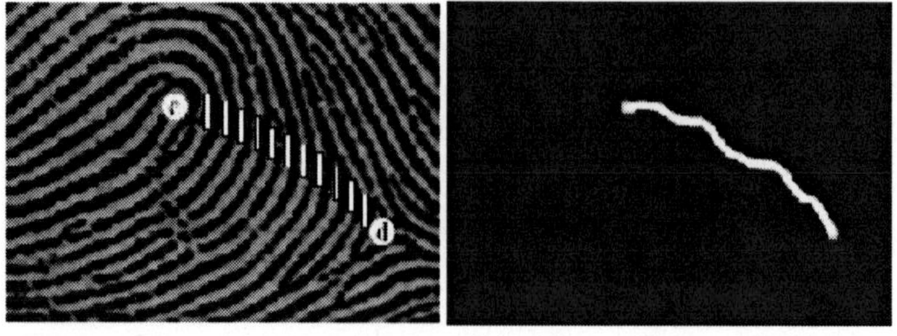

Figure 5. (a) Modified directional variances for left (L), right (R) and whorl (W) fingerprints (b) Graphs for left (L), right (R), whorl (W) and tented arch (T) fingerprints (Neuhaus, & Benke, 2005)

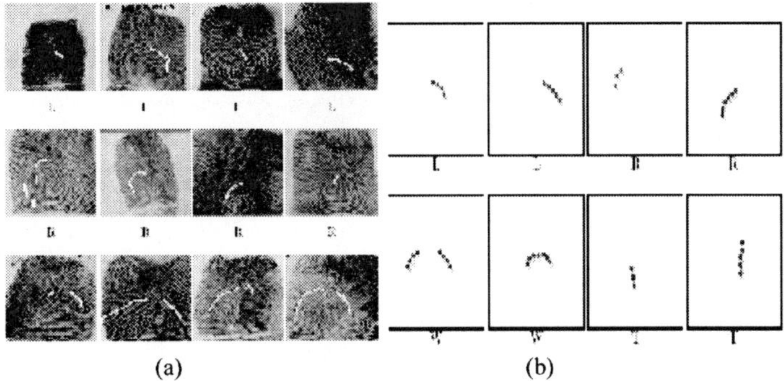

(a)　　　　　　(b)

Elastic Bunch Graph Matching (EBGM) based face recognition in (Wiskott, et. al., 1997) considers the fact that face images can be translated, rotated, scaled and deformed in the image plane. Each face is represented by a labeled graph where edges and nodes are labeled with distance information and wavelet responses respectively. Wavelet responses are locally bundled in jets (Wiskott, et. al., 1997). During matching, model graphs are matched to face graph generated from query faces. EBGM technique (Wiskott, et. al., 1997) uses wavelets for local features representation that are robust to partial lighting changes and small shifts and deformations. Constructed model graphs (Wiskott, et. al., 1997) can be used to translate, rotate, scale and deform the face im-

ages during the matching process for getting the best possible match. Figure 6 obtained through EBGM technique shows grids for face findings and for face recognition.

Usefulness of EBGM technique has been extended further in various face recognition approaches. In (Zhang, & Ma, 2005), grid based parallel elastic graph matching is used to obtain a face recognition system. Illumination invariant face recognition with the help of elastic bunch graph matching has been discussed in (Kela, et. al., 2006). An improved EBGM based face recognition has been discussed in (Liu, & Liu, 2005) where fuzzy fusion based on fuzzy measure and fuzzy integral is used with EBGM.

Figure 6. Grids for face finding and grids for face recognition (Wiskott, et. al., 1997)

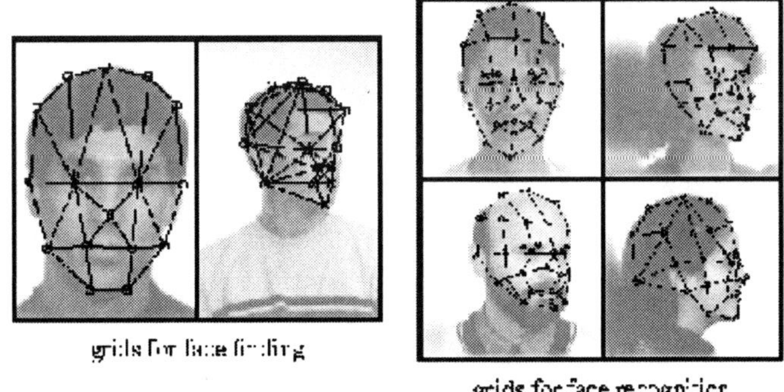

To speed up EBGM technique in the manner of local graph matching, a face recognition has been developed in (Senaratne, et. al., 2009) where Particle Swarm Optimization (PSO) technique is used with EBGM. To locate a landmark point, Gabor wavelet is used as bunch of jets and matching process of EBGM is optimized by particle swarm optimization. For feature extraction, Local Landmark Model (Senaratne, & Halgamuge, 2006) is extended by combining Gabor wavelets with gray-level profiles. Gray-level profiles provide intensity information which is unavailable in jets. The PSO based face recognition is composed of four steps: (a) face bunch graph (FBG) creation, (b) face finding, (c) landmark finding and (d) recognition. The second and third steps are shown in Figure 7 and Figure 8 respectively.

2D face recognition (Fazi-Ersi, et. al., 2007) uses a labeled graph to represent each face image drawn on 3-tuple of feature points characterized by local feature analysis technique. The method builds a graph for each individual and matching is performed between the graphs extracted from a probe face image and the gallery model graphs.

Iris Recognition using Graphs

Iris recognition is regarded as the accurate, authentic and most reliable biometric trait. The first iris recognition system has been introduced in (Daugman, 1993). However, there exists several iris recognition systems developed in the last few years (Wildes, 1997; Ma, et. al., 2004; Lim, et. al., 2001). Any iris system generally comprises four basic steps such as iris segmentation, normalization, feature extraction and matching.

A graph cut based iris recognition system has been discussed in (Mehrabian, & Heshemi-Tari, 2007). Pupil has been detected using graph cut algorithm to segment the pupil portion from the background image. In iris recognition, pupil segmentation and its detection is an important part of recognition process and most of the pupil segmentation algorithms detect pupil area by fitting a circle to the boundary of the pupil. By considering off angle imaging effects, an efficient pupil segmentation algorithm (Mehrabian, & Heshemi-Tari, 2007) has been discussed using graph cut theory for iris recognition. It segments the pupil area using gray level pixels to compute weights for the relational links in graph. Graph cut (Mehrabian, & Heshemi-Tari, 2007) has two parts as terminals – one terminal is used to detect pupil area and the other terminal is used for background of the image. The iris recognition system consists of three steps – (a) segmentation of eye images, (b) graph cut implementation for segmentation of pupil and (c) implementation of iris recognition using graph cut based pupil detection.

Figure 7. (a) Face finding; (b) Landmark finding (Senaratne, et. al., 2009)

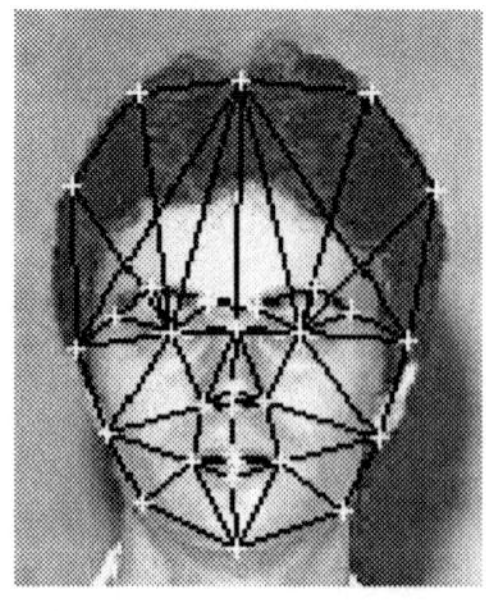

(a)   (b)

Figure 8. Face finding with particle swarm optimization at the end of 1st, 2nd, 3rd, 4th, 5th, 8th, 12th, 16th and 20th iterations (Senaratne, et. al., 2009)

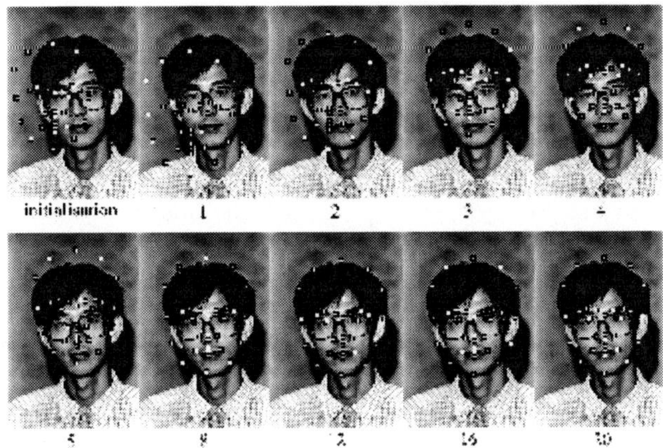

INVARIANT FACE RECOGNITION USING GRAPH TOPOLOGY

This section presents a face recognition system (Kisku, et. al., 2007) which uses graph topology drawn on SIFT (Scale Invariant Feature Transform) (Lowe, 1999; Lowe, 2004) extracted from face images. To recognize and classify objects efficiently, feature points from objects can be extracted to make a robust feature descriptor or representation of the objects. David Lowe (Lowe, 1999; Lowe, 2004) introduced a technique to extract features from images, which are called Scale Invariant Feature Transform (SIFT). These features are invariant to scale, rotation, partial illumination and 3D projective transform and they are shown to provide robust matching across a substantial range of affine distortion, change in 3D viewpoint, addition of noise, and change in illumination. SIFT image features provide a set of features of an object that are not affected by occlusion, clutter, and unwanted "noise" in the image. In addition, the SIFT features are highly distinctive in nature which have accomplished correct matching on several pair of feature points with high probability between a large database and a test sample. Following are the four major filtering stages of computation used to generate the set of image feature based on SIFT.

Scale-Space Extrema Detection

This filtering approach attempts to identify image locations and scales that are identifiable from different views. Scale space and Difference of Gaussian (DoG) functions (Lowe, 1999; Lowe, 2004) are used to detect stable keypoints. Difference of Gaussian is used for identifying key-points in scale-space and locating scale space extrema by taking difference between two images, one

Figure 9. Eye image, graph cut and pupil boundary (left to right) (Mehrabian, & Heshemi-Tari, 2007)

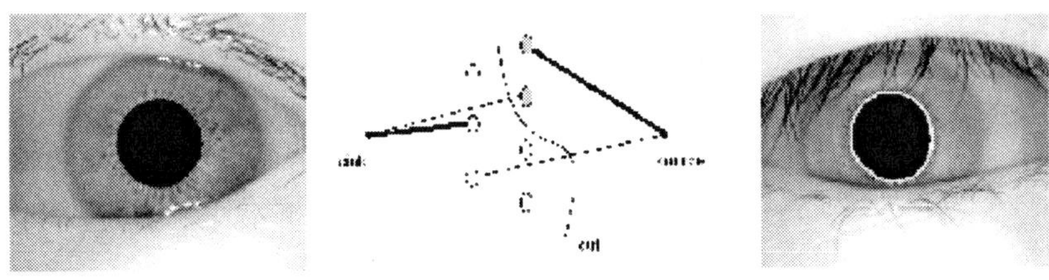

with scaled by some constant times of the other. To detect the local maxima and minima, each feature point is compared with its 8 neighbors at the same scale and in accordance with its 9 neighbors up and down by one scale. If this value is the minimum or maximum of all these points then this point is an extrema.

Localization of Keypoints

To localize keypoints (Lowe, 1999; Lowe, 2004), a few points after detection of stable keypoint locations that have low contrast or are poorly localized on an edge are eliminated. This can be achieved by calculating the Laplacian space. After computing the location of extremum value, if the value of difference of Gaussian pyramids is less than a threshold value the point is excluded. If there is a case of large principle curvature across the edge but a small curvature in the perpendicular direction in the difference of Gaussian function, the poor extrema is localized and eliminated.

Orientation Assignment

This step aims to assign consistent orientation (Lowe, 1999; Lowe, 2004) to the key-points based on local image characteristics. From the gradient orientations of sample points, an orientation histogram is formed within a region around the key-point. Orientation assignment is followed by key-point descriptor which can be represented relative to this orientation. A 16x16 window is chosen to generate histogram. The orientation histogram has 36 bins covering 360 degree range of orientations. The gradient magnitude and the orientation are pre-computed using pixel differences. Each sample is weighted by its gradient magnitude and by a Gaussian-weighted circular window.

Key-Point Descriptor

In the last step, the feature descriptors (Lowe, 1999; Lowe, 2004) which represent local shape distortions and illumination changes, are computed. After candidate locations have been found, a detailed fitting is performed to the nearby data for the location, edge response and peak magnitude. To achieve invariance to image rotation, a consistent orientation is assigned to each feature point based on local image properties. The histogram of orientations is formed from the gradient orientation at all sample points within a circular window of a feature point. Peaks in this histogram correspond to the dominant directions of each feature point. For illumination invariance, 8 orientation planes are defined. Finally, the gradient magnitude and the orientation are smoothened by applying a Gaussian filter and then are sampled over a 4 x 4 grid with 8 orientation planes.

Graph Matching Constraints for Face Recognition

Three face matching constraints (Kisku, et. al., 2007) are presented which are implemented using graph taxonomy and they are Gallery Image based Match Constraint (GIbMC) (Kisku, et. al., 2007), Reduced Point based Match constraint (RPbMC) (Kisku, et. al., 2007) and Regular Grid based Match Constraint (RGbMC) (Kisku, et. al., 2008). These techniques can be applied to find the corresponding sub-graph in the probe face image for a given complete graph in the gallery image. The correspondence graph problem (Gross, & Yellen, 2005) is to find a match between two structural descriptions, i.e., a mapping function between elements of two set of feature points which preserve the maximum matching proximity between feature relations of face images. Detail definition of the directional correspondences between two feature points is given in and based on these two definitions this graph matching constraints have

Figure 10. Corresponding points of first face image mapped into Second Face image (Kisku, et. al., 2007)

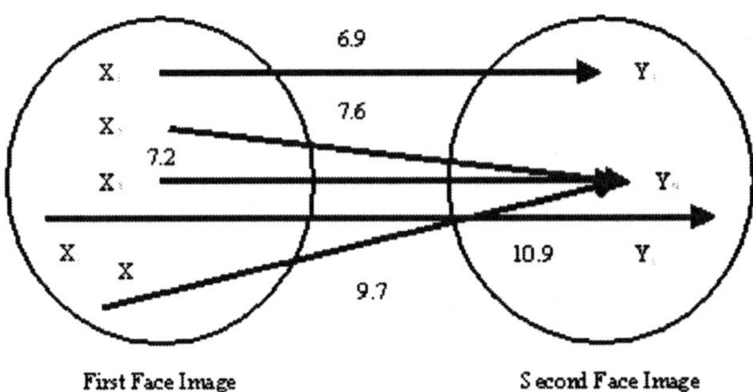

been developed. This face recognition system uses SIFT operator (Lowe, 1999; Lowe, 2004) for feature extraction and each feature point composed of four different types of information such as spatial location, key point descriptor, scale and orientation.

Gallery Image Based Match Constraint

Gallery Image based Match Constraint (Kisku, et. al., 2007) has been developed based on the assumption that matching points can be found around similar positions i.e., fiducial points on the face image. While establishing correspondence between two feature sets extracted from two face images, more than one feature points on the gallery face may correspond to a single point on the probe face and vice versa. To eliminate false matches and to consider the only minimum pair distance from a set of pair distances for making a correspondence, first it needs to verify the number of feature points that are extracted from the gallery and probe faces. When the number of feature points on the gallery face is less than that of the probe face, many points of interest from the probe face would be discarded. If reverse is possible, i.e., if the number of points of interest on the gallery face is more than that of the probe face, then a single interest point on the probe face may act as a match point for many points of interest of gallery face. Moreover, many points of interest on the gallery face may have correspondences to a single point of interest on the probe face. In both the cases, single point of interest on the probe face may correspond to many points on the gallery face. After computing all distances between points of interest of gallery and probe faces that have made correspondences, only the minimum pair distance is paired (see Figure 10 and 11 for illustration). The distances are computed as the hausdorff distance

Figure 11. Feature points and their matches for a pair of faces (Kisku, et. al., 2007)

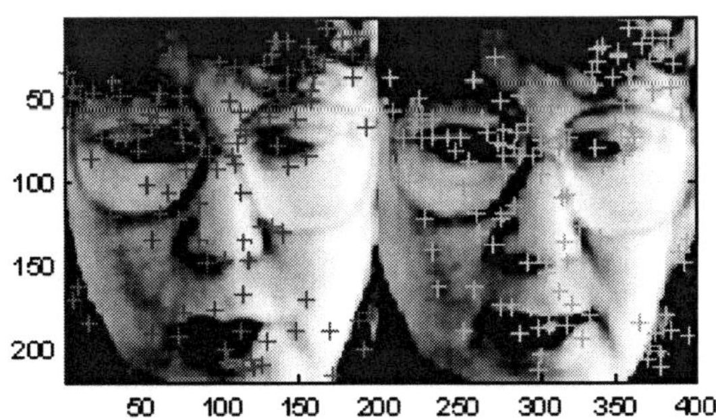

Figure 12. Elimination of false matches (Kisku, et. al., 2007)

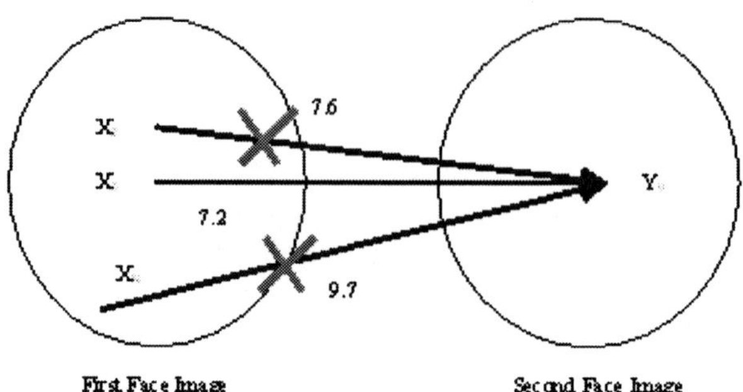

using Euclidean distance metric and dissimilarity scores are computed between all pairs of vertices of two face images after constructing complete graphs on the interest points.

Reduced Point Based Match Constraint

Multiple assignments determined in Gallery Image based Match Constraint (GIbMC) (Kisku, et. al., 2007) are removed and the technique is furthermore extended in Reduced Point based Match Constraint (RPbMC) (Kisku, et. al., 2007). It has been observed that in the Gallery Image based Match Constraint there can be some false matches. Usually, these false matches are obtained due to multiple assignments while more than one point are assigned to a single point on another face, or due to existence of one way assignments (see Figure 12). The false matches due to multiple assignments are eliminated by pairing the points

with the minimum distance. The false matches due to one way assignments are eliminated by removing the correspondence links that do not have any corresponding assignment from the other face. The graph on gallery face and the corresponding graph on the probe face have been shown in Figure 13. All matches computed from left face to right face are shown in Figure 13(a) while resulted graphs with few false matches are shown in Figure 13(b).

These false matches can be eliminated with the application of another constraint, namely, the Reduced Point based Match Constraint (Kisku, et. al., 2007) which guarantees that each assignment from an image to another image would have a corresponding assignment from the second image to the first image. With this consideration, the false matches due to multiple assignments are eliminated by choosing the match pair with the minimum distance. The false matches due to one

Figure 13. Reduced point based match constraint (Kisku, et. al., 2008)

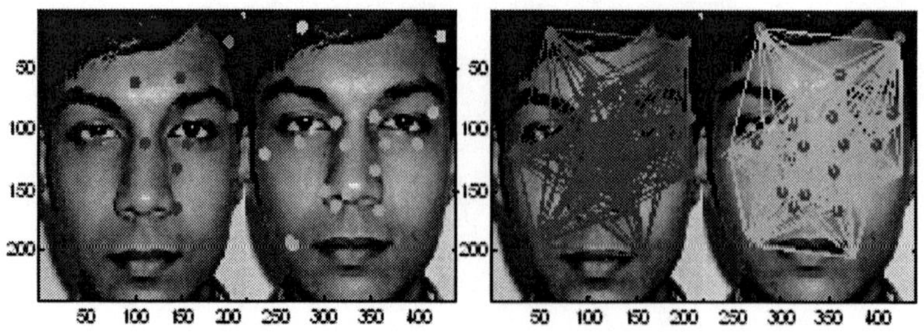

way assignments are eliminated by removing the links which do not have any corresponding assignment from the other side. Examples showing the matches before and after applying the Reduced Point based Match Constraints (Kisku, et. al., 2007) are given in Figure 13.

False matches, due to multiple assignments, are removed by choosing the match with the minimum distance between two face images. The dissimilarity scores on reduced points between two face images for nodes and edges, are computed in the same way as for the gallery image based match constraint. Finally, the weighted average score is computed by using Gaussian Empirical Rule (Kisku, et. al., 2007). This graph matching technique is found to be more efficient than Gallery Image based Match Constraint since the matching is done on a very small number of feature points with very few floating feature points.

Regular Grid Based Match Constraint

The graph matching technique (Kisku, et. al., 2008) presented in this sub-section has been developed with the idea of matching of corresponding sub-graphs for a pair of face images. First the face image is divided into sub-images, using a regular grid with overlapping regions. The matching between a pair of face images is performed by comparing sub-images and by computing distances between all pairs of corresponding sub-image graphs in a pair of face images and finally by averaging the dissimilarity scores for a pair of sub-images. Final matching score is computed to be a weighted score. Weight assignment is performed by using Gaussian Empirical Rule discussed in (Kisku, et. al., 2007). From an experimental evaluation, it is found that if sub-images of dimensions 1/5 of width and 1/5 of height represent a good compromise between localization accuracy and robustness to registration errors on a face image. The overlapping has been set to 30%.

FACE RECOGNITION USING PROBABILISTIC GRAPHS

This section proposes a new local feature based face recognition technique (Kisku, et. al., in press) which makes use of dynamic (mouth) and static (eyes, nose) salient features of face obtained through SIFT operator (Lowe, 1999; Lowe, 2004). Differences in facial expression, head pose, illumination, and partly occlusion may result to variations of facial characteristics and attributes. To capture the face variations, face characteristics of dynamic and static parts are further represented by incorporating repetitive graph relaxations drawn on SIFT features (Lowe, 1999; Lowe, 2004) extracted from localized mouth, eyes and nose facial parts.

Salient Landmarks Selection and SIFT Features Extraction

Deformable objects are generally difficult to characterize with a rigid representation in feature spaces for recognition. With a large view of physiological characteristics in biometrics including iris, fingerprint, hand geometry, etc, faces are considered as highly deformable objects. Different facial regions, not only convey different relevant and redundant information on the subject's identity, but also suffer from different time variability due to motion or illumination changes. A typical example is the case of a talking face where the mouth part can be considered as dynamic facial landmark part. But eyes and nose can be considered as the static facial landmark parts which are almost still and invariant over time. As a consequence, the features extracted from the mouth area cannot be directly matched with the corresponding features from a static template. Moreover, single facial features may be occluded making the corresponding image area not usable for identification. To localize the major facial features such as eyes, mouth and nose, positions are automatically located by applying the technique in (Smeraldi, et.

al., 1999; Gourier, et. al., 2004). A circular region of interest (ROI) centered at each extracted facial landmark location is considered to determine the SIFT features [27] of the landmark. The face recognition system can use SIFT descriptor for extraction of invariant features from each facial landmark (Kisku, et. al., in press), namely, eyes, mouth and nose.

Graph Relaxation and Matching

In order to interpret the facial landmarks with invariant SIFT points (Lowe, 1999) and graph relaxation topology (Yaghi, & Krim, 2008), each extracted feature can be thought as a node and the relationship between invariant points can be considered as an edge between two nodes. At the level of feature extraction, invariant SIFT feature points are extracted. Relaxation graphs (Yaghi, & Krim, 2008) are then drawn on the features extracted from these landmarks. These relaxations are used for matching and verification. Thus, the graph (Gross, & Yellen, 2005) can be represented by $G=\{V,E,K,\zeta\}$ where V and E denote the set of nodes and set of edges, respectively and K denotes the set of keypoint descriptors associated with various nodes while ζ provides the relationship between two keypoint descriptors.

Suppose, $G_R=\{V_R, E_R, K_R, \zeta_R\}$ and $G_Q=\{V_Q, E_Q, K_Q, \zeta_Q\}$ are two graphs. These two graphs can be compared to determine whether they are identical or not. If it is found that $|V_R| = |V_Q|$ for the given two graphs, the problem is said to be exact graph matching problem. The problem is to find a one-to-one mapping $f: V_Q \rightarrow V_R$, such that $(u,v) \in E_Q$ iff $(f(u), f(v)) \in E_R$. This mapping f is called an isomorphism and G_Q is called isomorphic to G_R. In this case, isomorphism (Gross, & Yellen, 2005) is not possible because identical SIFT feature points may not be present on two different landmarks. Hence, it is forced to apply inexact graph matching problem in the context of probabilistic graph matching where either $|V_R| < |V_Q|$ or $|V_R| > |V_Q|$. This may occur when the number of SIFT keypoints or vertices in both the graphs is different.

The similarity measure for vertex and edge attributes can be defined as the similarity measure for nodes $v_R^i \in V_R$ and $v_Q^j \in V_Q$ as $s_{ij}^v = s(v_R^i, v_Q^j)$ where $v_R^i \in K_R \in V_R$ and $v_Q^j \in K_Q \in V_Q$, and the similarity between edges $e_R^{ip} \in E_R$ and $e_Q^{jq} \in E_Q$ can be denoted as $s_{ipjq}^e = s(e_R^{ip}, e_Q^{jq})$ where $e_R^{ip} \in \zeta_R \in E_R$ and $e_Q^{jq} \in \zeta_Q \in E_Q$.

Now, v_Q^j would be best probable match for v_R^i, when v_Q^j maximizes the posteriori probability (Yaghi, & Krim, 2008) of labeling. Thus for the vertex $v_R^i \in V_R$, we are searching the most probable label or vertex $v_R^{-i} = v_Q^j \in V_Q$ in the graph. Hence, it can be stated as

$$\overline{v}_R^i = \arg \max_{j,v_Q \in V_Q} P(\psi_i^{v_Q^j} \mid K_R, \varsigma_R, K_Q, \varsigma_Q) \qquad (4.1)$$

For efficient searching of matching probabilities from the query sample, we use relaxation technique which simplifies the solution of matching problem. Let $\overline{P}_{ij}^v$ denote the matching probability for vertices $v_R^i \in V_R$ and $v_Q^j \in V_Q$. Now, by reformulating Equation (4.1) one gets

$$\overline{v}_R^i = \arg \max_{j,v_{Qj} \in V_Q} \overline{P}_{ij}^v \qquad (4.2)$$

Equation (4.2) can be considered for searching the best labels for $\overline{v}_R^i$. This can be achieved by assigning prior probability $\overline{P}_{ij}^v$ proportional to $s_{ij}^v = s^v(k_R^i, k_Q^j)$. The iterative relaxation (Yaghi, & Krim, 2008) rule which can be used to define $\overline{P}_{ij}^v$ is given by

$$\hat{P}_{ij}^v = \frac{\overline{P}_{ij}^v . Q_{ij}}{\displaystyle\sum_{j,v_Q^j \in V_Q} \overline{P}_{ij}^v . Q_{ij}} \qquad (4.3)$$

where Q_{ij} is given by

$$Q_{ij} = \bar{P}_{ij}^v \prod_{v_i \in V_R} \sum_{v_j \in V_Q} s_{ij}^e . \bar{P}_{ij}^v \qquad (4.4)$$

In Equation (4.4), Q_{ij} conveys the support of the neighboring vertices and $\hat{P}_{ij}^v$ represents the posteriori probability. The relaxation cycles are repeated until the difference between prior probability $\bar{P}_{ij}^v$ and posteriori probabilities $\hat{P}_{ij}^v$ becomes smaller than certain threshold Φ and when this is reached, it is assumed that the relaxation process is stable. Hence, the best matched graph for query sample is established by using the posteriori probabilities of Equation (4.3).

Fusion Strategy of Invariant Features

The Dempster-Shafer decision theory (Bauer, 1996; Barnett, 1981; Bauer, 1997) which is applied to combine the matching scores obtained from individual landmark is based on combining the evidences obtained from different sources to compute the probability of an event. This is obtained by combining three elements: the basic probability assignment function (*bpa*), the belief function (*bf*) and the plausibility function (*pf*).

The *bpa* maps the power set to the interval $[0,1]$. The *bpa* of the empty set is *0* while the *bpa*'s of all the subsets of the power set is 1. Let m denote the *bpa* function and *m(A)* represent the *bpa* for a particular set *A*. Formally, the basic probability assignment function can be represented by the following equations

$$m: \breve{A} \rightarrow [0,1] \qquad (4.5)$$

$$m(\emptyset) = 0 \qquad (4.6)$$

$$\sum_{A \in \breve{A}} m(A) = 1 \qquad (4.7)$$

where $\breve{A}$ is the power set of A and $\emptyset$ is the empty set. From the basic probability assignment (Barnett, 1981; Bauer, 1997) the upper and lower bounds of an interval are bounded by two non-additive continuous measures, called Belief and Plausibility. The lower bound, Belief, for a set A is defined as the sum of all the basic probability assignments of proper subsets B of the set of interest A. The upper bound, Plausibility is the sum of all the basic probability assignments of the sets B that intersect A. Thus, Belief for a A, *Bel(A)* and Plausibility of A, *Pl(A)* can be defined as

$$Bel(A) = \sum_{B|B \subseteq A} m(B) \qquad (4.8)$$

$$Pl(A) = \sum_{B|B \cap A \neq \emptyset} m(B) \qquad (4.9)$$

An inverse function with the Belief measures can be used to obtain the basic probability assignment. Therefore,

$$m(A) = \sum_{B|B \subseteq A} (-1)^\gamma Bel(B) \qquad \because \gamma = \mid A - B \mid \qquad (4.10)$$

where $|A-B|$ is the difference of the cardinality between the two sets A and B. It is possible to derive Belief and Plausibility from each other with the help of following equation

$$Pl(A) = 1 - Bel(\bar{A}) \qquad (4.11)$$

where is the complement of A. In addition, the Belief measures can be written as:

$$Bel(\bar{A}) = \sum_{B|B \subseteq A} m(B) = \sum_{B|B \cap A = \emptyset} m(B) \qquad (4.12)$$

and

$$\sum_{B|B\cap A\neq\varnothing} m(B) = 1 - \sum_{B|B\cap A=\varnothing} m(B) = Pl(A)$$

$$(4.13)$$

Let $\Gamma^{left-eye}, \Gamma^{right-eye}, \Gamma^{nose}$ and Γ^{mouth} be the individual matching scores obtained from the four different matching of salient facial landmarks. It is illustrated in Figure 14. In order to obtain the combine matching score from the four salient landmarks pairs, Dempster combination rule (Barnett, 1981; Bauer, 1997) has been applied. First, we combine the matching scores obtained from the pairs of left-eye and nose landmark features and then the matching scores obtained from the pairs of right-eye and mouth landmark features are combined. Finally, the matching scores determined from the first and second processes are fused. Also, let $m(\Gamma^{left-eye})$, $m(\Gamma^{right-eye})$, $m(\Gamma^{nose})$ and $m(\Gamma^{mouth})$ be the *bpa* functions for the Belief measures $Bel(\Gamma^{left-eye})$, $Bel(\Gamma^{right-eye})$, $Bel(\Gamma^{nose})$ and $Bel(\Gamma^{mouth})$ for the four classifiers, respectively. Then the Belief probability assignments *(bpa)* $m(\Gamma^{left-eye}), m(\Gamma^{right-eye}), m(\Gamma^{nose})$ and $m(\Gamma^{mouth})$ can be combined together to obtained a Belief

committed to a matching score set using orthogonal sum rule

$$m(C_1) = m(\Gamma^{left-eye}) \oplus m(\Gamma^{nose}) =$$

$$\frac{\displaystyle\sum_{\Gamma^{left-eye}\cap\Gamma^{nose}=C_1} m(\Gamma^{left-eye})m(\Gamma^{nose})}{1 - \displaystyle\sum_{\Gamma^{left-eye}\cap\Gamma^{nose}=\varnothing} m(\Gamma^{left-eye})m(\Gamma^{nose})}, \quad C_1 \neq \varnothing.$$

$$(4.14)$$

$$m(C_2) = m(\Gamma^{right-eye}) \oplus m(\Gamma^{mouth}) =$$

$$\frac{\displaystyle\sum_{\Gamma^{right-eye}\cap\Gamma^{mouth}=C_2} m(\Gamma^{right-eye})m(\Gamma^{mouth})}{1 - \displaystyle\sum_{\Gamma^{right-eye}\cap\Gamma^{mouth}=\varnothing} m(\Gamma^{right-eye})m(\Gamma^{mouth})}, \quad C_2 \neq \varnothing.$$

$$(4.15)$$

$$m(C) = m(m(C_1)) \oplus m(m(C_2)) =$$

$$\frac{\displaystyle\sum_{m(C_1)\cap m(C_2)=C} m(m(C_1))m(m(C_2))}{1 - \displaystyle\sum_{m(C_1)\cap m(C_2)=\varnothing} m(m(C_1))m(m(C_2))}, \quad C \neq \varnothing$$

$$(4.16)$$

Figure 14. SIFT features of a pair of faces (Kisku, et. al., in press)

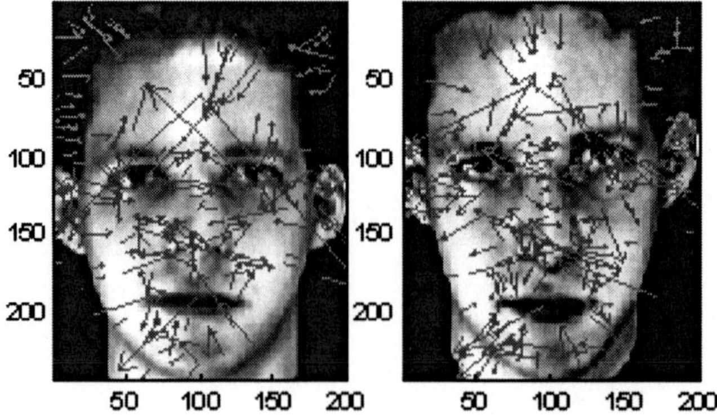

The denominator in equations (4.14), (4.15) and (4.16) are the normalizing factors which denote the art of Belief probability assignments $m(\Gamma^{left-eye})$, $m(\Gamma^{right-eye})$, $m(\Gamma^{nose})$ and $m(\Gamma^{mouth})$.

Let $m(m(C_1))$ and $m(m(C_2))$ be the two sets of matching scores obtained from the local and global matching strategies. They can be fused together recursively as

$$m(FMS) = m(m(C_1)) \oplus m(m(C_2)) \qquad (4.17)$$

where $\oplus$ denotes the Dempster combination rule (Barnett, 1981; Bauer, 1997). The final decision of user acceptance and rejection can be established by the following equation and by applying the threshold Ψ to the final match $m(FMS)$

$$decision = \begin{cases} accept, & if \quad m(FMS) \geq \Psi \\ reject, & otherwise \end{cases}$$

$$(4.18)$$

Practical illustration Sentz, K., & Ferson, S. (2002) of Dempster combination rule is given in Appendix.

BIOMETRICS EVIDENCE FUSION USING WAVELET DECOMPOSITION AND MATCHING USING MONOTONIC-DECREASING GRAPH

Multibiometric systems (Jain, & Ross, 2004) remove some of the drawbacks of the uni-modal biometric systems by acquiring multiple sources of information together in an augmented group which has richer detail. Utilization of these biometric systems depends on more than one physiological or behavioral characteristic for enrollment and verification/ identification. There exist multimodal biometrics (Ross, & Jain, 2003; Ross, & Govindarajan, 2005) with various levels of fusion, namely, sensor level, feature level, matching score level and decision level. Fusion at low level / sensor level by biometric image fusion may be an emerging area for biometric authentication. But, due to improper image registration it is quite impossible to achieve fusion at low level. Fusions on multisensor evidences are already used successfully in many applications (Stathaki, 2008) such as biomedical informatics, remote sensing imaging, and machine vision.

A multisensory based multimodal biometric system which fuses information at low level or sensor level of processing is expected to produce

Figure 15. SIFT features on facial landmarks (Kisku, et. al., in press)

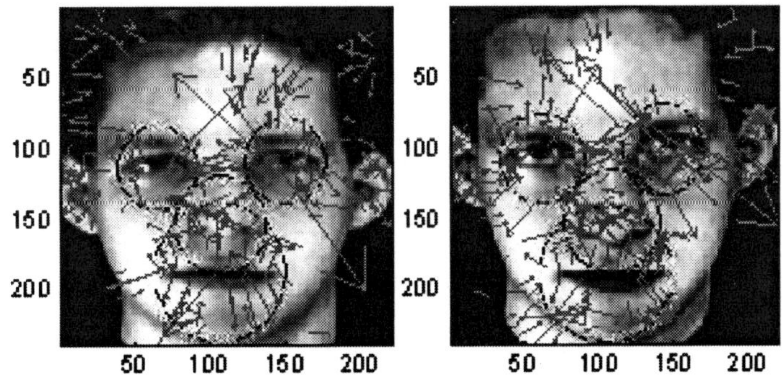

more accurate results than a system that integrates information at a later stages, namely, feature level, matching score level, because of the availability of more richer and relevant information.

In this section, a novel biometric sensor generated evidence fusion of face and palmprint images using wavelet decomposition is presented (Kisku, et. al., 2009). The approach of biometric image fusion at sensor or low level refers to a process that fuses images captured at different resolutions and by different biometric sensors to acquire richer and complementary information to produce a new fused image in spatially enhanced form. When the fused image is ready for further processing, SIFT operator (Lowe, 1999; Lowe, 2004) are then used for feature extraction and identity verification is performed by monotonic decreasing graph between a pair of fused images by searching the corresponding points using recursive descent tree traversal approach (Kisku, et. al., 2009; Lin, et. al., 1986).

Face and Palmprint Image Fusion using Wavelet Decomposition

Multisensor image fusion is performed with one or more images. However the fused image is considered as a unique single pattern from where the invariant keypoint features are extracted. The fused image should have more useful and richer information from individual images. The fusion of the two images (Stathaki, 2008; Liu, 2005) can take place at the signal, pixel, or feature level.

The method for evidence fusion (Kisku, et. al., 2009) presented in this subsection is based on the face and palmprint images decomposition into multiple channels depending on their local frequency. The wavelet transform (Stathaki, 2008; Liu, 2005) provides an integrated framework to decompose biometric images into a number of new images, each of them having a different degree of resolution. According to Fourier transform, the wave representation is an intermediate representation between Fourier and spatial representations.

It has the capability to provide good optimal localization for both frequency and space domains.

Basic Structure for Image Fusion using Wavelet Transform and Decomposition

The biometrics image fusion (Stathaki, 2008) extracts information from each source image and obtains the effective representation in the final fused image. The aim of image fusion technique is to fuse detailed information obtained from both the source images.

The approach fuses face and palmprint images having identical resolutions and the images are completely different with respect to texture information. The face and palmprint images are obtained from different sources. More formally, these images are obtained from different sensors. After re-scaling and registration (Stathaki, 2008; Liu, 2005), the images are fused together by using wavelet transform and decomposition (Stathaki, 2008). Finally, we obtain a completely new fused image where both the attributes of face and palmprint images are focused and reflected. The method for image fusion opposes the multi-resolution image fusion approach where multi-resolution images of same subject are collected from multiple sources.

Wavelet transforms (Stathaki, 2008) are determined from face and palmprint images. The wavelet transform contains low-high bands, high-low bands and high-high bands of the face and palmprint images at different scales including low-low bands of the images at coarse level. The low-low band has all positive transform values and remaining bands have transformed values which are fluctuating around zeros. The larger transform values in these bands respond to sharp changes in brightness and thus to the changes of salient features in the image such as edges, lines, and boundaries. This image fusion rule selects the larger absolute values of the two wavelet coefficients at each point. Therefore, a fused image is produced by performing an inverse

Figure 16. Generic structure of wavelet based fusion approach (Kisku, et. al., 2009)

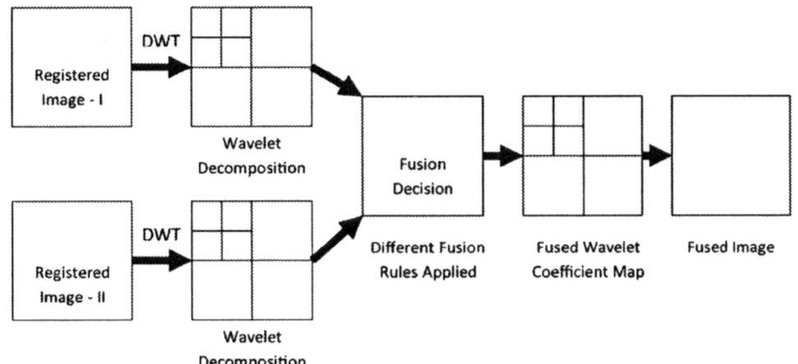

wavelet transform based on integration of wavelet coefficients corresponding to the decomposed face and palmprint images. The generic wavelet-based decomposition and image fusion approach is shown in Figure 16 and Figure 17.

The face and palmprint images are decomposed by a discrete wavelet transform (DWT), the wavelet coefficients are then selected using the 'maximum' fusion rule, and an inverse discrete wavelet transform (IDWT) is performed to reconstruct the fused image. More formally, wavelet fusion methods differ mostly in the fusion rule applied for selection of wavelet coefficients.

The wavelet based image fusion is applied to two-dimensional face and palmprint images at each level which is used "maximum" wavelet fusion rule. Detail description about the wavelet fusion rules is available in (Stathaki, 2008). In maximum fusion rule, maximum wavelet coefficients are selected during any decomposition.

SIFT Features Extraction from Fused Image

The scale invariant feature transform, called SIFT descriptor (Lowe, 1999), has been proved to be invariant to image rotation, scaling, partly illumination changes and the camera view. The fused image is normalized by histogram equalization and after normalization invariants SIFT features are extracted from the fused image. Each feature point is composed of four types of information – spatial location (x, y), scale (S), orientation (θ) and Keypoint descriptor (K). For the sake experiment, only keypoint descriptor information has been taken which consists of a vector of 128 elements representing neighborhood intensity changes of

Figure 17. Wavelet decomposition and fusion of face and palmprint images (Kisku, et. al., 2009)

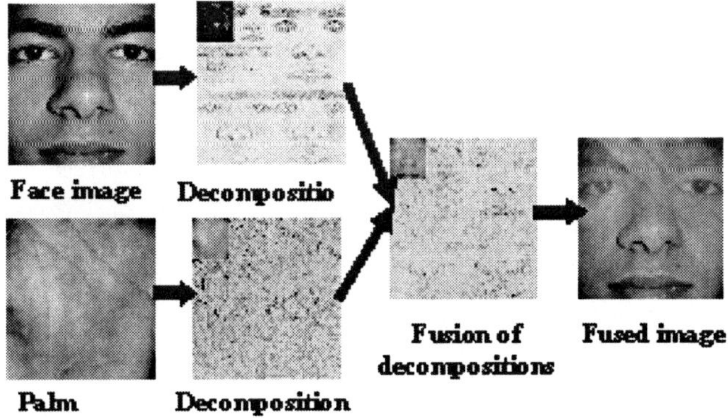

current points. SIFT features extraction a fused image is shown in Figure 18.

Interpretation of Fused Image using Monotonic Decreasing Graph and Matching

In order to establish a monotonic-decreasing graph based relation (Kisku, et. al., 2009; Lin, et. al., 1986) between a pair of fused images, a recursive approach based tree traversal algorithm (Kisku, et. al., 2009; Lin, et. al., 1986) is used for searching the feature points on the probe/query fused sample which are corresponding to the points on the database/gallery fused sample. Verification is performed by computing of differences between a pair of edges that are members of original graph on gallery sample and graph on probe sample, respectively.

The basic assumption is that the moving features points are rigid. Let $\{g_1, g_2 ..., g_m\}$ and $\{p_1, p_2, ..., p_n\}$ be two sets of feature points at the two time instances where $m=n$ or $m \neq n$. But, in 99% cases, it has been seen that identical set of feature points is not available from a pair of instances of a same user or from different users. So, the second case (i.e., $m \neq n$) is considered for the study.

The method is used based on the principle of invariance of distance measures under rigid body motion where deformation of objects does not occur. Using this strategy (Kisku, et. al., 2009),

maximal matching points and minimum matching error is obtained. First, we choose a set of three points, say g_1, g_2 and g_3 on a given fused gallery image which are uniquely determined. These three points are connected to form a triangle $\Delta g_1 g_2 g_3$ with three distances $d(g_1, g_2)$, $d(g_2, g_3)$ and $d(g_1, g_3)$. Now we try to locate another set of three points, p_i, p_j and p_k on a given fused probe image so that the triangle formed by these three points would be best match of the triangle $\Delta g_1 g_2 g_3$. Note that the best match would be possible when the edge (p_i, p_j) matches the edge (g_1, g_2), (p_j, p_k) matches (g_2, g_3) and (p_i, p_k) matches (g_1, g_3). This can be attained when these matches lie within a threshold ε. We can write,

$$\begin{cases} |\, d(p_i, p_j) - d(g_1, g_2)\,| \leq \varepsilon_1 \\ |\, d(p_j, p_k) - d(g_2, g_3)\,| \leq \varepsilon_2 \\ |\, d(p_i, p_k) - d(g_1, g_3)\,| \leq \varepsilon_3 \end{cases} \tag{5.1}$$

Equation (5.1) is used for making closeness between a pair of edges using edge threshold ε. Traversal would be possible when p_i may correspond to g_1 and p_j corresponds to g_2 or conversely, p_j to g_1 and p_i to g_2. Traversal can be started from the first edge (p_i, p_j) and by visiting the feature points, we can generate a matching graph $P' = (p'_1, p'_2, p'_3, ..., p'_m)$ on the fused probe image which should be a corresponding candidate

Figure 18. SIFT features from fused image (Kisku, et. al., 2009)

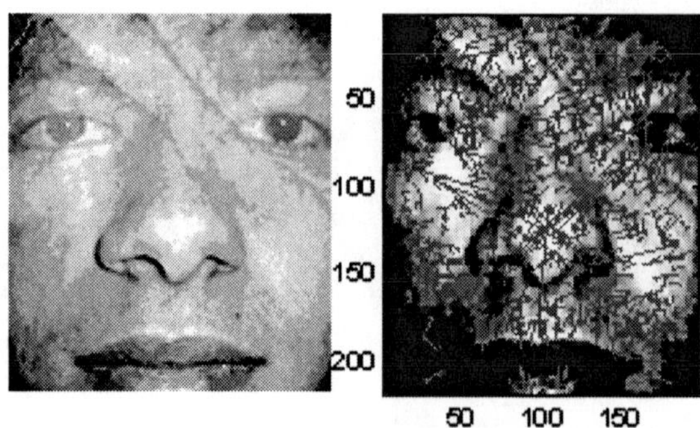

graph of G. In each recursive traversal, a new candidate graph P'_i is found. At the end of the traversal algorithm, a set of candidate graphs $P_{i=1...m}' = (p_{1i}', p_{2i}', p_{3i}', ..., p_{mi}')$ is found and all these graphs are having identical number of feature points.

For illustration, consider the minimal k^{th} order error from G. The final optimal graph P'' can be found from the set of candidate graphs P'_i and we can write,

$$| P''- G |_k \leq | P_i'- G |_k, \forall i$$

The kth order error between P'' and G can be defined as

$$| P''- G |_k = \sum_{i=2}^{m} \sum_{j=1}^{\min(k,i-1)} | d(p_i', p_{i-j}') - d(g_i, g_{i-j}) |,$$
$$\forall k, k = 1, 2, 3, ..., m$$

$$(5.2)$$

Equation (5.2) denotes sum of all differences between a pair edges corresponding to a pair of graphs. This sum can be treated as final dissimilarity value for a pair of graphs and also for a pair of fused images. It is observed that when k is large, the less error correspondence can be found. This is not always true as long as we have a good choice of the edge threshold ϵ. Although for the larger k, more comparison is needed. For identity verification of a person, client-specific threshold has been determined heuristically for each user and the final dissimilarity value is then compared with client-specific threshold and decision is made.

EXPERIMENTAL RESULTS

To verify the efficacy and robustness of graph matching techniques in biometric discussed in the chapter, several biometric databases such as BANCA (Kisku, et. al., 2007; Bailly-Baillire, et. al., 2003), FERET (Philips, et. al., 1998), ORL (formerly known as AT&T) (Samaria, & Harter, 1994), IIT Kanpur (Kisku, et. al., 2009) face databases and IIT Kanpur palmprint database (Kisku, et. al., 2009) are used. This chapter is described three identity verification and recognition techniques and they are invariant face recognition through complete graph topology, face recognition by fusion of invariant features of salient landmarks using probabilistic graphs and biometrics evidence fusion using wavelet decomposition where face and palmprint images are fused. Performance of each technique has been measured through ROC curve. The experimental results are given as follows.

Invariant Face Recognition Using Graph Matching

The graph matching technique has used the BANCA database (Kisku, et. al., 2007; Bailly-Baillire, et. al., 2003) with three matching constraints. BANCA face database is (Bailly-Baillire, et. al., 2003) a challenging, realistic and large face database that has variations of face instances. Face images have recorded in controlled, degraded and adverse conditions with over 12 different sessions spanning three months. In total, face images of 52 subjects are taken from 26 male participants and 26 female participants. For this experiment, the Matched Controlled (*MC*) protocol (Bailly-Baillire, et. al., 2003) is followed where the images from the first session are used for training and second, third, and fourth sessions are used for testing and generating client and impostor scores. Three graph matching constraints which are Gallery Image based Match Constraint (GIBMC) (Kisku, et. al., 2007), Reduced Point based Match Constraint (RPBMC) (Kisku, et. al., 2007) and Regular Grid based Match Constraint (RGBMC) (Kisku, et. al., 2008) have been tested with BANCA face database. The testing images are divided into two groups, *G1* and *G2*, of 26 subjects each. The Prior Equal Error Rate (*PEER*) (Kisku, et. al., 2007), Weighted Error Rate (*WER*) [16] and client-specific threshold are computed using the procedure presented in (Kisku, et. al., 2007).

Prior Equal Error Rates for *G1* and *G2* are presented in Table 1 showing the weighted equal error rates for three different values of *R* (*R* is defined as the cost ratio for three different operating points, namely, *R=0.1*, *R=1* and *R=10*). The corresponding ROC curves are shown in Figure 19. From Table 1 it can be seen that the WER for Reduced Point based Match Constraint (Kisku, et. al., 2007) determined on *G2* is very low while it is compared with other two match constraints. On the other hand, WER on *G1* determined with Regular Grid based Match Constraint (Kisku, et. al., 2008) shows low as it is compared with GIBMC (Kisku, et. al., 2007) and RPBMC (Kisku, et. al., 2007). For *G1*, Regular Grid based Match Constraint outperforms others and for *G2*, Reduced Point based Match Constraint performance better than other two techniques. Therefore, the significant number of features that forming better matched pair of SIFT feature points can be efficiently used in Reduced Point based Match Constraint (RPBMC) and Regular Grid based Match Constraint (RGBMC). Further RGBMC uses grids on face image are formed by dividing the image into 5×5 equal regions with the consideration of 30% overlapping of sub-region boundaries.

This technique is found to perform better than the previous work (Bicego, et. al., 2006) based on the SIFT features. The results show the capability of the system to cope for illumination changes and occlusions occurring in the database or the query face image. It can be compared with the Elastic Bunch Graph Matching technique (Wiskott, et. al., 1997) which is based on a straightforward comparison of image graphs. Identification experiments with the EBGM are reported on the FERET (Philips, et. al., 1998) database as well as the Bochum database (Lades, et. al., 1993) including recognition across different poses but the errors are found to be higher than those obtained from this system. A comprehensive illustration of performances of different techniques has been given in Table 2.

Face Recognition by Fusion of Invariant Features of Salient Landmarks

To investigate the effectiveness and robustness of the graph-based face matching strategy (Kisku, et. al., in press) using fusion of invariant features of salient landmarks, experiments have been carried out on the three face databases, namely FERET (Philips, et. al., 1998), ORL (Samaria, & Harter, 1994) and IITK (Kisku, et. al., in press) face databases.

Experiment with FERET Face Database

The FERET face database (Philips, et. al., 1998) is a collection of face images acquired by NIST. For this evaluation, 1396 face images are considered as training dataset out of which 200 images labeled as *bk*. For query set we have considered

Table 1. Weighted error rates for the GIBMC, RPBMC and RGBMC

Methods → WER ↓	GIBMC (%)	RPBMC (%)	RGBMC (%)
WER (R = 0.1) on G1 WER (R = 0.1) on G2	10.24 6.83	7.09 2.24	4.07 3.01
WER (R = 1) on G1 WER (R = 1) on G2	10.13 6.46	6.66 1.92	4.6 2.52
WER (R = 10) on G1 WER (R = 10) on G2	10.02 6.09	6.24 1.61	4.12 2.02

Table 2. Comparison of recognition rates for different graph-based face biometrics systems

Modality	Method	Database	Recognition rate (%)
Face Recognition	EBGM (Wiskott, et. al., 1997)	FERET (*fa/fb*)	99 (First 10 rank) 98 (First rank)
	Illumination invariant EBGM (Kela, et. al., 2006)	IIT Kanpur Database	93.32
	EBGM with fuzzy fusion (Liu, & Liu, 2005)	FERET (*ba/bj*) FERET (*ba/bk*)	98.9 (best one) 93.4 (best one)
	EBGM with PSO (fully automatic) (Senaratne, et. al., 2009)	FERET (*fb*) FERET (*dup1*)	92 50
	EBGM with PSO (partially automatic) (Senaratne, et. al., 2009)	FERET (*fb*) FERET (*dup1*)	96.1 59.3
	Local labeled graph (Fazi-Ersi, et. al., 2007)	ORL FERET	100 98.4
	MPD (R=0.1) with SIFT features EM (R=0.1) with SIFT features RG (R=0.1) with SIFT features (Non-graph method) (Bicego, et. al., 2006)	BANCA	92.6 (best one) 95.58 (best one) 96.96 (best one)
	GIBMC (R=10) with SIFT features	**BANCA**	**93.91 (best one)**
	RPBMC (R=10) with SIFT features	**BANCA**	**98.39 (best one)**
	RGBMC (R=10) with SIFT features	**BANCA**	**97.98 (best one)**
	SIFT-based graph matching with salient landmarks	**IIT Kanpur** **FERET** **ORL**	**93.63** **92.34** **97.33**

1195 images that are labeled as *fafb*. All these images have been downscaled to 140x100 from the original size of 150x130. For testing purpose, we take *fa* labeled dataset of 1195 and the *duplicate 1* dataset of 722 face images as probe set. In Figure 20, some sample face images are shown from the FERET database (Philips, et. al., 1998). Prior to processing, the faces are well registered to each other and the background effects are eliminated. Moreover, only the frontal view face images are used, which have natural facial expressions (*fa*)

Figure 19. ROC curves for GIBMC, RPBMC and RGBMC determined with BANCA face database (G1 and G2 groups) (Kisku, et. al., 2008)

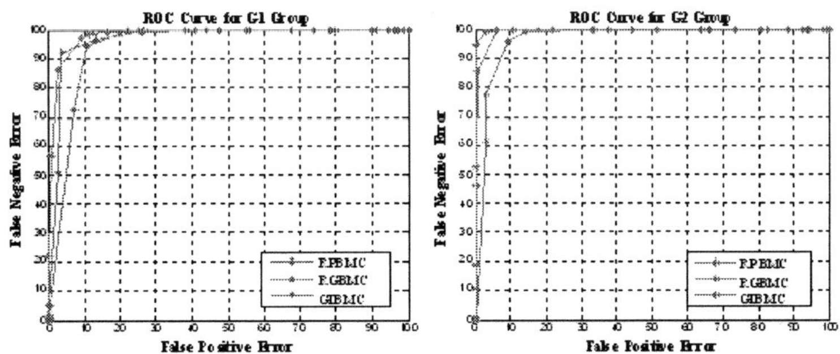

Figure 20. Sample face images of FERET face database. From left to right: from fa dataset, from fb dataset, from hr dataset and from hl dataset (Philips, et. al., 1998).

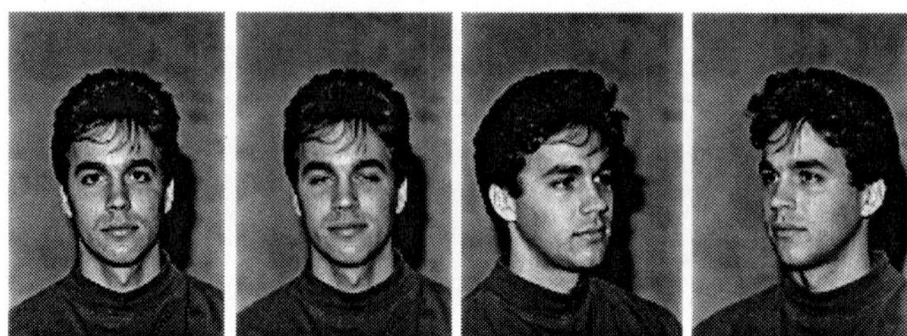

and the face images which have taken under different lighting conditions.

The result obtained from the FERET dataset is shown in Figure 21. The recognition accuracy of the system is found to be 92.34%. Consequently, the result proved to be an appropriate one for changing illumination and facial expression. In addition, the use of invariant SIFT features along with the graph relaxation topology has made this system robust and efficient.

Experiment with IIT Kanpur Database

The IITK face database (Kisku, et. al., in press) consists of 1200 face images with four images per person (300X4). These images are captured under control environment with ±20 degree changes of head pose and with at most uniform lighting and illumination conditions and with almost consistent facial expressions. For the face matching, all probe images are matched against all target images.

From the ROC curve in Figure 21 it has been observed that the recognition accuracy is 93.63%, with the false accept rate (FAR) of 5.82%.

Experiment with ORL Database

The ORL face database (Samaria, & Harter, 1994) consists of 400 images taken from 40 subjects. Out of these 400 images, 200 face images are considered for experiment. It has been observed that there exist changes in orientation in images which lying between -20^0 and 30^0. The face images are found to have the variations in pose and

Figure 21. ROC curves for different methods on different databases (Kisku, et. al., in press)

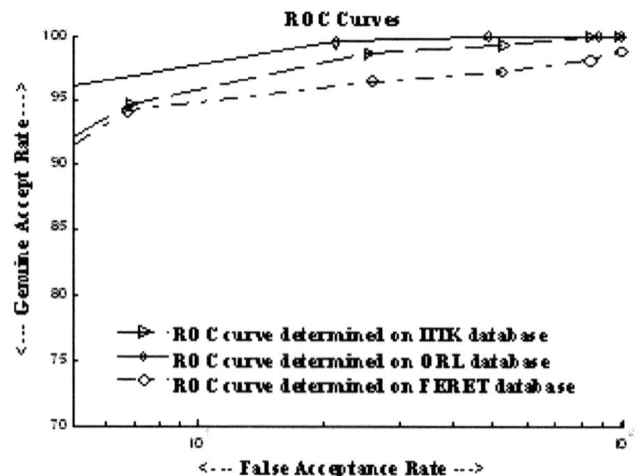

facial expression (smile/not smile, open/closed eyes). The original resolution of the images is 92 x 112 pixels. However, for the experiment, the resolution is set to 120×160 pixels.

From the ROC curve in Figure 21 it has been observed that the recognition accuracy for the ORL database (Samaria, & Harter, 1994) is 97.33%, yielding 2.14% FAR. The relative accuracy of matching strategy for ORL database increases of about 3% and 5% over the IITK database (Kisku, et. al., in press) and the FERET database (Philips, et. al., 1998) respectively.

It has been determined that when the face matching accomplishes with the whole face region, the global features (whole face) are easy to capture and they are generally less discriminative than localized features. In the face recognition method, local facial landmarks are considered for further processing. The optimal face representation using graph relaxation drawn on local landmarks allows matching the localized facial features efficiently by searching the correspondence of keypoints using iterative relaxation.

Biometrics Evidence Fusion by Wavelet Decomposition and Matching Using Monotonic-Decreasing Graph

The experiment of the third method (Kisku, et. al., 2009) is carried out on multimodal database (Kisku, et. al., 2009) of face and palmprint images collected at IIT Kanpur which consists of 750 face images and 750 palmprint images of 150 individuals. Face images are captured under control environment with $\pm 20^0$ changes of head pose and with at most uniform lighting and illumination conditions, and with almost consistent facial expressions. For the sake of experiment, cropped frontal view face has been taken covering face portion only. For the palmprint database, cropped palm portion has been taken from each palmprint image, which contains three principal lines, ridge and bifurcations. The multisensor

biometric evidence fusion method presented here is considered as a semi-sensor fusion approach with some minor adjustable corrections in terms of cropping and registration. Biometric sensors generated face and palmprint images are fused at low level by using wavelet decomposition and fusion of decompositions. After fusion of cropped face and palmprint images of 200×220 pixels, the resolution for fused image has been set to 72 dpi. The fused image is then pre-processed by using histogram equalization. Finally, the matching is performed between a pair of fused images by structural graphs drawn on both the gallery and the probe fused images using extracted SIFT keypoints.

The matching is accomplished for the method and the results show that fusion performance at the semi-sensor level / low level is found to be superior when it is compared with other two monomodal methods, namely, palmprint verification and face recognition drawn on same feature space. Multi-sensor biometric fusion produces 98.19% accuracy while face recognition and palmprint recognition systems produce 89.04% accuracy and 92.17% accuracy respectively, as shown in the Figure 22. The ROC curves shown in Figure 22 illustrate the trade-off between accept rate and false accept rate. Further, it shows that the increase in accept rate is accompanied by decrease in false accept rate happens in each modality, namely, multisensor biometric evidence fusion, palmprint matching and face matching. The theoretical model for multimodal fusion (Poh, & Kittler, 2008) can be treated to produce the same effects as multisensor biometrics fusion and it uses the error bounds to optimize the cost of the multibiometrics system.

Comparison of Different Techniques

In this section, some well known graph matching techniques for biometrics authentication and recognition are compared with the techniques discussed in this chapter. Results of some graph based face recognition techniques are presented

Figure 22. ROC curves for dfferent methods (Kisku, et. al., 2009)

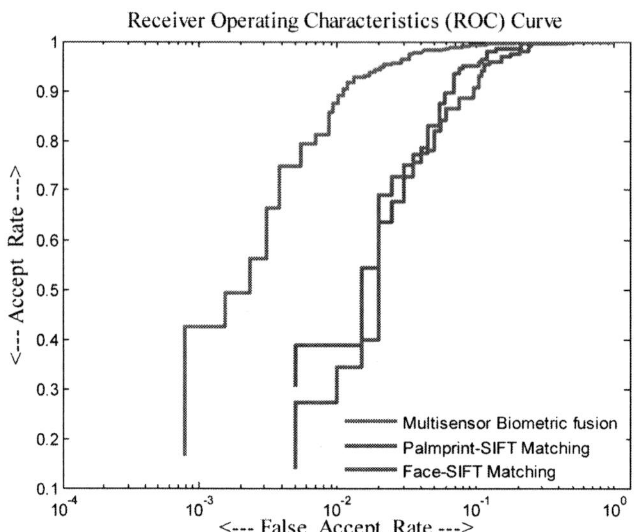

with respect to recognition rates as well as databases used by the techniques. The recognition rates for different techniques are given in Table 2. The first method known as Elastic Bunch Graph Matching technique (Wiskott, et. al., 1997) uses Gabor jets matching and it is tested on FERET database (Philips, et. al., 1998). In this experiment, different poses of face images are used, viz. frontal view with neutral expression (*fa*), frontal view with different facial expression (*fb*), half-profile right (*hr*) or left (*hl*) (rotated by about 40^0 to 70^0) and profile right (*pr*) or left (*pl*). However, recognition results are shown for *fa* and *fb* faces only. For the first rank and for the first 10 ranks, 98% and 99% accuracies are obtained respectively. It shows better accuracies than the techniques (i.e., GIBMC, RPBMC, RG-BMC and salient landmarks methods) discussed in this chapter. However, the traditional EBGM technique is tested on frontal view face images with neutral expression and frontal view face images with different facial expressions. However it does not deal with changes due to illumination. Three techniques; namely, GIBMC, RPBMC and RGBMC are tested on BANCA database and deal with illumination problem as well as variations of

facial expressions. The second method illustrates illumination invariant EBGM (Kela, et. al., 2006) technique for face recognition which achieves 93.32% accuracy and the obtained recognition accuracy is less than that of GIBMC, RPBMC, RGBMC and salient landmarks techniques. These techniques consider the problem occurred on face images due to illumination changes. It is seen that the difference of recognition accuracy between illumination invariant EBGM technique and the salient landmarks technique is about 0.31% which is ignorable. The third technique uses EBGM with fuzzy fusion (Liu, & Liu, 2005) strategy where the recognition performance is found to be compatible with the graph based face recognition techniques presented in this chapter. The fourth technique mentioned in Table 2 uses Particle Swarm Optimization technique for improving EBGM technique (Senaratne, et. al., 2009). Two different variations of EBGM-PSO techniques are presented, namely, fully automatic face recognition and partially automatic face recognition. In order to use the EBGM-PSO technique (Senaratne, et. al., 2009) for face recognition in real time environment, fully automatic system is more useful than partial one. However, the performance of partially automatic system is found to be much better than that of fully automatic one in terms of recognition accuracy. These two experimental variations are tested on FERET database with *fb* and *dup1* datasets. Fully automatic system achieves 92% and 50% recognition accuracies while partially automatic system achieves 96.1% and 59.3% accuracies with *fb* and *dup1* datasets respectively. Experimentally, irrespective of methodological criteria and classifiers used, the EBGM-PSO technique and the Salient Landmarks methods are found to be very similar. However, the salient landmarks method is found to be superior to that of EBGM-PSO method and also its computational complexity is less than that of EBGM-PSO method because of use of less complicated feature extraction and classifiers in salient landmarks method. Other face recognition methods, viz. GIBMC, RPBMC and RGBMC are discussed in this chapter outperform the EBGM-PSO method. The fifth method (Fazi-Ersi, et. al., 2007) describes a face recognition method using local labeled graph drawn on each face and the technique uses two-stage feature matching for recognition. On the other hand, the methods which are presented in this chapter are implemented with single-stage feature matching for recognition. The performance of local labeled graph matching is found to be superior to the later ones while FERET and ORL databases are used. On ORL database 100% recognition accuracy is obtained and in contrast, 98.4% recognition accuracy is obtained on FERET database. However, due to the use of two-stage feature matching criteria, its computational complexity is higher than that of the face recognition methods (GIBMC, RPBMC, RGBMC and salient landmarks method).

The graph based face recognition techniques (GIBMC, RPBMC, RGBMC and salient landmarks) are also compared with the non-graph based face recognition methods (Bicego, et. al., 2006), viz. MPD, EM and RG (see Table 2). Both these graph based and non-graph based face recognition techniques are implemented with SIFT features. From the table, it can be seen that non-graph based

methods are performed well while regular grids are used on the whole face. However, recognition results of the graph based methods are found to be superior to that of non-graph based methods as indicated in Table 2. The bold face letters denote the techniques that are discussed in this chapter.

SUMMARY

Graphs offer an extremely useful and powerful feature representation technique in pattern recognition and classification, machine learning and computer vision fields. There exist many other feature representation techniques used in computer and machine vision fields such as appearance based, feature based and model based techniques. These techniques specially have been used in biometric recognition. However, graph representation of feature space not only provides good representation capability but also provides robustness to the system. It often requires in the field of biometrics that the matching of relational structures becomes an important task of solving the identity verification and identification problem. The matching of relational structures can be transformed into the matching problem of two graphs in biometrics which is proved to be useful. In graph based biometrics authentication, extracted features are encoded in the form of graph which is further used for matching of two graphs and compute the matching proximity of corresponding two biometric samples. The encoding scheme using graphs reflect the topological relations between the feature points. While matching is performed between two graphs, one graph is mapped to another graph and amount of deflection occurred to the feature points is computed. When the deflection of feature points is less for a pair of graphs, best match is found.

This chapter discusses the graph matching algorithms exploited to biometrics recognition. Despite the graph based biometric systems, an automatic SIFT feature detection through staged filtering approach is presented. Section 1 and 2 briefly introduces overview of biometric systems along with the state-of-the-art graph based biometric systems. Graph techniques used in different biometric traits including fingerprint, face and iris recognition are discussed. Different state-of-the-art graph based fingerprint systems such as relational graph based fingerprint verification, fuzzy bipartite weighted graph based fingerprint system and directional variance with graph matching are discussed while EBGM technique for face recognition and Particle Swarm Optimization based graph matching technique used in face recognition are also discussed. Further, a graph based iris recognition system is discussed in this section where graph cut algorithm is used for pupil detection from the background.

Section 3 discusses SIFT-based face recognition where complete graph topology has been presented for graph matching. Three variations of the technique are used for identity verification, namely, Gallery Image based Match Constraint (GIBMC), Reduced Point based Match Constraint (RPBMC) and Regular Grid based Match Constraint (RGBMC). Graphs are drawn on SIFT features which are extracted from face images. Then based on to the graph matching constraints, graphs are being drawn on extracted SIFT feature points and matching is performed. GIBMC uses all of the feature points which are extracted from face image and the corresponding points are also determined on the second face image. Very small number of SIFT points are used for matching of faces and a graph on these points is drawn. The matching constraint RGBMC makes use of the grids of faces. Initially, face image is divided into 25 sub-regions of equal size and then graphs are drawn on the sub-regions of faces. Finally, matching is performed between two graphs corresponding to a pair of sub-regions.

Next section has been discussed a face recognition by fusion of invariant SIFT features extracted from salient facial parts of a face. Both the eyes, nose and mouth parts are considered as salient facial regions from where the SIFT features are extracted and on these SIFT feature points probabilistic graphs are drawn for individual salient parts. Matching are then performed between salient parts correspond to a pair of faces. The matching scores are obtained from each matching components are then fused using Dempster-Shafer decision theory and finally, acceptance or rejection decision is made.

Section 5 addresses a biometrics evidence fusion through palmprint and face images using wavelet decomposition and monotonic-decreasing graph. Monotonic-decreasing structural graphs are used for fused image representation and matching. SIFT features are extracted from the fused image and graph is then drawn on these feature points. By recursive descent tree traversal algorithm, the most probable graph is determined and matching is performed.

Section 6 discusses experimental results of the graph based face recognition techniques, viz. gallery image based match constraint, reduced point based match constraint, regular grid based match constraint, salient landmarks. A comparison of the graph based face recognition techniques with the graph based and non-graph based techniques is also presented in this section.

Therefore, the graph representation and matching algorithms are proved to be useful to biometrics authentication and recognition. Along with the graph matching algorithms, SIFT descriptor is also proved to be a useful tool for invariant feature extraction. SIFT features are invariant to rotation, scaling, partial illumination and 3D projective transform. In the present days, the use of graphs in biometrics is essential part of identity verification. The graph algorithms are comparable with other pattern recognition algorithms in terms of computational complexity and accuracy. The experimental results show robustness and efficacy of the biometric systems discussed in this chapter.

REFERENCES

Abuhaiba, I. S. I. (2007). Offline signature verification using graph matching. *Turk Journal of Electronic Engineering, 15*(1), 89–104.

Bailly-Baillire, E., Bengio, S., Bimbot, F., Hamouz, M., Kitler, J., Marithoz, J., et al. (2003). The BANCA database and evaluation protocol. *Proceedings of International Conference on Audio – and Video-Based Biometric Person Authentication* (pp. 625 – 638).

Barnett, J. A. (1981). Computational methods for a mathematical theory of evidence. Proceedings of *International Conference on Artificial Intelligence* (pp. 868-875).

Bauer, M. (1996). Approximation algorithms and decision-making in the dempster-shafer theory of evidence—An empirical study. *International Journal of Approximate Reasoning, 17,* 217–237. doi:10.1016/S0888-613X(97)00013-3

Bicego, M., Lagorio, A., Grosso, E., & Tistarelli, M. (2006). On the use of SIFT features for face authentication. *Proceedings of IEEE International Workshop on Biometrics, in association with CVPR.*

Conte, D., Foggia, P., Sansone, C., & Vente, M. (2003). Graph matching applications in pattern recognition and image processing, *Proceedings of International Conference on Image Processing.*

Daugman, J. (1993). High confidence visual recognition of persons by a test of statistical independence. *IEEE Transactions on Pattern Analysis and Machine Intelligence, 15*(11), 1148–1161. doi:10.1109/34.244676

Fan, K.-C., Liu, C.-W., & Wang, Y.-K. (1998). A fuzzy bipartite weighted graph matching approach to fingerprint verification, *IEEE International Conference on Systems, Man and Cybernetics* (pp. 4363-4368).

Fazi-Ersi, E., Zelek, J. S., & Tsotsos, J. K. (2007). Robust face recognition through local graph matching. *Journal of Computers, 2*(5), 31–37.

Gourier, N., James, D. H., & Crowley, L. (2004). Estimating face orientation from robust detection of salient facial structures. *FG Net Workshop on Visual Observation of Deictic Gestures.*

Gross, J. L., & Yellen, J. (2005). *Graph theory and its applications.* Boca Raton, FL: Chapman & Hall/CRC.

Jain, A. K., Flynn, P., & Ross, A. (2007). *Handbook of biometrics.* New York: Springer.

Jain, A. K., & Ross, A. (2004). Multibiometric systems. *Communications of the ACM, 47*(1), 34–40. doi:10.1145/962081.962102

Jain, A. K., Ross, A., & Pankanti, S. (2006). Biometrics: A tool for information security. *IEEE Transactions on Information Forensics and Security, 1*(2), 125–143. doi:10.1109/TIFS.2006.873653

Jain, A. K., Ross, A., & Prabhakar, S. (2004). An introduction to biometric recognition. *IEEE Transactions on Circuits and Systems for Video Technology, Special Issue on Image- and Video-Based Biometrics, 14*(1), 4-20.

Kela, N., Rattani, A., & Gupta, P. (2006). Illumination invariant elastic bunch graph matching for efficient face recognition. In *Proceedings of Conference on Computer Vision and Pattern Recognition Workshop.*

Kisku, D. R., Gupta, P., & Sing, J. K. (in press). Face recognition by fusion of invariant facial landmarks.

Kisku, D. R., Gupta, P., & Sing, J. K. (in press). Fusion of multiple matchers using SVM for offline signature identification, *International Conference on Security Technology (SecTech).*

Kisku, D. R., Rattani, A., Grosso, E., & Tistarelli, M. (2007). Face identification by SIFT-based complete graph topology, *5th IEEE International Workshop on Automatic Identification Advanced Technologies (AutoId)* (pp. 63—68).

Kisku, D. R., Rattani, A., Tistarelli, M., & Gupta, P. (2008). Graph application on face for personal authentication and recognition. *Proceedings of 10th IEEE International Conference on Control, Automation, Robotics and Vision* (pp. 1150—1155).

Kisku, D. R., Sing, J. K., Tistarelli, M., & Gupta, P. (2009). Multisensor biometric evidence fusion for person authentication using wavelet decomposition and monotonic-decreasing graph. In *Proceedings of 7th IEEE International Conference on Advances in Pattern Recognition* (pp. 205—208).

Kokiopoulou, E., & Frossard, P. (2009). Video face recognition using graph based semi-supervised learning, *International Conference on Multimedia and Expo* (pp. 1564-1565).

Lades, M., Vorbrüggen, J. C., Buhmann, J., Lange, J., von der Malsburg, C., Würtz, R. P., & Konen, W. (1993). Distortion invariant object recognition in the dynamic link architecture. *IEEE Transactions on Computers, 42*(3), 300–311. doi:10.1109/12.210173

Li, S. Z., & Jain, A. K. (Eds.). (2005). *Handbook of face recognition.* New York: Springer.

Lim, S., Lee, K., Byeon, O., & Kim, T. (2001). Efficient iris recognition through improvement of feature vector and classifier. *ETRI Journal, 23*(2), 61–70. doi:10.4218/etrij.01.0101.0203

Lin, Z. C., Lee, H., & Huang, T. S. (1986). Finding 3-D point correspondences in motion estimation. *Proceedings of International Conference on Pattern Recognition* (pp.303 – 305).

Liu, J., & Liu, Z.-Q. (2005). EBGM with fuzzy fusion on face. *Advances in Artificial Intelligence. LNCS, 3809,* 498–509.

LiuZ. (2005). http://www.eecs.lehigh.edu/SPCRL/IF/image_fusion.htm

Lowe, D. G. (1999). Object recognition from local scale invariant features. *International Conference on Computer Vision* (pp. 1150–1157).

Lowe, D. G. (2004). Distinctive image features from scale invariant keypoints. *International Journal of Computer Vision, 60*(2), 91–110. doi:10.1023/B:VISI.0000029664.99615.94

Ma, L., Tan, T., Wang, Y., & Zhang, D. (2004). Efficient iris recognition by characterizing key local variations. *IEEE Transactions on Image Processing, 13*(6), 739–750. doi:10.1109/TIP.2004.827237

Maltoni, D., Maio, D., Jain, A. K., & Prabhakar, S. (Eds.). (2003). *Handbook of fingerprint recognition.* Springer.

Mehrabian, H., & Hashemi-Tari, P. (2007). *Pupil boundary detection for iris recognition using graph cuts* (pp. 77–82). Image and Vision Computing New Zealand.

Neuhaus, M., & Benke, H. (2005). *A graph matching based approach to fingerprint classification using directional variance, Audio and Video based Biometric Person Authentication (Vol. 3546,* pp. 191–200). LNCS.

Phillips, P. J., Wechsler, H., Huang, J., & Rauss, P. (1998). The FERET database and evaluation procedure for face-recognition algorithms. *Image and Vision Computing Journal, 16*(5), 295–306. doi:10.1016/S0262-8856(97)00070-X

Poh, N., & Kittler, J. (2008). On Using Error Bounds to Optimize Cost-sensitive Multimodal Biometric Authentication, *17th International Conference on Pattern Recognition* (pp. 1 – 4)

Ross, A., & Govindarajan, R. (2005). Feature Level Fusion Using Hand and Face Biometrics, In. *Proceedings of SPIE Conference on Biometric Technology for Human Identification, II,* 196–204.

Ross, A., & Jain, A. K. (2003). Information Fusion in Biometrics. *Pattern Recognition Letters, 24,* 2115–2125. doi:10.1016/S0167-8655(03)00079-5

Samaria, F., & Harter, A. (1994). Parameterization of a stochastic model for human face identification. In *Proceedings of IEEE Workshop on Applications of Computer Vision.*

Senaratne, R., & Halgamuge, S. (2006). Optimized landmark model matching for face recognition. In *Proceedings of 7th International Conference on Automatic Face and Gesture Recognition* (pp. 120–125).

Senaratne, R., Halgamuge, S., & Hsu, A. (2009). Face recognition by extending elastic bunch graph matching with particle swarm optimization. *Journal of Multimedia, 4*(4), 204–214. doi:10.4304/jmm.4.4.204-214

Sentz, K., & Ferson, S. (2002). Combination of Evidence in Dempster–Shafer Theory, Sandia National Laboratories SAND 2002-0835.

Smeraldi, F., Capdevielle, N., & Bigün, J. (1999). Facial features detection by saccadic exploration of the gabor decomposition and support vector machines. *Proceedings of the 11th Scandinavian Conference on Image Analysis* (pp. 39-44).

Stathaki, T. (2008). *Image fusion – algorithms and applications.* United Kingdom: Academic Press.

Tarjoman, M., & Zarei, S. (2008). Automatic fingerprint classification using graph theory, World Academy of Science. *Engineering and Technology, 47,* 214–218.

Wildes, R. P. (1997). Iris recognition: An emerging biometric technology. *Proceedings of the IEEE, 85,* 1348–1363. doi:10.1109/5.628669

Wiskott, L., Fellous, J. M., Kruger, N., & von der Malsburg, C. (1997). Face recognition by elastic bunch graph matching. *IEEE Transactions on Pattern Analysis and Machine Intelligence, 19*(7), 775–779. doi:10.1109/34.598235

Yaghi, H., & Krim, H. (2008). Probabilistic graph matching by canonical decomposition. *Proceedings of the IEEE International Conference on Image Processing* (pp. 2368 – 2371).

Zhang, H., & Ma, H. (2005). Grid-based parallel elastic graph matching face recognition. [LNCS.]. *Proceedings of International Workshop on Web-Based Internet Computing for Science and Engineering, 3842,* 1041–1048.

KEY TERMS AND DEFINITIONS

Biometrics: Techniques for identifying or verifying people based on their physiological and/or behavioral characteristics.

Graphs: A collection of objects where objects are connected by links or simple paths.

Authentication: A process by which we can establish the identity of a person who he claims to be.

Identification: A process by which a captured biometric sample is compared with a biometric database in attempt to identify an unknown person.

SIFT: Known as Scale Invariant Feature Transform which is used to detect and extract the useful invariant features from the objects. These keypoint features are invariant to rotation, scaling, partial illumination and 3D projective transform.

APPENDIX

Suppose two experts are consulted regarding a system failure. The failure could be caused by Component A, Component B or Component C. The first expert believes that the failure is due to Component A with a probability of 0.99 or Component B with a probability of 0.01 (denoted by $m1(A)$ and $m1(B)$, respectively). The second expert believes that the failure is due to Component C with a probability of 0.99 or Component B with a probability of 0.01 (denoted by $m2(C)$ and $m2(B)$, respectively). The distributions can be represented by the following:

Expert 1:

$m1(A) = 0.99$ (failure due to Component A)

$m1(B) = 0.01$ (failure due to Component B)

Expert 2:

$m2(B) = 0.01$ (failure due to Component B)

$m2(C) = 0.99$ (failure due to Component C)

The combination of the masses associated with the experts is summarized in Table 3.

Table 3. An Example of Dempster Combination rule (Sentz, & Ferson, 2002)

			Expert 1			
			A	B	C	Failure Cause
			0.99	0.01	0	m_1
Expert 2	Failure Cause	m_2				
	A	0	$m_1(A)m_2(A) = 0$	$m_1(B)m_2(A) = 0$	$m_1(C)m_2(A) = 0$	
	B	0.01	$m_1(A)m_2(B) = 0.0099$	$m_1(B)m_2(B) = 0.0001$	$m_1(C)m_2(B) = 0$	
	C	0.99	$m_1(A)m_2(C) = 0.9801$	$m_1(B)m_2(C) = 0.0099$	$m_1(C)m_2(C) = 0$	

Chapter 11

Biometric Identity Based Encryption:
Security, Efficiency and Implementation Challenges

Neyire Deniz Sarier
Bonn-Aachen International Center for Information Technology, Germany

EXECUTIVE SUMMARY

In this chapter, we evaluate the security properties and different applications of Identity Based Encryption (IBE) systems. Particularly, we consider biometric identities for IBE, which is a new encryption system defined as fuzzy IBE. Next, we analyze the security aspects of fuzzy IBE in terms of the security notions it must achieve and the prevention of collusion attacks, which is an attack scenario specific to fuzzy IBE. In this context, we present a new method that avoids the collusion attacks and describe the currently most efficient biometric IBE scheme that implements this new method. Also, we investigate implementation challenges for biometric IBE systems, where fuzzy IBE could be a potential cryptographic primitive for biometric smartcards. Due to the limited computational power of these devices, a different solution for biometric IBE is considered, which is the encryption analogue of the biometric identity based signature system of Burnett et al. (2007). Finally, we state the future trends for biometric IBE systems and conclude our results.

INTRODUCTION

Cryptography consists of set of mathematical techniques to achieve the goals of confidentiality, data integrity, entity authentication, and data origin authentication in order to provide information security in theory and in practice. These cryptographic goals can be summarized as follows (Sarier, 2007).

- *Confidentiality:* Confidentiality is the protection of transmitted data from passive attacks. Other aspect of confidentiality is the protection of traffic flow from analysis.
- *Authentication:* It is concerned with assurance of identity. It ensures that the origin of a message or electronic document is

DOI: 10.4018/978-1-60960-015-0.ch011

correctly identified, and the identity is not false. When a sales clerk compares the signature on the back of a credit card with the signature on a sales slip, the clerk is using the handwritten signatures as an authentication mechanism, to verify the person presenting the credit card is the person the card was sent to by the issuing bank.

- *Data Integrity*: assures that data has not been modified since the signature was applied. In other words, it ensures that only authorized parties are able to modify computer system assets and transmitted information. While a handwritten signature does not in itself provide data integrity services, digital signatures provide excellent data integrity services by virtue of the digital signature value being a function of the message digest; even the slightest modification of digitally signed messages will always result in signature verification failure.

- *Non-repudiation*: It prevents either sender or receiver from denying a transmitted message and could provide evidence to a third-party (like a judge, or jury, for example). The buyer's signature on the credit card sales slip provides evidence of the buyer's participation in the transaction, and protects the store and the card-issuing bank from false denials of participation in the transaction by the buyer.

- *Access Control:* It is the ability to limit and control the access to host systems and applications via communications links.

- *Availability:* It requires that computer system assets be available to authorized parties when needed.

Encryption tries to solve the problem of secure communication over an insecure channel, where apart from the sender and the receiver, an adversary may involve controlling the channel. The two types of encryption schemes are called as symmetric and asymmetric encryption, where the basic difference is the same secret key that is shared in the former one, whereas a pair of keys called public and secret key take part in the latter one. In addition, in symmetric encryption, the shared secret key must be transferred through a secure channel while asymmetric encryption does not require a secure channel to pass the encryption key at the cost of *authentication of public* keys. This way the sender A is sure that he is encrypting under the legitimate public key of the receiver.

The setting of public-key cryptography (PKC) is asymmetric in key information held by the parties, since one party (Bob) has a secret key while another (Alice) uses the public key that matches this secret key. This is in contrast to symmetric encryption, where both parties share the same key. Asymmetric encryption is thus another name for public-key encryption. Bob generates the pair of public/secret keys that belong to him and sends his public key over an authenticated channel to Alice, so that Alice can encrypt a message with Bob's public key to be sent to him. The only person, who is able to read the message, is Bob, since only he possesses the secret key, which cannot be recovered in polynomial time. The authenticated channel is necessary to assure Alice that the public key of Bob really belongs to Bob. One difference between the symmetric and the asymmetric setting is the channel over which the keys are distributed. Instead of a secure channel, an authenticated channel is sufficient for PKC. On the other hand, PKC requires much more computational resources as the number-theoretic operations in these schemes are computationally costly relative to symmetric key cryptography (SKC), which should considered for energy-constrained ad hoc network devices. Hence, to minimize the amount of data to which these number-theoretic operations are applied, public key cryptography is used only to encrypt small data (short strings), namely symmetric encryption keys and digital signatures.

Besides, key management is easier in PKC since authenticity of public key through certificates is sufficient to encrypt any message with it, their secrecy is not needed. However, an on-line trusted server i.e. a certificate authority (CA) is required for verifying the identity of the receiver and issuing a tamper resistant and non-spoofable digital certificate for participants. Such certificates are signed data blocks stating that this public key belongs to that receiver. The trusted server is part of every secure message transmission, there is high server traffic and the sender and central server have to be online to provide secure communication.

To avoid the disadvantages of PKC, a special form of public key cryptography is defined as Identity Based Encryption (IBE) which does not require the binding of the peer identity and its public key through the certification by a trusted third party. Since the public key of an entity can be his email address, IP address or his identity, there is no need for a Public Key Infrastructure (PKI), CA and CA hierarchy, key directory, centralized online authority and pair wise pre-shared secrets among all involved parties. Only an offline authority called Private Key Generator (PKG) is necessary for keying and for adding a timestamp or a sequence number to the identity (namely his public key) proposed by the node when joining the system, to avoid collisions in name space.

BACKGROUND

Identity based encryption (IBE) scheme consists of four algorithms: Setup, Extract, Encrypt and Decrypt.

- *Setup:* Given a security parameter k, setup generates the parameters of the scheme, master public key M_{pk} and the master secret key M_{sk}, where M_{sk} is only known to PKG. In addition, the description of a finite message space M as M= $\{0, 1\}^l$ and the description of a finite ciphertext space C are part of the scheme parameters.

- *Extract:* Given an arbitrary identifier string $ID_i = \{0, 1\}^*$ of entity i, M_{sk} and the system parameters the algorithm returns the private key d_i associated to the given identity. Considering the ID_i as a public key, the algorithm returns its private key.
- *Encrypt:* Given the system parameters, a message m ε M and an identity ID, the algorithm returns a ciphertext c ε C
- *Decrypt:* Given a ciphertext c ε C, and a private key d of identity ID, the algorithm returns the message m.

To be consistent, an IBE scheme must satisfy the following condition for all messages in M.

$\forall$ m εM Decrypt(M_{pk}, c, d) = M where c = Encrypt(M_{pk}, ID, m)

Most of the IBE schemes make use of a bilinear pairing, which is implemented using a weil or a tate pairing on elliptic curves. Let G and F be two cyclic groups of the same prime order q, where G is an additive group of points of an elliptic curve and F is a multiplicative group of a finite field (Sarier, 2007). IBE depends on a special type of function called a bilinear map, which is a pairing with the property Pair (a • P, b • Q) = Pair (b • P, a • Q). For IBE, the operator "•" represents the multiplication of integers with points on elliptic curves. While multiplication itself (e.g., calculating a•P) is easy, the *inverse* operation (finding a from P and a•P) is practically impossible due to the elliptic curve discrete logarithm problem, which is explained as follows. If E is an elliptic curve over a finite field and P is a point on E, then the discrete log problem on E to the base P is finding an integer a such that aP= Q, given a point Q on E and if such an integer exists.

A map ê: GxG→F is called an admissible bilinear map satisfying the following properties.

- *Bilinear:* The map ê: GxG→F is bilinear if ê (aP, bQ) = ê (P,Q)^{ab} $\forall$ P,Q ε G and $\forall$ a,b ε Z.

- *Non-degenerate:* Given a point $Q \varepsilon G$, $\hat{e}(Q, R) = 1_F \ \forall \ R \ \varepsilon \ G$ iff $Q=1_G$, which implies that if P is a generator of G then $\hat{e}(P, P)$ is a generator of F.
- *Computable:* $\hat{e}(Q, R)$ is efficiently computed $\forall \ Q, R \ \varepsilon \ G$

Consequently, any bilinear map defined as above is symmetric: $\hat{e}(Q, R) = \hat{e}(R, Q)$ if Q=sP and R=hP where s, $h \ \varepsilon \ Z$ and P a generator

$$\hat{e}(Q, R) = \hat{e}(sP, hP) = \hat{e}(P, P)^{sh} = \hat{e}(hP, sP) = \hat{e}(R, Q)$$

A NEW PRIMITIVE: FUZZY IBE

In Eurocrypt'04, Sahai and Waters proposed a new Identity Based Encryption (IBE) system called fuzzy IBE, which provides error tolerance property in IBE in order to use biometric attributes as the identity instead of an arbitrary string like an email address. This new system combines the advantages of IBE with using biometrics as an identity, where IBE avoids the need for an online Public Key Infrastructure (PKI), which is the most inefficient and costly part of public key encryption. The use of biometrics as the identity in the framework of IBE simplifies the process of key generation at the Private Key Generator (PKG). Since biometric information is unique, unforgettable and non-transferable, the user only needs to provide his biometrics at the PKG to obtain his secret key instead of presenting special documents and credentials to convince the PKG about his identity. Also, biometrics is attached to the user; hence the user does not need to remember any password, to use any public key or even an e-mail address since the public key of the user is always with him to be used for encryption during an ad hoc meeting. Finally, biometric data could be easily integrated with fuzzy IBE due to its error tolerance property, which is required for the noisy nature of biometrics. The main feature of fuzzy IBE is the construction of the secret key based on the biometric data of the user which can decrypt a ciphertext encrypted with a slightly different measurement of the same biometrics. Specifically, fuzzy IBE allows for error tolerance in the decryption stage, where a ciphertext encrypted with the biometrics w could be decrypted by the receiver using the private key corresponding to the biometrics w', provided that w and w' are within a certain distance of each other. Besides, fuzzy IBE could be applied in the context of Attribute-Based Encryption (ABE), where the sender encrypts data using a set of attributes such as {university, faculty, department} and the ciphertext could only be decrypted if the receiver has the secret key associated to all of these attributes or sufficient number of them (Sarier, 2010).

In current fuzzy IBE schemes, the private key components are generated by combining the values of a unique polynomial evaluated on each attribute with the master secret key. This way, different users, each having some portion of the secret keys associated to the attributes of a given ciphertext c cannot collude to decrypt c, which guarantees collusion resistance. The basic fuzzy IBE schemes guarantee a weak level of security for identity based setting i.e. Indistinguishability against Chosen Plaintext Attack (IND-sID-CPA), but they could be combined with well-known generic conversion systems to obtain a high level of security i.e. Indistinguishability against Chosen Ciphertext Attack (IND-sID-CCA). Besides, the biometrics is considered as public information; hence the compromise of the biometrics does not affect the security of the system. Thus, in existing systems, biometrics w of the receiver is sent together with the corresponding ciphertext.

RELATED WORK

The first fuzzy IBE scheme is described by Sahai & Waters (2005) and its security is reduced to the MBDH problem in the standard model, where the size of the public parameters is linear in the size of the attribute space U or the number of attributes of a user n. Piretti et al. (2006) achieved a more efficient fuzzy IBE scheme with short public parameter size by employing the Random Oracle Model (ROM). Baek et al. (2007) described two new fuzzy IBE schemes with an efficient key generation algorithm and proved the security in ROM based on the DBDH assumption. Also, in (Liesdonk, 2007), an anonymous fuzzy IBE scheme is described based on the Boneh Franklin IBE scheme (Boneh & Franklin, 2003), where anonymity guarantees that an adversary cannot tell who the recipient is by looking at the ciphertext, which could be used to thwart traffic analysis. The main disadvantage of the schemes in (Piretti et al., 2006; Baek et al., 2007) is the use of the MapToPoint hash function, which is inefficient compared to the ordinary hash functions. Recently, Sarier (2008) described a new biometric IBE scheme called as BIO-IBE, which is more efficient compared to the existing fuzzy IBE schemes due to the replacement of the MapToPoint hash function with an ordinary hash function. Besides, Burnett et al (Burnett et al., 2007) described a biometric Identity Based Signature (IBS) scheme called BIO-IBS, where they used the biometric information as the identity and construct the public key of the user using a fuzzy extractor (Dodis et al., 2004), which is then used in the modified SOK-IBS scheme. Although another biometric IBE scheme based on Baek et al's scheme is described in (Shi et al., 2009) by using fuzzy extractor to construct the public key (identity) of a user similar to the BIO-IBS/BIO-IBE approach, still MaptoPoint hash function is required for the construction.

DEFINITION OF FUZZY IBE

A **fuzzy IBE** scheme consists of four algorithms: Setup, Extract, Encrypt and Decrypt.

- **Setup**: Given a security parameter k, setup generates the parameters of the scheme, master public key M_{pk} and the master secret key M_{sk}, where M_{sk} is only known to PKG. In addition, the description of a finite message space M as $M= \{0, 1\}^l$ and the description of a finite ciphertext space C are part of the scheme parameters. Finally, U denotes the feature space of biometrics.

- **Extract**: Given the biometric vector $w= w_1, ..., w_n \in U$ and the system parameters the algorithm returns the private key D associated to the given user.

- **Encrypt**: Given the system parameters, a message $m \varepsilon M$ and the receivers biometrics w', it returns a ciphertext $c \varepsilon C$

- **Decrypt**: Given a ciphertext $c \varepsilon C$, and a private key D for w, the algorithm chooses a set $S \subset w \cap w^*$ such that $|S|=d$ and using Lagrange Interpolation in the exponents of the d bilinear pairings, it returns the message m. Here, d denotes the error tolerance parameter of the fuzzy IBE scheme.

To be consistent, an IBE scheme must satisfy the following condition for all messages in M.

$\forall\ m\ \varepsilon M$ Decrypt $(M_{pk}, c, d) = M$ where c = Encrypt (M_{pk}, w', m)

SECURITY MODEL OF FUZZY IBE

Most of the fuzzy IBE systems described achieve the notion of IND-sID-CPA, where selective identity attack is a weak model, but they could be combined with well-known generic conversion systems to obtain a high level of security i.e. Indistinguishability against Chosen Ciphertext Attack (IND-sID-CCA).

Basically, a fuzzy IBE scheme is IND-sID-CPA secure, if no polynomially bounded adversary A has a non-negligible advantage against the Challenger in the following IND-sID-CPA game.

- *Select:* The adversary A selects a target identity $w^* \in U$

- *Setup:* The challenger runs the Setup algorithm with the security parameter k and returns the adversary the system parameters and the master public key M_{pk}.
- *Phase 1:* The adversary issues private key extraction and the challenger responds with the private keys corresponding to the public key $|w \cap w^*| < d$
- *Challenge:* The adversary outputs equal length plaintexts m_0, m_1 εM provided that it was not queried in Phase 1. The challenger picks a random bit $b\varepsilon$ $\{0, 1\}$ and sends the adversary the encryption of m_b under w^* and M_{pk} as the challenge.
- *Phase 2:* The adversary issues adaptively extraction as in Phase 1, with the restriction that identities of $|w \cap w^*| > d$ cannot be queried.
- *Guess:* The adversary outputs a guess b' ε $\{0, 1\}$ and wins the game if b'=b.

Such an adversary is called an IND-sID-CPA adversary A, who successfully breaks the fuzzy IBE scheme if he guesses the random bit correctly with a probability significantly better than just random guessing and its advantage ε against the scheme with security parameter k is defined as below. The random bits used by the adversary and challenger defines the probability and negl(k) denotes the negligible function.

$Adv_{\varepsilon,A}$ (k)=| Pr[b=b']- ½ | <negl(k)

COLLUSION ATTACKS

Any biometric IBE/IBS scheme requires the biometric measurement of the receiver or the signer, respectively. For this purpose, the biometrics of the user is

captured using a sensor and the raw biometric data is further processed to extract the feature vector and to obtain the biometric template b of the user. In a biometric encryption scheme, feature extraction is applied on the raw biometric data to obtain the feature vector (or the attributes) and then, each attribute is associated with a unique integer $w_i \varepsilon Z_p$ to form the identity $w = (w_1, ...,w_n)$ (Piretti, 2006). Here, n denotes the size of the attributes of each user. Since some of the attributes could be common in some users, a unique polynomial is selected for each user and included in the key generation algorithm to bind the private key to the user. This way, different users cannot collude in order to decrypt a ciphertext that should only be decrypted by the real receiver.

In the biometric cryptosystems such as BIO-IBS (Burnett et al., 2007) and BIO-IBE of (Sarier, 2008), the biometric template b is computed using the feature vector and the hash of b is used as the identity ID. Here, the template b is assumed to be a fixed length binary string, so each feature forming the original biometric template (namely the feature vector) are quantized to generate multiple bits per feature that are concatenated to obtain the binary template b. Particularly, the framework for biometric template generation consists of (1) extracting features; (2) quantization and coding per feature and concatenating the output codes; (3) applying error correction coding (ECC) and hashing. During this process, many quantizers produce and use side-information, which could be published to be used later in the reconstruction of the binary template b'.

As different from existing fuzzy IBE systems, the BIO-IBE (Sarier, 2008) requires the use of the biometric template b obtained from the feature vector of the user, where feature extraction is the most costly part of the biometric template generation.

Since feature extraction is already performed in any fuzzy IBE scheme, one can easily apply a robust fuzzy extractor on the feature vector to bind the private key components to the user's identity and thus avoid collusion attacks. Instead of choosing a unique polynomial for each user, we use the robust fuzzy extractor to obtain a unique biometric string ID via error correction codes from the biometric template b of the user in such a way that an error tolerance t is allowed. In other words, we will obtain the same biometric string ID even if the fuzzy extractor is applied on a different b' such that dis (b,b')< t. Here, dis() is the distance metric used to measure the variation in the biometric reading and t is the error tolerance parameter of the fuzzy extractor.

FUZZY EXTRACTOR

Formally, an (M, l, t) fuzzy extractor is defined as follows (Burnett et al., 2007).

Let $M = \{0, 1\}^v$ be a finite dimensional metric space with a distance function

dis(): $M \times M \rightarrow Z^+$. Here, b ε M and dis() measures the distance between b and b', where b, b' ε M. An (M, l, t) fuzzy extractor consists of functions Gen and Rep.

- *Gen:* A probabilistic generation procedure that takes as input b ε M and outputs an biometric identity string ID ε $\{0, 1\}^l$. and a public parameter PAR, that is used by the Rep function to regenerate the same biometric string ID from b' such that dis(b, b') $\leq$ t.
- *Rep:* A deterministic reproduction procedure that takes as input b' and the publicly available value PAR, and outputs ID if dis(b, b') $\leq$ t.

In (Burnett ct al. 2007), the authors describe a concrete **fuzzy extractor** using a [n, k, 2t +1] BCH error correction code, Hamming Distance metric and a one-way hash function H: $\{0, 1\}^n \rightarrow \{0, 1\}^l$. Specifically,

- The Gen function takes the biometrics b as input and returns ID = H(b) and public parameter PAR = b $\oplus$ C(ID), where C is a one-to-one encoding function.

- The Rep function takes a biometric b' and PAR as input and computes

ID' = D(b' $\oplus$ PAR) = D(b $\oplus$ b' $\oplus$ C(ID)). ID = ID' if and only if dis(b, b') $\leq$ t. Here D is the decoding function that corrects the errors upto the threshold t.

BIOMETRIC IDENTITY GENERATION

In this section, we present a concrete example on the biometric identity (ID) generation using a fuzzy extractor and the biometric template b of the decryptor. We note that the public key generation phase of the BIO-IBS scheme is identical to the biometric identity (ID) generation of our system.

Specifically, the public key in standard IBE is based on the identity of the receiver of the ciphertext. In the case of biometric IBE, the public key of the receiver is derived from his biometric. First the biometric reader extracts the biometric feature vector, which is used in the computation of the biometric template b of the receiver identical to the java based implementation of the public key extraction of BIO-IBS. We refer to the concrete example in (Burnett et al., 2007), where the template b is obtained from the fingerprint as below:.

b = D4 44 5C <u>B3</u> 71 D8 47 A1 20 5B <u>5D</u> AD 37 06 82 E0......

Next, b is input to the fuzzy extractor to obtain the biometric identity

ID = 15 2A 1E 68 B1 90 27 5C 5C 9C 58 AB 4F C8 0E AE 26 43 CE 38.

When the sender wants to encrypt a message to the receiver, the sender first extracts the feature vector of the receiver's fingerprint and computes the biometric template b' as below:

b' = D4 44 5C <u>FB</u> 71 D8 47 A1 20 5B <u>58</u> AD 37 06 82 E0.....

As one can notice, due to the biometric measurement errors, the template differs from the previous measurement b at the underlined places. Next, the encryptor inputs b' in to the fuzzy extractor to obtain the same public key ID if dis(b, b′) ≤ t.

Namely, these are the errors that are corrected by the fuzzy extractor to generate the original identity of

ID' = 15 2A 1E 68 B1 90 27 5C 5C 9C 58 AB 4F C8 0E AE 26 43 CE 38.

The system of (Burnett et al., 2007) uses the BCH parameters [n, k, 2t + 1] =

(905, 160, 201) in this error correction procedure for fingerprint based biometric IBS scheme.

PREVENTING COLLUSION ATTACKS

In the anonymous fuzzy IBE scheme of (Liesdonk, 2007), collision attacks are avoided by combining each biometric feature w_i with the identity (i.e. Name, e-mail) of the user. However, this approach is against the nature of fuzzy IBE, where the identities should only consist of the biometric data of the user. Besides, an important privacy property that we will present in the next section is not satisfied despite the anonymity of the scheme (Sarier, N. D., (in press)). One can correct this fuzzy IBE scheme with a similar approach introduced in (Sarier, 2008), namely, the identity is obtained from the biometric information of the user using a feature extraction algorithm followed by a fuzzy extraction process, where the result of the former procedure (i.e. w = (w_1, ...,w_n)) is combined with the output of the latter (i.e. ID) to obtain the biometric attribute set BID = <H(w_1, ID), ...,H(w_n, ID)> to be used in the key generation phase. This way, the privacy of biometric-identity relation and the resistance against collusion attacks is maintained. Here, H is a cryptographic hash function.

A concrete application of this biometric identity structure is presented in Figure 1 and Figure 2, which is also currently the most efficient fuzzy IBE scheme provably secure in the Random Oracle Model as shown in Figure 3. Basically, the author presents a new biometric identity based encryption

scheme using the Sakai Kasahara Key Construction (Sarier, 2008) and achieve better efficiency compared to the existing fuzzy IBE schemes in terms of the key generation and decryption algorithms. This scheme has a structurally simpler key generation algorithm compared to (Piretti et al., 2006; Baek et al., 2007), since an ordinary one-way hash function is used instead of a MaptoPoint hash function and the number of exponentiations in the group G is reduced from 3n as in (Piretti, 2006) (and from 2n as in (Baek et al., 2007)) to n. Also, the decryption algorithm requires d bilinear pairing computations and d exponentiations, whereas the existing schemes require d + 1 bilinear pairing computations and 2d exponentiations. The security of this new scheme reduces to the well exploited k-BDHI computational problem in the random oracle model.

The main difference of biometric IBE scheme is the structure of the key generation algorithm, where a unique biometric identity string ID obtained from the biometric attributes is used instead of picking a different polynomial for each user and computing the private key components for each attribute using this polynomial, the master key and the attributes. Thus, the scheme is constructed using a different approach compared to the existing fuzzy IBE schemes. Besides, the scheme of (Sarier, 2008) allows for a combination of different biometric modalities as fusing multiple biometrics will improve wider coverage of population who may not be able to provide a single biometrics and also improve security of the systems in terms of spoof attacks in addition to the higher level of accuracy performance not feasible with a single biometrics today. An example of multi-biometrics based BIO-IBE scheme is presented in Figure 1.

BIO-IBE scheme of (Sarier, 2008) requires the public storage of the value PAR, which is the information needed for error-tolerant reconstruction of the biometric identity string ID and subsequent fuzzy extraction. Since the encryption is performed by combining each biometric feature w_i with the

Figure 1. The flow diagram of BIO-IBE for multi biometrics

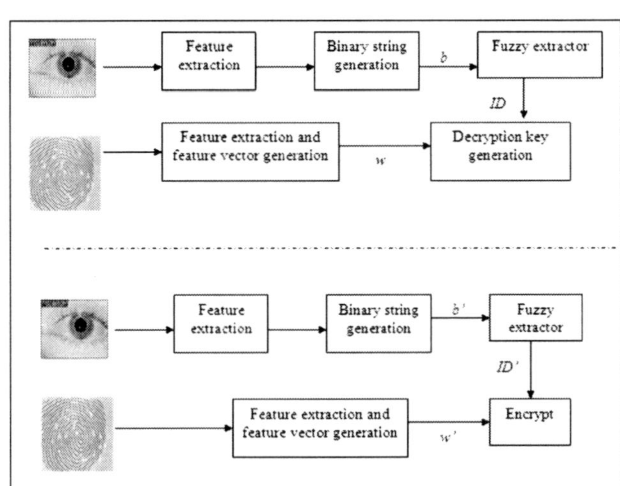

biometric identity ID of the receiver, the presence of an active adversary who maliciously alters the public string PAR leads the sender to use a wrong public key for the encryption due to a different identity string computed by the fuzzy extractor. By the malicious modification of the public value PAR, an adversary cannot gain any secret information but the receiver of the ciphertext either cannot decrypt it or he obtains a wrong plaintext upon decryption. In order to prevent this Denial of Service (DoS) attack, BIO-IBE is modified in (Sarier, 2010) by requiring the PKG to sign the public value PAR using an efficient pairing based IBS scheme and publish both values. The

flow diagram for encryption and decryption of modified BIO-IBE is shown in Figure 2. Similar to BIO-IBE, the modified scheme is applicable for multi-biometrics. The abbreviations used in Figure 3 are summarized in Table 1.

BIOMETRIC IBE FOR WEAK COMPUTATIONAL DEVICES

Currently, there exists remote biometric authentication schemes designed for weak computational devices such as biometric smartcards that implements biometric feature extraction and lightweight

Figure 2. The flow diagram of modified BIO-IBE (Sarier, 2010)

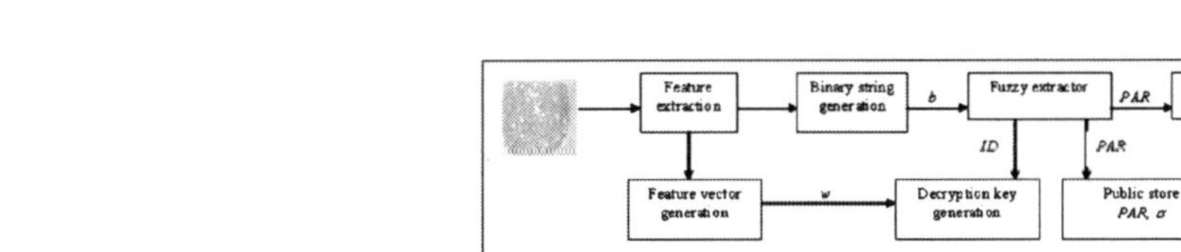

Figure 3. Comparison of different fuzzy IBE systems (Sarier, 2008)

Scheme	Piretti et al [2]	Baek et al [4]	Baek et al [4]	BIO-IBE [1]
Size of secret key	$2n\,l_1$	$2n\,l_1$	$2n\,l_1$	$n\,l_1$
Size of ciphertext	$(n+1)\,l_1 + l_2$	$(n+1)\,l_1 + l_2$	$(n+1)\,l_1 + l_2$	$n\,l_1 + l_2$
Key Generation	$n(T_H + T_m + 3T_e)$	$n(T_H + 2T_e)$	$n(T_H + T_m + 2T_e)$	$n(T_e + T_i) + FE_{ID}$
Encrypt	$n(T_H + T_e) + 2T_e + T_p + T_m$	$n(T_m + T_e + T_H) + 2T_e + T_p + T_m$	$n(T_H + T_e) + 2T_e + T_p + T_m$	$n(T_m + 2T_e) + T_p + FE_{ID}$
Decrypt	$d(T_m + 2T_e + T_p) + T_p + T_i' + T_m$	$d(T_m + 2T_e + T_p) + T_p + T_i' + T_m$	$d(T_m + 2T_e + T_p) + T_p + T_i' + T_m$	$d(T_e + T_p)$

cryptographic primitives (Atallah, 2005). The same procedures could be used for biometric IBE using smartcards, if efficient biometric IBE systems could be described applicable for energy constrained devices. In order to evaluate various IBE schemes, the authors of (Ateniese & Gasti, 2009) implement different anonymous IBE schemes to present the average times of encryption of a short session key. Using these values presented in (Ateniese & Gasti, 2009), we can compute any pairing based fuzzy IBE system as shown in Table 2. For simplicity, we use different variables to represent the approximate times, where x and y denote the encryption and decryption times for Boneh-Franklin IBE (Boneh & Franklin, 2003) scheme implemented for a unique identity (non-biometric) such as an e-mail address. Specifically, x is the time to compute two exponentiations within their respective groups if the bilinear pairing is precomputed and y is the time for one pairing computation, which is the dominant operation in terms of computation cost. For fuzzy IBE systems, since the identity is represented as a feature vector of length n such that $20 < n < 100$ depending on the biometric modality, the required times are computed as multiples of x and y. Although bilinear pairings could be computed efficiently, new biometric encryption systems should be designed for practical use which does not require bilinear pairings (or a few pairing computations) and thus

Table 1. Abbreviations used in Table 1

$\lvert S \rvert$	bit size of an element in the set S
N	number of features of a user
D	error tolerance parameter
T_e	time for a single exponentiation in G
T'_e	time for a single exponentiation in F
T_H	time for MaptoPoint hash function
T_m	time for a single multiplication in G
T'_m	time for a single multiplication in F
T_i	time for a single inverse operation in Z_p
T'_i	time for a single inverse operation in F
T_p	time for a single pairing operation
FE	time for the fuzzy extraction process
k_1	output size of the hash function

the system could be implemented for lightweight computational devices such as biometric smartcards. In this context, a simple solution could be obtained by implementing the biometric identity structure of (Burnett et al., 2007), which is used in the design of biometric identity based signature schemes as described in section Collision Attacks.

This way, the unique biometric identity of the receiver could be input to any standard IBE scheme such as Sakai Kasahara IBE scheme, which could be implemented efficiently in smartcards. Although the biometric IBE scheme of (Shi et al., 2009) could also be implementable for smart cards, their scheme employs the time-consuming MapToPoint hash function, which is inefficient and probabilistic and there is no deterministic polynomial time algorithm for it so far. Therefore, using general cryptographic hash function instead of the MapToPoint function can improve the efficiency of biometric IBE schemes as in the case of our proposal.

The only assumption for this new construction is that the biometric modality chosen could be error corrected practically and thus input to fuzzy extractor as in the case of a 2048 bit Iris code. In Table 2, we present the comparison of the encryption and decryption times of different IBE schemes, where the first scheme is based on non-biometric identities i.e. Name or e-mail address. The remaining IBE schemes are implemented for biometric identities. Here, FE denotes the time for fuzzy extraction of a unique biometric identity string ID, where the time for fuzzy extraction could be omitted if ID is precomputed. Again, n denotes the size of the feature vector and d is the

error tolerance parameter of the pairing based fuzzy IBE scheme.

FUTURE TRENDS

Currently, the secrecy of biometric data is viewed with skepticism since it is very easy to obtain biological information such as fingerprint, iris or face data through fingerprint marking or using a camcorder. However, biometrics is sensitive information, as in the case of biometric remote authentication, it should not be easy to obtain the biometric data by compromising the central server, where the biometrics of each user is often associated with his personal information. In particular, a user could use its biometrics on a number of applications such as identification, authentication, signing, etc. Thus, the secrecy of identity-biometrics relation should be maintained, which is defined as identity privacy (Bringer & Chabanne 2007b, 2008). Current fuzzy IBE and biometric IBE systems do not consider anonymity and privacy of user biometrics at the same time; hence, it is vital to describe an efficient and anonymous error-tolerant encryption system for biometric identities in order to avoid traceability of the user's actions. Although the fuzzy IBE scheme of (Liesdonk, 2007), provides anonymity, the scheme combines each biometric attribute with the identity (i.e. Name, e-mail address) of the user to avoid the collusion attacks. This approach is not only against identity privacy but also against the main principle of fuzzy IBE or biometric IBE, where the identity of the user should only consist of his biometric data.

Table 2. Comparison of the time complexity of biometric IBE schemes

	Encryption Time	Decryption Time
Bonch Franklin IBE	x	y
Pairing based Fuzzy IBE	nx	dy
Our solution	x + FE	y+FE

CONCLUSION

Fuzzy IBE is a new cryptographic tool which provides error tolerance property for biometric identities. There exists a number of pairing based schemes that require the decryptor to compute d bilinear pairings, where d is the error tolerance parameter of the fuzzy IBE scheme. However, for weak computational devices, more practical solutions such as systems requiring one or two bilinear pairing computations for each encryption process should be designed. In this chapter, we propose to use the encryption analogue of the biometric IBS scheme of Burnett et al., which is applicable to some biometric modalities that are suitable for error correction process such as a Iris template, which can be represented as a 2048 bit string (Bringer & Chabanne, 2007b). Although biometrics is assumed as public data, in current fuzzy IBE systems, the privacy of biometrics is not considered and the receiver's biometric data is attached to the ciphertext, which enables an adversary to trace users' actions via traffic analysis. Consequently, we need to describe efficient biometric IBE schemes that are anonymous and provide identity privacy.

REFERENCES

Advances in Cryptology - EUROCRYPT 2005: Vol. 3494. LNCS (pp. 457–473). Heidelberg, Germany: Springer.

Atallah, M. J., Frikken, K. B., Goodrich, M. T., & Tamassia, R. (2005). Secure biometric authentication for weak computational devices. In A.S. Patrick, M. Yung (Ed.), *FC 2005: Vol. 3570. LNCS* (pp. 357–371). Heidelberg, Germany: Springer.

Ateniese, G., & Gasti, P. (2009). Universally anonymous IBE based on the quadratic residuosity assumption. *CT-RSA '09: Vol. 5473. LNCS* (pp. 32–47). Heidelberg, Germany: Springer.

Baek, J., Susilo, W., & Zhou, J. (2007). New constructions of fuzzy identitybased encryption. *ACM Symposium on Information, Computer and Communications Security - ASIACCS'07* (pp. 368–370). New York: ACM.

Boneh, D., & Franklin, M. K. (2003). Identity-Based Encryption from the Weil Pairing. *SIAM Journal on Computing, 32*(3), 586–615. doi:10.1137/S0097539701398521

Bringer, J., & Chabanne, H. (2008). An Authentication Protocol with Encrypted Biometric Data. *AFRICACRYPT'08: Vol. 5023. LNCS* (pp. 109–124). Heidelberg, Germany: Springer.

Bringer, J., Chabanne, H., Cohen, G., Kindarji, B., & Zemor, G. (2007a). Optimal Iris Fuzzy Sketches. [IEEE Computer Society.]. *BTAS, 07*, 1–6.

Bringer, J., Chabanne, H., Izabach`ene, M., Pointcheval, D., Tang, Q., & Zimmer, S. (2007b). *An Application of the Goldwasser-Micali Cryptosystem to Biometric Authentication. ACISP'07, 4586. LNCS* (pp. 96–106). Heidelberg, Germany: Springer.

Burnett, A., Byrne, F., Dowling, T., & Duffy, A. (2007). A Biometric Identity Based Signature Scheme. *International Journal of Network Security, 5*(3), 317–326.

Dodis, Y., Reyzin, L., & Smith, A. (2004). Fuzzy Extractors: How to Generate Strong Keys from Biometrics and Other Noisy Data. *Advances in Cryptology - EUROCRYPT'04: Vol. 3027. LNCS* (pp. 523–540). Heidelberg, Germany: Springer.

Pirretti, M., Traynor, P., McDaniel, P., & Waters, B. (2006). Secure Attribute-Based Systems. *ACM Conference on Computer and Communications Security* (pp. 99–112). New York: ACM.

Sahai, A., & Waters, B. (2005). Fuzzy Identity-Based Encryption.

Sarier, N. D. (2007). Identity Based Encryption: *Security notions and new identity based encryption schemes based on Sakai-Kasahara's Key Construction*. Unpublished Master's thesis. RWTH Aachen.

Sarier, N. D. (2008). A New Biometric Identity Based Encryption Scheme. *The 2008 International Symposium on Trusted Computing - TrustCom 2008* (pp. 2061-2066). IEEE Computer Society.

Sarier, N. D. (2010). *A New Biometric Identity Based Encryption Scheme secure against DoS Attacks. Special Issue on "Trusted Computing and Communications". Journal of Security and Communication Networks SCN*. Wiley Interscience.

Sarier, N. D. (in press). Generic Constructions of Biometric Identity Based Encryption Systems. *WISTP'10*. Heidelberg, Germany: Springer.

Shi, W., Jang, I., & Yoo, H. S. (2009). Chosen Ciphertext Secure Fuzzy Identity-Based Encryption Scheme with Short Ciphertext. [IEEE Computer Society.]. *ICCIT, 09*, 1036–1040.

van Liesdonk, P. P. (2007). *Anonymous and fuzzy identity-based encryption*. Unpublished Master's Thesis. Technische Universiteit Eindhoven.

Chapter 12
Spam Detection Approaches with Case Study Implementation on Spam Corpora

Biju Issac
Swinburne University of Technology (Sarawak Campus), Malaysia

EXECUTIVE SUMMARY

Email has been considered as one of the most efficient and convenient ways of communication since the users of the Internet has increased rapidly. E-mail spam, known as junk e-mail, UBE (unsolicited bulk e-mail) or UCE (unsolicited commercial e-mail), is the act of sending unwanted e-mail messages to e-mail users. Spam is becoming a huge problem to most users since it clutter their mailboxes and waste their time to delete all the spam before reading the legitimate ones. They also cost the user money with dial up connections, waste network bandwidth and disk space and make available harmful and offensive materials. In this chapter, initially we would like to discuss on existing spam technologies and later focus on a case study. Though many anti-spam solutions have been implemented, the Bayesian spam detection approach looks quite promising. A case study for spam detection algorithm is presented and its implementation using Java is discussed, along with its performance test results on two independent spam corpuses – Ling-spam and Enron-spam. We use the Bayesian calculation for single keyword sets and multiple keywords sets, along with its keyword contexts to improve the spam detection and thus to get good accuracy. The use of porter stemmer algorithm is also discussed to stem keywords which can improve spam detection efficiency by reducing keyword searches.

INTRODUCTION

Over the last years, unsolicited bulk mail, better known as spam, has become one of the most annoying problems of the Internet. The increase of

spam emails uses bandwidth and fills up databases and therefore the global network becomes more crowded and less useful. Even though spam emails do not damage the data in the way that viruses do, they do harm the business intentions. For example, spam emails wastes user's time since the users devoid of anti-spam protection have to

DOI: 10.4018/978-1-60960-015-0.ch012

check which email is spam manually and then delete it. Sometimes, users can easily overlook or delete important email because of confusing it with spam. Email spamming often contains deceptive, worthless content or even a virus attachment.

Spam emails are getting better in its ability to break anti-spam filters and it would take a great deal of research to get it fully eradicated by coming up with very intelligent anti-spam filters. Spammers are also becoming more innovative, so that the anti-spam research is having a great relevance these days. There are various anti-spam techniques that have been created and implemented since spam started infiltrating user's inboxes. The most popular and direct way to prevent spam is the anti-spam filters. Anti-spam filters are the software tools that block spam messages automatically. These filters vary in functionality from black list (spammer list) and white list (trusted user list) to content-based filters. There are a lot of anti-spam filters or spam detection schemes available in the market.

The spammer's methods of avoiding detection evolve constantly, differing significantly from what has been used in the past. For every techniques created for filtering the emails, a new method to spread spam also comes out, making the battle between the spammers and mail agent even more challenging. We would like to introduce a Bayesian approach to the anti-spam solution, considering the context of keywords found. First we implement a simple Bayesian filter based on single keyword sets. Then we improve that by using multiple keyword sets and assigning a higher weightage to them. Finally, we further refine the anti-spam filter by using context matching technique along with the previous steps. The keywords are mapped to a keyword context, which is a collection of other keywords where the specific keyword is found.

The spam relayed by different countries in second quarter of 2007 is shown as a graph in Figure 1 (E-mail spam, na). This gives a good indication that some selected countries are the top

relay points of spam emails. The actual spammer may or may not be sending spam emails from the country of his residence or may use compromised PCs elsewhere, even in other countries.

EXISTING AND RELATED WORKS

A number of research works are happening in the field of spam detection techniques. Some are listed below. Sasaki and Shinnou proposed a new spam detection technique using the text clustering based on vector space model. Their method computes disjoint clusters automatically using a spherical k-means algorithm for all spam/non-spam mails and obtains centroid vectors of the clusters for extracting the cluster description. For each centroid vectors, the label (`spam' or `non-spam') is assigned by calculating the number of spam email in the cluster. When new mail arrives, the cosine similarity between the new mail vector and centroid vector is calculated. Finally, the label of the most relevant cluster is assigned to the new mail (Sasaki & Shinnou, 2005). When classifying emails as spam and ham (which is a valid email), a false positive is the valid email that was erroneously classified as spam and a false negative is the spam email that was erroneously classified as valid email. For email classification as spam or non-spam, naive bayes classification was used in several systems (Kiritchenko & Matwin, 2001; Chan & Poon, 2004; Schneider, 2003; Androutsopoulos et al., 2000). Chiu et al. presents an alliance-based approach to classify, discovery and exchange interesting information on spam mails. The spam filter is built based on the mixture of rough set theory, genetic algorithm and XCS (eXtended Classifier System) classifier system (Chiu, Chen, Jeng, & Lin, 2007). Sirisanyalak et al. uses an email feature extraction technique for spam detection based on artificial immune systems that extracts a set of four features that can be used as inputs to a spam detection model (Sirisanyalak & Sornil, 2007). Dhinakaran et al. collected 400

Figure 1. E-mail spam relayed by country in Quarter 2, 2007

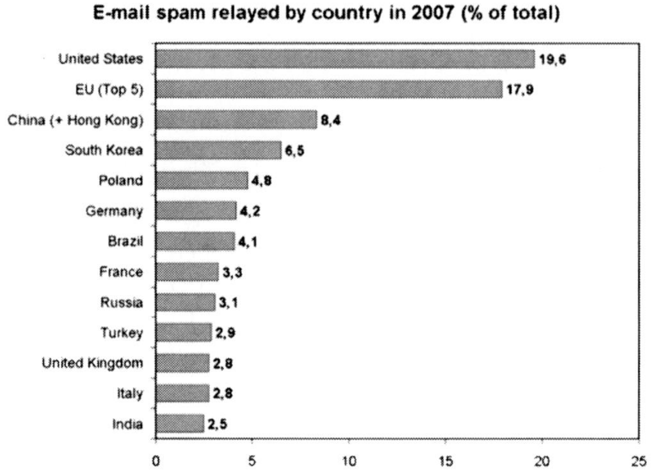

E-mail spam relayed by country in 2007 (% of total)

thousand spam mails from a spam trap set up in a corporate mail server for a period of 14 months form January 2006 to February 2007, which is a sample of world wide spam traffic. Studying the characteristics of this sample helps to better understand the features of spam and spam vulnerable e-mail accounts. They believe that this analysis is highly useful to develop more efficient anti spam techniques. In their analysis they classified spam based on attachment and contents (Dhinakaran, Lee & Nagamalai, 2007).

Zhou et al. explains on Good Word Attack that thwarts spam filters by appending to spam messages sets of "good" words, which are common in legitimate e-mail but rare in spam. They present a counterattack strategy that first attempts to differentiate spam from legitimate e-mail in the input space, by transforming each email into a bag of multiple segments, and subsequently applies multiple instance logistic regression on the bags. They treat each segment in the bag as an instance. An e-mail is classified as spam if at least one instance in the corresponding bag is spam, and as legitimate if all the instances in it are legitimate (Zhou, Jorgensen & Inge, 2007). Gao et al. propose a system using a probabilistic boosting tree to determine whether an incoming image is a spam or not based on global image features, i.e. color and gradient orientation histograms. The system identifies spam without the need for OCR and is robust in the face of the kinds of variation found in current spam images (Gao, Yang, Zhao, Pardo, Pappas & Choudhary, 2008). Balakumar et al. uses ontology for Statistical based filtering: understanding the content of the email and Bayesian approach for making the classification (Balakumar & Vaidehi, 2008). Ali et al. investigates current approaches for blocking spam and proposes a new spam classification method by using adaptive boosting algorithm. Experiment was carried out to evaluate the results of spam filtering and the results were supporting adaptive boosting algorithm (Ali & Xiang, 2007). Lan et al. present a filtering mechanism applying the idea of preference ranking. This filtering mechanism will distinguish spam emails from other email on the Internet. The preference ranking gives the similarity values for nominated emails and spam emails specified by users, so that the ISP/end users can deal with spam emails at filtering points. They designed three filtering points to classify nominated emails into spam email, unsure email and legitimate email (Lan & Zhou, 2005). Ming et al. used a method of spam behaviour recognition filtering. The method identifies the spam according to the behaviour of mail sent, set up the model by Bayes technique, and in the mail filtering application to filter the spam by stages (Ming, Yunchun & Wei, 2007).

Other more prevalent anti-spam methods are listed below. Word filters are a quite an easy and effective way to block obvious spam mails. Word filters simply identify any email that contains certain key words, like "viagra, penis enlargement" that are commonly found in spam mails. Rule-based scoring systems are more complex. As word filters simply just block emails that contain certain key words, rule-based scoring systems use rules to analyze emails and assign scores to each key word it finds. Bayesian filters can adapt automatically to changes in spam mails. To determine the likelihood that an email is spam, these filters use Bayesian analysis to compare the words or phrases in the email to the frequency of the same words or phrases in the intended recipient's past emails (both regular and spam). Black list IP is a common spam blocking technique that simply involves organizations to manually keep a list of the IP addresses of known spammers (a "black list") so that emails from those addresses are blocked. RBLs (Realtime Blackhole List), also known as DNSRBLs, check every incoming email's IP address against a list of IP addresses in the RBL. If the IP address is part of the RBL, then the email is identified as spam and blocked. Black List Sender Email Addresses is a simple spam blocking technique where users create a black list from addresses that should be prevented from entering the network and reaching the user's inbox (Barracuda Networks, 2004). There are different types of spam filters that are available today.

Let's look at some of the different kinds of spam filters that are available (Types of Spam Filters, na) and they are discussed as follows.

Content Based Filters

These are the traditional type of spam filters that analyze the message subject, headers and content searching for specific words or phrases, or other indicators of spam. Whenever an unsolicited mail comes into your mail box, the user can create a new filter by choosing certain words, or phrases from the message that indicate it is spam. But spammers know that their messages were being marked by these content filters and have resorted to counter the content filter through words with special characters inserted like "Vi@gra", "p.0.r.n", "L|0|a|n|$" etc. This effort is getting increasingly popular that previous versions of content-based filters are not delivering well in terms of performance. But as one can perform wildcard searches and has the ability to see the spammer's attempts at obfuscating the words such as in the examples shown above, the mails can be classified as spam. A vast majority of spam emails are less legible because of their effort to bypass the content-based filters. The content based approach nevertheless is quite flexible. We can easily specify the filtering to the exact type of spam message that is in question and avoid regular words that we use daily communication. But on the downside, it requires more effort and hands on tuning, along with regular updation. As spammers look to novel approaches to circumvent the filters, the filters need to be modified to deal with them.

Bayesian Based Filters

Thomas Bayes developed an approach that allowed one to find the probability of an event occurring based on the probabilities of two or more independent events. Bayesian filters are based on this approach using Bayes equation. These filters when implemented as software, have to be trained from a set of known good and bad e-mails. During training they extract tokens (which are keywords) and store them in a data store. When the filter analyze an email message, the message is split into tokens and the presence of such tokens is attributed a value according to the following criteria such as – the frequency of the token in spam messages, the frequency of the token in good messages, the number of spam messages, and the number of good messages. After applying Bayes equation, a spamicity value is extracted that gives the probability of an email message being spam or not. The Bayesian based filters require little maintenance and follow-up than the other filters. Once the filter has been trained, it is quite self reliant as it can self-adapt automatically to changing trends in spam. The Bayesian filters are self learning in nature and it will continue to learn from newly arrived email messages. But on the downside, its filtering is only as good as the messages on which the filter is trained. Many filters based on this approach comes as pre-trained, but not on the email messages received by the user. It will thus require some time before the filter can reach its optimum levels of performance, after being trained by user's incoming mail pattern.

Whitelist or Blacklist Filters

These are very simple and elementary types of filters which are not used independently, but can be used as part of an integrated email filtering system. Whitelist filters will not accept e-mail from any address outside the list of known good e-mail addresses. On the contrary, Blacklist filters allow messages from any address except the list of known bad email addresses. The blacklists can be locally kept and administered or accessed through the Internet. The readily available Blacklists on the Internet are known as RBLs or Realtime Blackhole Lists. Even though whitelists are guaranteed to thwart e-mail from unwanted sources, it is a drastic measure with very little flexibility. Sometimes the people that compile RBLs - the realtime blacklists available on the Internet put entire ranges of IP addresses on their blacklist even though previous abuse occurred only on a certain part of that range. This results in a situation where wrong people get blocked as a result of stopping the spammer and is a debatable issue.

Challenge/Response Filters

Challenge/Response filters features the option to automatically send a response to an anonymous sender by asking them to act further so that their message will be received. This approach is referred to as a "Turing Test" – named after a test devised by British scientist Alan Turing to determine if machines can possibly think. Of late, we can see the appearance of some Internet services that does perform this Challenge/Response function for the user and require the sender of an e-mail to visit their web site to facilitate the receipt of their message.

Community Filters

These types of filters work on the basis of "community knowledge" of spam and this knowledge is resident on a central server. When a user receives a spam message, they simply mark it and inform the server. Based on the information given to the central server, a message fingerprint is added to the database. When a number of people have identified the message as spam, it will be stamped as spam and would be stopped from user's inboxes in future. On the positive side, it is easy to set up and minimal administration is needed. On the down side, before enough people identify the email as spam, somebody will be receiving the spam messages. Different people can have different view points on what spam mail is and so some good mails may be stopped, thus increasing the possibility of false positives.

CASE STUDY OF CONTENT BASED BAYESIAN ANTI-SPAM FILTER

We would be looking into a content based Bayesian anti-spam filter. Bayesian filtering works on the principle that the probability of an event occurring in the future can be inferred from the previous occurrences of that event (Graham, 2003).

The Bayesian method has some advantages. It takes the whole email message into consideration. It notes the keywords that identify spam, but it also notes words that denote valid mail. The advantage of the Bayesian method is that it considers the most interesting or specific key words and comes up with a probability that a message is spam. Thus Bayesian filtering is an efficient and intelligent approach because it examines all aspects of an email message, compared to keyword checking that stamps a mail as spam on the basis of a single word. Bayesian type of filter is constantly self-adapting and self-learning. By learning from new email spam and new valid emails, the Bayesian filter evolves and adapts to new spam techniques as it automatically notices spammer's tactics. This technique is also sensitive to the user as it learns the email habits of the company and understands that. Another interesting aspect is that the Bayesian method is multi-lingual and international. A Bayesian anti-spam filter, being adaptive, can be used for any language required. The self adaptive nature and the evolving intelligence enable such the filter to catch more spam. This filter is difficult to break compared to a keyword filter.

Spam emails can be processed through Bayesian filters using keywords, is widely known. Single keyword or multiple keyword combinations can be used to decide on spam score. Along with the keywords, we used keyword contexts. Making a spam decision by merely using keywords cannot be that accurate. Once the keyword is checked using its context, the picture becomes clearer and a more accurate decision can be taken in classifying a mail as spam. Context is a set of remaining keywords that is mapped to every keyword chosen as shown

in Figure 2. For example, if the [keyword 1] has a context of [keyword 2, keyword 3 … keyword n], then [keyword 2] has a context of [keyword 1, keyword 3 … keyword n] etc. Generally, the keywords chosen can be uncommon or critical nouns (or combinations), along with acronyms, names etc. An exemption text file of common words can be used during implementation, to avoid classifying those common words as keywords.

The anti-spam algorithm can be described as follows. Accept the incoming mails and extract keywords from subject line and email contents as one-keyword (k_{1i}), two-keyword (k_{2i}), three-keyword (k_{3i}) or multi keyword sets. Form contexts C_{ij} for content keywords (k_{1i}), two-keyword (k_{2i}) and three-keyword (k_{3i}) sets. The context for any keyword is a set that contains all other keywords except itself. Thus a keyword or keyword combinations can have more than one context, as different spam can contain different sets of keyword combinations. Use the identified keywords to assign a Bayesian probability related score. The keyword contexts are compared to the set of existing keywords, to find a context matching percent (CMP).

Three approaches are discussed here—Bayesian using single keywords, Improved Bayesian with multiple keywords and Improved Bayesian with keyword context matching (Graham, 2003; Issac & Raman, 2006).

Bayesian Approach with Single keywords

This approach is done in many spam filters, as one part of the implementation. The commercial spam filters are mostly composite products which implements more than one idea. The Bayesian probability *p(k)* for keyword *k* is given as in Equation 1:

$$p(k) = \frac{s(k)}{s(k) + ns(k)}$$

(1)

Figure 2. The keyword and context relationship

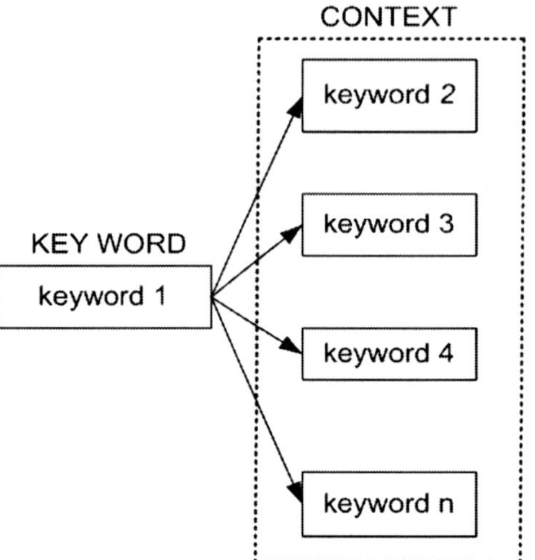

where, *s(k)* is the number of spam emails with keyword *k* and *ns(k)* is the number of non-spam emails with keyword *k*. The overall weighted spam score is calculated as follows. The Bayesian score for single keywords and multi-keywords are calculated and no weights are assigned to multi-keywords. The keyword scores are totaled to get the spam score for a given mail.

The Bayesian probability *p(sk)* for single keyword set *sk*,

$$p(sk) = \frac{s(sk)}{s(sk) + ns(sk)}$$

(2)

where, *s(sk)* is the number of spam emails with all single keyword set *sk* and *ns(sk)* is the number of non-spam emails with all single keyword set *sk*. Similar approach is adopted for multi-keywords.

Improved Bayesian Approach with Multiple Keywords

The previous approach treats all the keywords, whether single or multiple words in the same manner. In comparison to the previous method, here weights are assigned to multiple keywords, giving it more importance in the spam score calculation. Weights associated with one, two and three keywords (or multiple keywords) are denoted as Wk_{1i}, Wk_{2i} and Wk_{3i}, respectively, where i = 1 to n (where $Wk_{1i} < Wk_{2i} < Wk_{3i}$). Spam score for one, two and three keywords are denoted as Sk_{1i}, Sk_{2i} and Sk_{3i} respectively, where i = 1 to n. Bayesian calculation is done with weights and keywords scores are determined, which are eventually added to get the spam score.

The Bayesian probability *p(mk)* for multi-keyword set *mk,*

$$p(mk) = \frac{s(mk)}{s(mk) + ns(mk)}$$

(3)

where, *s(mk)* is the number of spam emails with all multi-keyword set *mk* and *ns(mk)* is the number of non-spam emails with all multi-keyword set mk. In the simulation done, the multiple keywords present are assigned different weights in spam score calculation as follows: Two keywords can be assigned a weight of MK_WEIGHT*2 (constant value), three keywords are assigned a weight of

MK_WEIGHT*3, four keywords or more are assigned a weight of MK_WEIGHT*4. Single keywords are not assigned any weights.

Improved Bayesian with Keyword-Context Approach

To further improve the accuracy, we added the keyword context score or context matching percent score to the improved Bayesian score, which sensed multiple keywords. Spam score for one, two and three keywords with corresponding keyword contexts are Skc_{1i}, Skc_{2i} and Skc_{3i} respectively, where i = 1 to n. This score is calculated with respect to the matches spam mail keywords contexts find in the existing database of keywords. For example, consider a keyword [viagra] that has a context of [word 1, word 2, word 3, word 4] in a mail received. Matching percentage can be given as $x\%$ for keyword context match. If two words match out of four, then matching percentage would be 50%. The keyword context score (Skc_{ij}) would be a function of this matching percentage. This spam score for keyword-context pairs can have a greater contribution in the overall score. This is effected by W_1 and W_2, where W_1 is the weight (say, 70%) associated with keyword score and W_2 (say, 30%) is associated with keyword-context score component in Equation 4. These values can be fine-tuned for best results. Weights associated with contexts that corresponds to one, two and three keywords are Wkc_{1i}, Wkc_{2i} and Wkc_{3i} respectively, where i = 1 to n (where $Wkc_{1i} < Wkc_{2i} < Wkc_{3i}$).

The Total Spam Score = Total weighted Bayesian score for all keywords found + Total weighted score based on matching percent for all keyword-contexts found, corresponding to all keywords. That can be mathematically expressed as in Equation 4:

$$S_{total} = \sum_{i=1;j=1}^{i=n;j=n} W_1(Sk_{ij} \times Wk_{ij}) + W_2(Skc_{ij} \times Wkc_{ij})$$

(4)

For each keyword, the corresponding contexts are formed. The presence of spam keyword itself doesn't guarantee a good spam score, but keywords with contexts if present, can give a good spam score. Threshold and weight factors should be fine tuned in different stages (Issac & Raman, 2006; Androutsopoulos, Koutsias, Chandrinos, Paliouras & Spyropoulos, 2000).

A number of so-called stemming Algorithms, or stemmers, have been developed, which attempt to reduce a word to its stem or root form. Thus, the key terms of a query or document are represented by stems rather than by the original words. This not only means that different variants of a term can be conflated to a single representative form – it also reduces the dictionary size, that is, the number of distinct terms needed for representing a set of documents. A smaller dictionary size results in a saving of storage space and processing time. We will be using one such approach called Porter stemming algorithm (Porter, 1980) in our implementation to reduce dictionary size and thus better efficiency.

IMPLEMENTATION AND ANALYSIS

The implementation program was written in Java and the software once developed was trained and tested using two public spam corpuses – Ling-spam Corpus (small size) and Enron-spam Corpus (big size) as found in (Software and data – Natural Language Processing Group, na).

The text based spam detector was implemented in Java for the three approaches outlined, with single and multi-keyword detection capability. The code has extensive features to process text from the emails and to extract keywords. The following steps were done to develop the software into its working mode.

1. A ignore word list was formed with common words that should be ignored as keywords. These are the common words in English.

2. The mails files were read from the spam corpus one by one during training session and two files were created. One file with single keywords and multiple keywords and another file with only single keywords. The multiple keywords are those continuous words that can be found in any mail text (e.g. best selling pills).

3. The two files created are sorted in ascending order. The file names of the keyword origin are appended at the end of every line.

4. Using TreeSet class in Java, multiple entries were removed, as a set doesn't store duplicate entries. Now the two files contain only unique words along with its file name, where it is found. The file names were later removed as in Figure 3 and 4 and it shows the captured key words.

5. Based on the above files, the count or frequencies of all these keywords in these two files are taken separately. This gives the number of mails where these single keywords or multiple keywords were found.

6. During the testing phase, the mails are checked for single and multiple keywords by reading those files. Binary search is used on sorted files.

7. The frequencies of all single keywords are added in spam and non-spam to find the bayesian score. Similarly, the frequencies of all multiple keywords are added in spam and non-spam to find the bayesian score.

8. Weights are used (rather multiplied) if necessary, especially for multiple keyword frequency to improve the overall score accuracy.

9. Context matching percent is also calculated for all keywords, based on how many single or multiple keyword match is found during testing phase.

Ling-spam corpus is a mixture of 481 spam messages and 2412 messages sent via the Linguist list, a moderated (hence, spam-free) list about the profession and science of linguistics. Attachments, HTML tags, and duplicate spam messages received on the same day are not included. The corpus contains 10 directories with a combination of non-spam and spam mails amounting to 2893 total mails.

Figure 3. The file showing multiple (yet unique) spam keywords in different spam emails captured during testing session on spam corpus

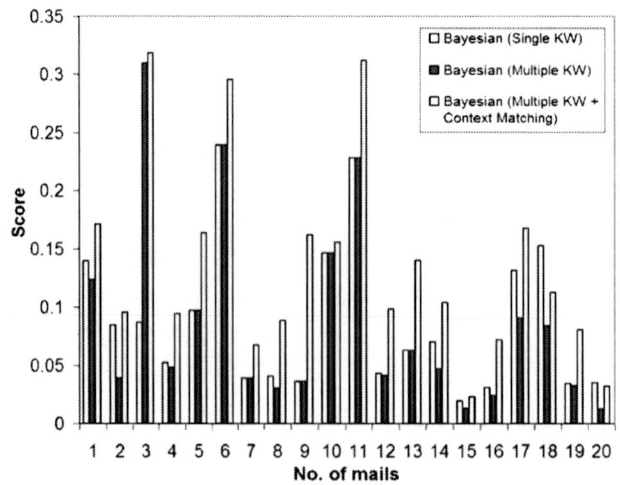

Figure 4. The file showing multiple (yet unique) non-spam keywords in different spam emails captured during testing session on spam

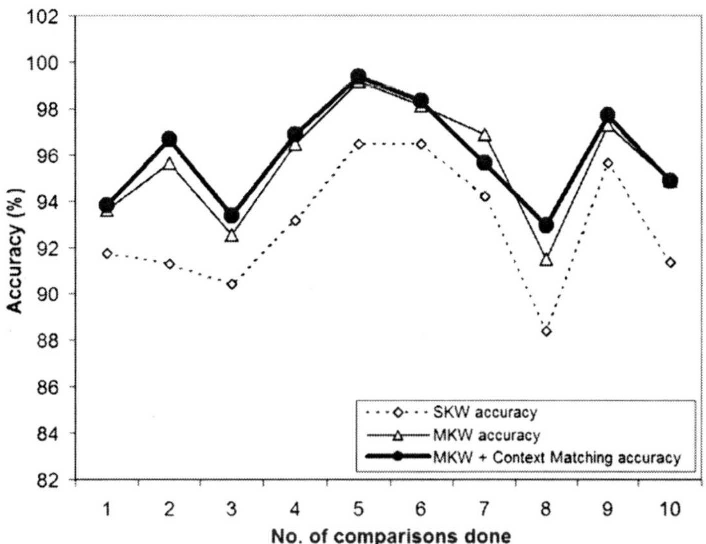

Enron-spam corpus contains preprocessed and raw forms of Enron-Spam datasets, amounting to 33716 total messages. The "preprocessed" directory contains the messages in preprocessed format. Attachments, HTML tags, and duplicate spam messages received on the same day are not included. The "raw" directory contains the messages in their original form. Spam messages in non-Latin encodings, ham messages sent by the owners of the mailboxes to themselves (sender in "To:", "Cc:", or "Bcc" field), and a handful of virus-infected messages have been removed, but no other modification has been made. The corpus is arranged into 6 directories that contains a combination of non-spam and spam messages.

In the Ling-spam corpus used (under bare directory), it contained contains 10 subdirectories (part1, ... part10). These correspond to the 10 partitions of the corpus that were used in the experiment. The 9 parts (part1 to part 9) were used for training and one part was used for testing (part 10). Later, all possible combinations of folders were used – nine for training and one for testing. Each one of the 10 subdirectories contains

spam and legitimate messages, one message in each file. In Enron corpus, it was organized into 6 folders. Each time five folders are used for training and the remaining one was used for testing. In our implementation, we extracted only the first 100 keywords from all the mails for spam score analysis. Figure 5 shows the scores during Ling-spam testing.

The average number of training and testing mails used in each of the 10 runs in Ling-spam corpus were as follows:

No. of Training Non-Spam mail = 2171
No. of Training Spam mail = 432
No. of Testing Non-Spam mail = 242
No. of Testing Spam mail = 49

The spam thresholds set were as follows: Bayesian with single keywords (0.15), Bayesian with multiple keywords (0.15) and Bayesian with multiple keywords and context matching (0.24). Table I shows the comparison of all possible combinations on folders in Ling-spam. You can see the three implemented Bayesian approaches

Figure 5. The graph showing the spam scores for emails during testing session on Ling-Spam corpus

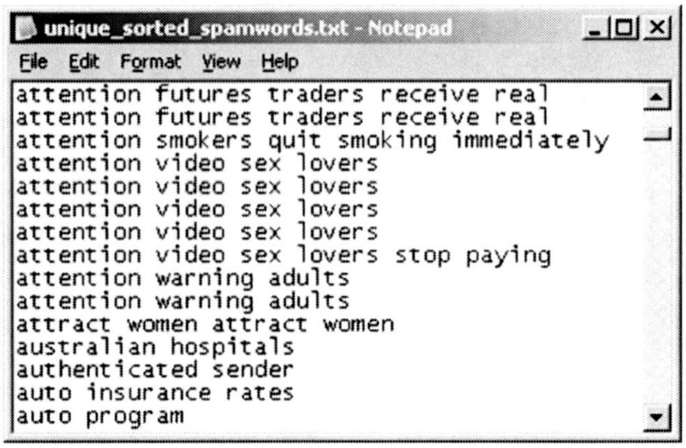

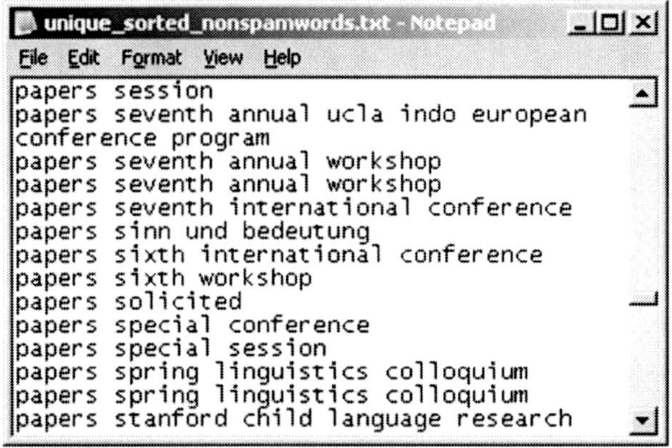

Figure 6. The graph for Ling-spam corpus showing the spam score accuracy for the three approaches (single keyword, multiple keyword, multiple keyword with context matching)

and the corresponding false positives and false negatives. Thus the average spam detection accuracy was around 96%. The accuracy graphs for all approaches are shown in Figure 6.

The average number of training and testing mails used in each of the 6 runs in Enron-spam corpus were as follows:

No. of Training Non-Spam mail = 12533
No. of Training Spam mail = 15671
No. of Testing Non-Spam mail = 4012
No. of Testing Spam mail = 1500

Figure 7 shows the scores during Enron-spam corpus testing. The spam thresholds set were as follows: Bayesian with single keywords (0.57), Bayesian with multiple keywords (0.59) and Bayesian with multiple keywords and context matching (0.70). Table II shows the comparison of all possible combinations on folders on Enron.

Generally the false positives and false negatives are getting lower for the third case with context matching. Thus, the false positives (non-spam as spam) and false negatives (spam as non-spam) percentage is lesser for the third category, that we

Table 1. Comparison table for ling-spam corpus

Bayesian with single keyword		Bayesian with multiple keywords		Bayesian with multiple keywords and context matching		
False positive %	False negative %	False positive %	False negative %	False positive %	False negative %	Train and Test folders
16.53	0	12.81	0	12.40	0	2-10 and 1
15.35	2.08	6.64	2.08	6.64	0	1, 3-10 and 2
12.86	6.25	8.71	6.25	7.05	≈ 6.25	1-2, 4-10 and 3
13.69	0	7.05	0	6.22	0	1-3, 5-10 and 4
7.02	0	1.65	0	1.24	0	1-4, 6-10 and 5
2.90	4.17	1.66	2.08	1.24	≈ 2.08	1-5, 7-10 and 6
11.62	0	6.22	0	4.56	≈ 4.17	1-6, 8-10 and 7
23.24	0	17.01	0	14.11	0	1-7, 9-10 and 8
8.71	0	5.39	0	4.56	0	1-8, 10 and 9
9.09	8.16	2.07	8.16	2.07	≈ 8.16	1-9 and 10
*12.10	*2.07	*6.92	*1.86	*6.01	*2.07	

Note: *Average

Figure 7. The graph showing the spam scores for emails during testing session on Enron spam corpus

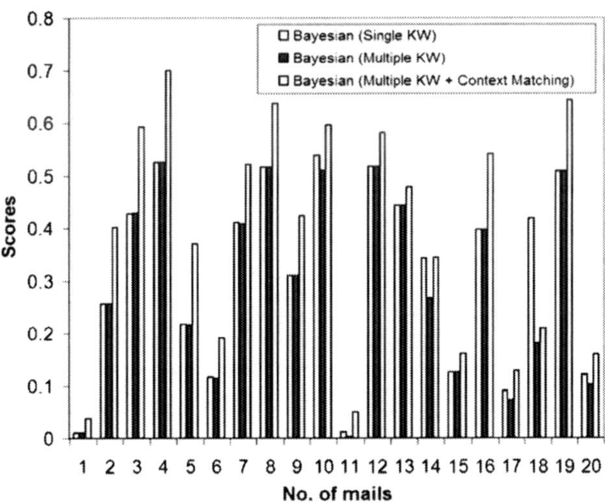

proposed. Thus the average spam detection accuracy was around 92%. The accuracy graphs for all three approaches are shown in Figure 8.

We wanted to check the effect of Porter stemming algorithm (Porter, 1980) on spam detection. The Porter stemming algorithm (or 'Porter stemmer') is a process for removing the commoner morphological and inflexional endings from words in English. Its main use is as part of a term normalization process that is usually done when setting up Information Retrieval systems. We used this algorithm to do spam detection using stem keywords, rather than using full keywords, on the above two corpuses and it yielded the results as

Table 2. Comparison table for enron-spam corpus

Bayesian with single keyword		Bayesian with multiple keywords		Bayesian with multiple keywords and context matching		
False positive %	**False negative %**	**False positive %**	**False negative %**	**False positive %**	**False negative %**	**Train and Test folders**
9.01	17.33	6.43	14.40	5.39	13.80	2-6 and 1
16.37	13.23	10.41	5.15	11.42	1.60	1, 3-6 and 2
9.72	8.80	5.38	5.13	5.96	4.73	1-2, 4-6 and 3
3.33	30.07	2.27	25.04	1.87	24.62	1-3, 5-6 and 4
2.80	31.18	2.00	20.02	1.20	13.71	1-4, 6 and 5
5.93	28.4	3.67	19.87	3.13	18.22	1-5 and 6
*7.86	*21.50	*5.03	*14.94	*4.83	*12.78	

Note: *Average

Figure 8. The graph for Enron corpus showing the spam score accuracy for the three approaches (single keyword, multiple keyword, multiple keyword with context matching)

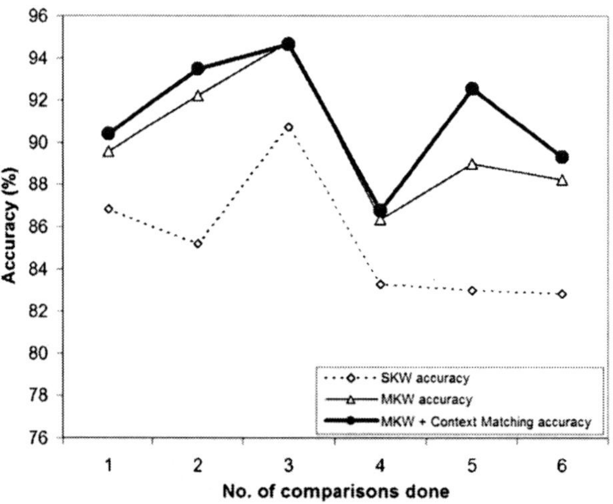

follows in table III and IV. You can see the three implemented Bayesian approaches and the corresponding false positives and false negatives. We did not observe considerable amount of improvement in spam detection, though there is improvement in keyword search efficiency. With porter stemmer approach the number of keywords would be smaller, as we consider only the stem keywords. Enron corpus (large corpus) spam detection average is better for all cases combined (89.9% accu-

racy compared to 88.8%) with Porter stemmer. With context matching sub-case, it is 91.7% accuracy compared to 91.2%. So that is an encouraging sign. Figure 9 shows the flow chart of the spam detection scheme that was implemented.

We also want to show the spam detection results of some commercial Bayesian filters available and the test results have been taken from an external source (Spam Filter Reviews, na). The sample size used in all cases is generally quite

Table 3. Comparison table for ling-spam corpus using porter stemmer algorithm

Bayesian with single keyword		Bayesian with multiple keywords		Bayesian with multiple keywords and context matching		
False positive %	False negative %	False positive %	False negative %	False positive %	False negative %	Train and Test folders
13.22	2.08	9.50	4.17	6.61	13.22	2-10 and 1
12.03	4.17	5.81	6.25	6.22	12.03	1, 3-10 and 2
7.88	2.08	6.22	0.00	4.98	7.88	1-2, 4-10 and 3
11.62	2.08	7.88	0.00	7.05	11.62	1-3, 5-10 and 4
2.89	2.08	1.65	2.08	0.83	2.89	1-4, 6-10 and 5
2.49	2.08	0.83	2.08	1.66	2.49	1-5, 7-10 and 6
6.22	0.00	4.15	2.08	4.98	6.22	1-6, 8-10 and 7
15.77	0.00	10.37	0.00	11.20	15.77	1-7, 9-10 and 8
6.22	6.25	3.73	4.17	3.32	6.22	1-8, 10 and 9
5.79	10.20	2.89	12.24	2.89	5.79	1-9 and 10
*8.41	*3.10	*5.31	*3.31	*4.97	*8.41	

Note: *Average

Table 4. Comparison Table for Enron-Spam Corpus using porter stemmer algorithm

Bayesian with single keyword		Bayesian with multiple keywords		Bayesian with multiple keywords and context matching		
False positive %	False negative %	False positive %	False negative %	False positive %	False negative %	Train and Test folders
9.31	16.20	7.00	12.53	3.76	16.20	2-6 and 1
14.72	11.23	11.10	3.34	7.20	3.01	1, 3-6 and 2
8.85	8.87	6.16	4.40	3.49	5.60	1-2, 4-6 and 3
3.00	27.98	2.33	21.12	0.93	25.43	1-3, 5-6 and 4
3.87	28.27	2.67	12.82	1.80	13.66	1-4, 6 and 5
5.73	25.09	3.80	14.64	2.40	16.62	1-5 and 6
*7.58	*19.61	*5.51	*11.48	*3.26	*13.42	

Note: *Average

less compared to what the author had done, especially with Enron corpus. Some of them use hybrid schemes along with other anti-spam approaches. The author had not verified the results himself. See the false positive and false negative values as compared to author's findings and some of which looks compatible.

STEPS TO FURTHER IMPROVE SPAM DETECTION

Some other additional steps that can improve the overall spam detection capability can be added as follows:

1. Check for any embedded hyperlinks within the email text, with the centralized hyper-

Table 5. Comparison Table for different commercial Bayesian anti-spam filters

Type of filter	Message count	Spam	False positive	False negative
Outlook spam filter	1361	89.05%	3.53%	2.87%
IHateSpam filter	2030	89.95%	3.74%	6.4%
SpamBully filter	695	89.86%	2.43%	1.14%
InBoxer filter	2588	86.13%	.97%	9.51%
MailWasher Pro filter	1407	91.61%	0.71%	18.27%
SpamWeed	739	82.95%	2.98%	27.20%

Figure 9. The flow chart of the Bayesian spam detection scheme with stemming and keyword contact matching

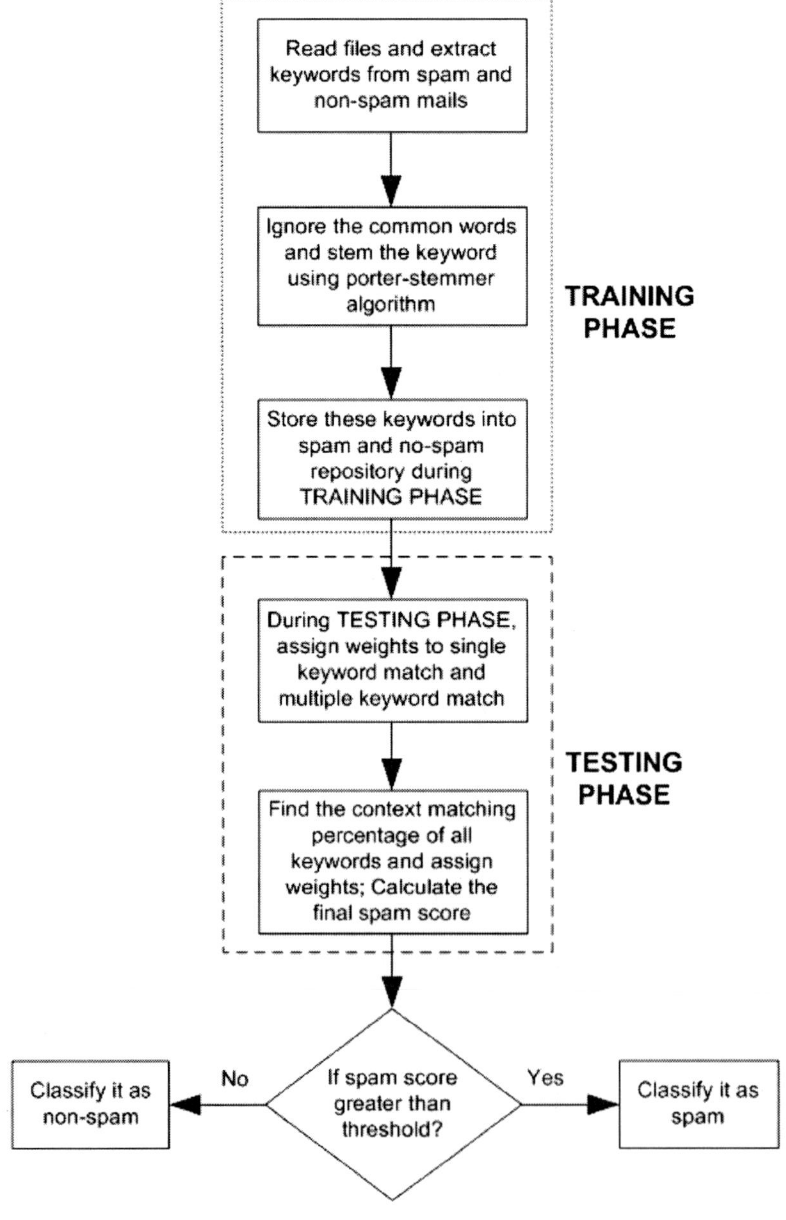

link blacklist. Stamp it as spam, if the link is found in hyperlink blacklist. This single step if positive, can override other spam score calculations.

2. The user software interface can have a "Report Spam" option, to report the anti spam server software, on the status of the new incoming emails. This ensures automatic on-going training in real time. The reported spam details are used for training and fed to database, once minimum n users have reported it as spam.

3. Special characters (like \$, -, *, digits 1-9, ', ", -#, etc.) introduced by spammers to confuse spam filters can be extracted/removed or replaced (say, 0 with o) from keywords to improve filtering.

4. Growing White List and Black Lists can be maintained as a local (or global) online repository that could be checked for existing spam signatures. Implement a white-list, which is a list of "fully permitted" email addresses. Black-listed email addresses will also be ranked based on how many people reported it as spam or phishing addresses.

5. Securing of SMTP Server is another option. SMTP servers from registered static IP address only should be allowed. It should support SMTP user authentication and be standardized to work only in this way. No SMTP relays should be allowed. SMTP servers should not be allowed to run from a dynamic IP address, as spammers could run their own SMTP servers from dial-up connections. Optionally, digital signatures can be gradually made mandatory in email-ing systems so that sender identity cannot be forged. This will prevent further email messages with spoofed sender addresses as such emails would be rejected. Only a valid sender can now send emails.

6. Implementing Grey Listing is a good option too. The Grey listing approach proposed by Harris (Harris, 2004) looks at three pieces of information that form a signature – the IP address of the host attempting the delivery, the envelope sender address and the envelope recipient address. If the receiving side has never seen this signature, the email would be rejected for the first time and it would become a bounced email. It would be allowed in only a second time (when the sender resends), after a delay of 25 minutes to 4 hours. Generally, this would stop spam emails to a great extent, since spammers may not resend (most of the time) their emails with the same signature.

7. Matching DNS names can improve the scenario. The web links in spam emails are also checked for veracity with the original organizations web domain, through a DNS query. If it is a concocted website link and a domain, the link can immediately be notified to the user and the central server database can be updated with the details. For example, consider a spam email with Citibank details, asking the user to click a web link to update Citibank account details. The first 2 octets in IP address of Citibank in decimal dot notation is 192.193 and this can be checked with the forged domain's IP address.

8. Email authentication can ensure that message is sent by the intended person who is the sender of the mail. The attacker normally forges the return address and would send email from a similar-looking domain to that of an original domain. There are different approaches proposed for email authentication, as of now. Return address forgery can be tackled by Sender-ID and SPF by checking DNS records to ensure whether the IP address of the sending MTA (Mail Transfer Agent) is an authorized sender. Domain level cryptographic signatures can also be used to provide authentication through Domain keys by cross-checking the DNS record. Cryptographically signed emails can be a

good option especially if signing becomes a normal way of sending emails.

CONCLUSION

Spam emails are also known as junk mails and most of the time, the spam is about commercial advertising or some fake get-rich-quick schemes etc. This chapter discusses some existing work on spam detection research and focuses on a case study done on two spam corpora. The spam detection implementation in Java and the subsequent analysis on two independent spam corpuses (Ling-spam and Enron-spam) shows that the Bayesian approach taking into account multiple keywords and keyword contexts looks very promising. The idea is very practical and can be implemented with much promise. The inclusion of porter stemmer algorithm to stem keywords can improve spam detection efficiency, as the search happens with a lower number of stem keywords. Thus the experimental results show that the proposed method is quite efficient and useful in identifying spam emails. Like in most anti-spam approaches, the filter needs to be trained with known spam and non-spam mails, so that it can classify the spam mails correctly later.

REFERENCES

Ali, S., & Xiang, Y. (2007). Spam Classification Using Adaptive Boosting Algorithm, *6th IEEE/ACIS International Conference on Computer and Information Science* (pp.972 – 976). Australia: IEEE Computer Society.

Androutsopoulos, I., Koutsias, J., Chandrinos, K. V., Paliouras, G., & Spyropoulos, C. D. (2000). An Evaluation of Naive Bayesian Anti-Spam Filtering. *Workshop on Machine Learning in the New Information Age, 11th European Conference on Machine Learning* (pp. 9-17). Spain: LNCS Springer.

Androutsopoulos, I., Paliouras, G., Karkaletsis, V., Sakkis, G., Spyropoulos, C., & Stamatopoulos, P. (2000). Learning to filter spam e-mail: A comparison of a naive bayesian and a memory-based approach, *4th PKDD's Workshop on Machine Learning and Textual Information Access*. France: LNCS Springer.

Balakumar, M., & Vaidehi, V. (2008). Ontology based classification and categorization of email, *Conference on Signal Processing, Communications and Networking* (pp.199-202). USA: IEE Computer Society.

Barracuda Networks. (2004). *An Overview of Spam Blocking Techniques*, White paper.

Chan, K. J., & Poon, J. (2004). Co-training with a single natural feature set applied to email classification, *IEEE International Conference on Web Intelligenc*. China: IEEE Computer Society.

Chiu, Y., Chen, C., Jeng, B., & Lin, H. (2007). An Alliance-based Anti-Spam Approach, *Third International Conference on Natural Computation* (pp.203-207). China: IEEE Computer Society.

Dhinakaran, C. Lee J. K., & Nagamalai, D. (2007). An Empirical Study of Spam and Spam Vulnerable email Accounts, *Conference on Future generation communication and networking* (pp.408-413). Korea: IEEE Computer Society. E-mail spam (na). *Wikipedia article*, Retrieved January 20, 2010, from http://en.wikipedia.org/wiki/Anti_spam_filter

Gao, Y., Yang, M., Zhao, X., Pardo, B., Pappas, Y. W., & Choudhary, T. N. (2008). Image spam hunter, *IEEE International Conference on Acoustics, Speech and Signal Processing* (pp.1765-1768). USA: IEEE.

Graham, P. (2003). *Better Bayesian Filtering.* Retrieved May 25, 2006 from http://www.paulgraham.com/ better.html

Harris, E. (2004). The Next Step in the Spam Control War: Greylisting, Retrieved February 25, 2009 from http://projects.puremagic.com/ greylisting/whitepaper. htm

Issac, B., & Raman, V. (2006). Implementation of Spam Detection on Regular and Image based Emails - A Case Study using Spam Corpus, *MMU International Symposium on Information and Communication Technologies* (pp.431-436). Malaysia: Multimedia University.

Kiritchenko, S., & Matwin, S. (2001). *Email classification with co-training* in the Centre for Advanced Studies on Collaborative Research (pp.1-8). Ontario, Canada.

Lan, M., & Zhou, W. (2005). Spam filtering based on preference ranking, Fifth International Conference on Computer and Information Technology (pp.223-227). China: IEEE Computer Society.

Ming, L., Yunchun, L., & Wei, L. (2007). Spam Filtering by Stages, *International Conference on Convergence Information Technology* (pp. 2209-2213).

Porter, M. F. (1980). An algorithm for suffix stripping. *Program, 14*(3), 130–137.

Sasaki, M., & Shinnou, H. (2005). Spam detection using text clustering, *International Conference on Cyberworlds* (pp.1-4). Singapore: IEEE Computer Society

Schneider, K. (2003). A comparison of event models for naive bayes anti-spam e-mail filtering, *11th Conference of the European Chapter of the Association for Computational Linguistics.* Hungary: ACM

Sirisanyalak, B., & Sornil, O. (2007). An artificial immunity-based spam detection system, *IEEE Congress on Evolutionary Computation* (pp.3392-3398). Singapore: IEEE.

Software and data (n.d.). *Software and data – Natural Language Processing Group.* Retrieved March 20, 2009 from http://nlp.cs.aueb.gr/software.html

Spam Filter Reviews. (n.d.). *Spam Filter Reviews.* Retrieved January 25, 2010, from http://www. whichspamfilter.com /Reviews/ SpamFilterReviews.htm

Types of Spam Filters. (n.d.). *Types of Spam Filters.* Retrieved January 25, 2010 from http:// www.whichspamfilter.com/ TypesOfFilters.htm

Zhou, Y., Jorgensen, Z., & Inge, M. (2007). Combating Good Word Attacks on Statistical Spam Filters with Multiple Instance Learning. *IEEE International Conference on Tools with Artificial Intelligence* (pp.298-305). France: IEEE Computer Society.

KEY TERMS AND DEFINITIONS

Spam: Spam emails are unwanted and unsolicited emails send by a person for commercial advertising and to breach security of computers with virus attachments.

Ham: Ham emails are regular and valid emails.

False Positive: When classifying emails as spam and ham, a false positive is the valid email that was erroneously classified as spam.

False Negative: When classifying emails as spam and ham, a false negative is the spam email that was erroneously classified as valid.

Bayesian Classifier: Bayesian Classifier puts incoming email into two or three groups – spam and ham (and sometimes "not-sure" which is a mail that isn't clearly spam or ham and hence is grouped into the third category).

Email Filtering: It is the processing of e-mail to organize it according to the automatic processing of incoming messages. The term also applies to the intervention of human intelligence in addition to the anti-spam techniques.

Chapter 13
On The Design of Secure ATM System

Lawan Ahmed Mohammed
King Fahd University of Petroleum & Minerals, Saudi Arabia

EXECUTIVE SUMMARY

Over the past three decades, consumers have been largely depending on and trust the Automatic Teller Machine, better known as ATM machine to conveniently meet their banking needs. ATM is a data terminal, it has to be connected to, and communicate through, a host processor. The host processor may be owned by a bank or any financial institution, or it may be owned by an independent service provider. Moreover, an ATM can support multiple ATM cards owned by different financial institutions or banks. Most host processors can support leased-line or dial-up machines. However, despite the numerous advantages of ATM system, ATM fraud has recently become more widespread. Recent occurrences of ATM fraud range from techniques such as shoulder surfing and card skimming to highly advanced techniques involving fraudulent mobile alerts, and account takeover via stolen information and call centers, software tampering and/or hardware modifications to divert, or trap the dispensed currency. In this chapter, we provide a comprehensive overview of the possible fraudulent activities that may be perpetrated against ATMs and investigates recommended approaches to prevent or deter these types of frauds. In particular we develop a model for the utilization of biometrics equipped ATM to provide security solution against must of the well-known breaches associated with the current ATM system practice.

INTRODUCTION

An automated teller machine (also known as Cash Machine), is a computerized device that provides the customers of a financial institution with the ability to perform financial transactions without the need for a human clerk or bank teller. Most modern ATMs identify the customer by the plastic card that the customer inserts into the ATM. The plastic card can contain a magnetic stripe or a chip that contains a unique card number and some security information, such as an expiration date

DOI: 10.4018/978-1-60960-015-0.ch013

and card validation code (CVC). When using an ATM, customers can access their bank accounts in order to make cash withdrawals (or credit card cash advances) and can check their account balances as well as purchasing mobile phone prepaid credit, paying bills and so on. ATM, was first introduced in 1960 by City Bank of New York on a trial basis, the concept of this machine was for customers to pay utility bills and get a receipt without a teller (NetWorld Alliance, 2003). It allows financial institutions to provide their customers with a convenient way, round the clock, to carry out varying transactions which included withdrawal of funds, made deposits, check account balance, and later on included features to allow customers pay bills, etc. There was no need for a cashier to be present or for a customer to physically visit the financial institutions premises to carry out such transactions. ATMs are not only located at banks but also increasing numbers of businesses, especially retailers for both customer convenience and a new revenue stream. Similarly this will reduce the cost of transactions as transactions that normally would require a bank employee's time and paperwork can be managed electronically by the customer with a card. A global ATM market forecast research conducted by Retail Banking Research Limited (RBR, 2010) shows that there are 1.8 million ATMs deployed around the world today and the figure is forecast to reach 2.5 mil-

lion by 2013. In a similar research by European ATM Security Team (EAST), the total number of ATMs in Europe continues to show year on year growth as shown in the Figure 1. In addition, there are 84,500 ATMs in Russia, which are not shown in the figure.

Authentication methods for ATM cards have little changed since their introduction in the 1960's. Typically, the authentication design involves a trusted hardware device (ATM card or token). The card holder's Personal Identification Number (PIN) is usually the only means to verify the identity of the user. Further, many existing designs based on such devices use a delegation technique whereby the device acts on behalf of the user by deploying its strong cryptographic capability. Typical ATM authentication process is depicted in Figure 3.

However, due to the limitations of such design, an intruder in possession of a user's device can discover the user's PIN with brute force attack. For instance, in a typical four digits PIN, one in every 10,000 users will have the same number.

As ATM card becomes widely used, it produces new kinds of crime, mostly derived from the security pitfalls of the magnetic media. The data in the magnetic stripe is usually coded using two or three tracks. The standard covering this area is ISO 7811. The technique for writing to the tracks is known as F/2F. The reason is that it is not that

Figure 1. Number of ATMs in Europe (excluding Russia) from 2005 - 2009

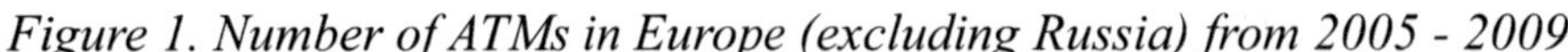

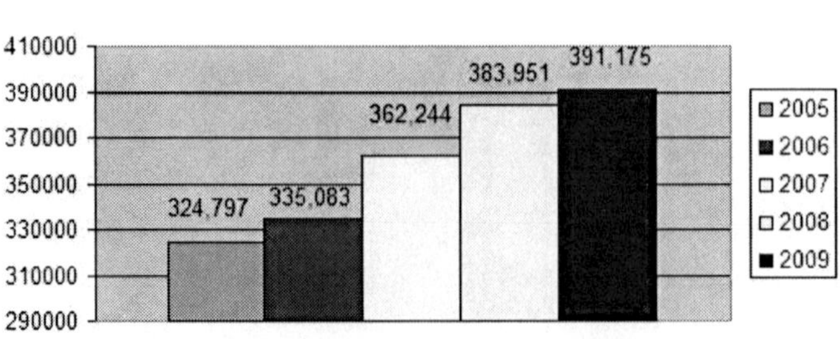

Figure 2. ATM authentication process

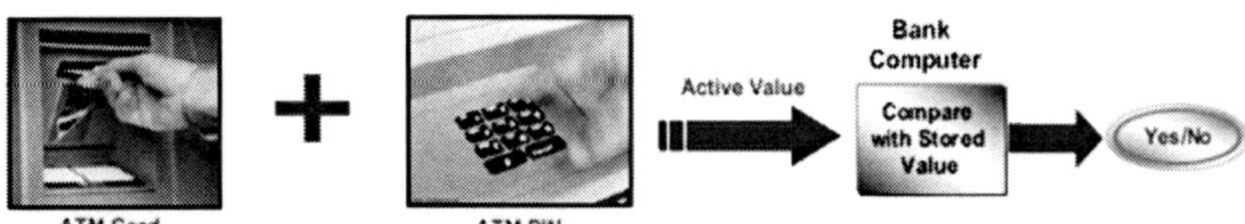

difficult and/or expensive to have the equipment to encode magnetic stripes. In fact, any type of coded badge can be decoded and duplicated if you devote enough money and talent to the task. The major encoding techniques, from the easiest to duplicate to the hardest are: *Electric circuit code, Magnetic stripe code, Magnetic code, Metallic stripe code, Capacitance code, Passive electronic code, Active electronic code.*

The first two are very easy to duplicate; the last five are significantly more difficult. When the code data are cryptographically encoded or contain other internal checks. Counterfeiting then would require both decoding and understanding the internal check algorithm. Some sensitive applications are using two main ways of encoding; the use of a magnetic material called high-coercivity (HiCo), and the low-coercivity (LoCo) material. The HiCo material requires stronger magnetic fields to encode in it. Any card reader can read any one of these materials, since the encoding technique (F/2F) is the same. The security resides in the fact that not many encoding machines in the market can handle the HiCo material, and are definitely more expensive than those to encode LoCo material. The manufacturers of these encoders will certainly want to know why someone may be interested in purchasing such a device. A good reason for using the HiCo material is that it is better suited to avoid local disturbances on the stripe due to magnetic fields and heat. Fortunately, magnetic stripe weakness has been partly addressed by the introduction in Europe of EMV smartcards (also known as Chip and PIN cards or Chip cards) - a standard for the interoperation of smart cards and enabled POS terminals and ATM's, for authenticating credit and debit card payments. EMV specification addresses issues such as *Application Independent, ICC to terminal Interface Requirements, Security & Key Management, Application Specification, Cardholder, Attendant, and Acquirer, Interface*

Figure 3. Percentages of ATM EMV compliance in Europe from 2005 - 2009

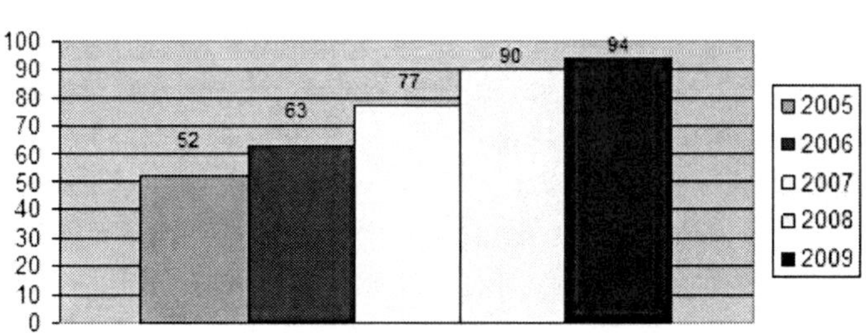

Requirements, Cardholder Verification, ICC Authentication. Details of these specifications can be found in (Diebold, 2003). The name EMV comes from the initial letters of Europay, MasterCard and VISA, the three companies which originally cooperated to develop the standard. EMV rollout in all countries in the Single Euro Payments Area (SEPA) is expected to be completed within this year (2010). Figure 3 shows the percentages of ATM EMV compliance from 2005 to 2009.

Despite security measures based on EMV specification, cases of ATM crimes continue to occur globally. Incidents have been reported in Asia-Pacific, the Americas, Africa, Russia and the Middle East. Some examples include:

- USD 500,000 were stolen from an Australian bank using a skimming device attached to an ATM in Melbourne (atmmarketplace, 2009(a)).
- Devices capable of scanning bank and credit cards details were placed on cash machine outside a supermarket in UK (BBC News, 2009).
- Ten ATMs were used to clone cards and steal more than USD 1 million from banking accounts in Melbourne (atmmarketplace, 2009(b)).
- USD 500,000 were stolen from more than 250 victims in Staten Island by placing cameras directly onto the ATM keypad and filming victims typing in their PIN codes (DailyNews, 2009).
- On November, 2009, a coordinated attack on 130 ATM machines in 49 cities enabled 'cashers' - low-level operatives probably recruited by higher-level criminals - to take $9m using cloned cards. The attack happened just two days before the Royal Bank of Scotland subsidiary discovered the data breach, focusing on data from its payroll and open loop giftcard business. The stolen data enabled the criminals to clone the cards. Cashers operated in cities from the US through to Russia and Asia (inforsecurity, 2009).
- More recently, in January 2010, a Boston area man was arrested for using cameras and skimming devices to steal over $100,000 from the account of ban customers (snopes, 2004).
- Similarly, the European ATM Security Team (https://www.european-atm-security.eu/) has announced the publishing of its first European Fraud Update report for 2010. According to the report, which is based on country crime updates from 19 European countries, found that ATM skimming, despite the wide launch of EMV/chip-and-PIN technology, remains a primary security issue in the European Union, with repeat attacks at single ATMs continuing to take place.

ATM ATTACK TECHNIQUES

ATMs are attractive to criminals because they provide direct access to currency, bank notes, and in some cases even user's personal information which can be used for identity theft. While an ATM may contain a significant amount of currency, bank cards themselves can give thieves access to customers'bank accounts which can easily exceed the value of the money contained in a single ATM. In the last few years, there have been many reports of hacking into the electronic ATM system and caused billion dollars of losses in the banking company itself. Oracle attack on authentication protocols and breaches affecting the ATM machine such as cloning of cards and hacking of PIN code have been reported increasingly. The U.S. Secret Service estimate annual losses associated with credit card fraud to be in the billions of dollars. Although it is commonly called the credit card statute, this law also applies to other crimes involving access devices including debit cards, ATM cards, computer passwords, personal identification numbers, credit card or debit card account numbers, long-distance access codes, and the Subscriber Identity Module (SIM) contained within cellular telephones that assign billing (http://www.secretservice.gov/criminal.shtml). These are increasing the need for further research in the design of ATM security systems as our modern society depends largely on electronic banking technologies. Details of some popular frauds/attacks are explained below in the following subsection.

Skimming Attack

This is the most popular breach in ATM transaction. In this case, criminal are taking advantage of technology to make counterfeit ATM cards by using a skimmer. Skimmers are devices used by crooks to capture data from the magnetic stripe on the back of an ATM card. These devices resemble a hand-held credit card scanner and are often fastened in close proximity to or over top of an ATM's factory-installed card reader. When removed from the ATM, a skimmer allows the download of personal data belonging to everyone who used it to swipe an ATM card. A single skimmer can retain information from than 200 ATM cards before being re-used. Example of skimmer is shown in Figure 4.

Figure 4. ATM skimmer

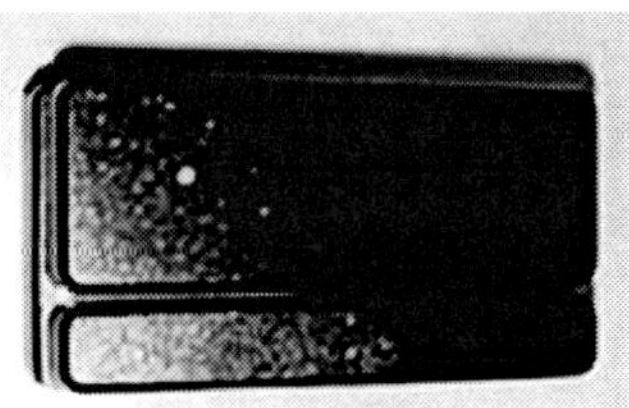

Skimming has risen substantially, and these high-tech bandits are fast gaining in their technical finesse, including buying their own ATM machines to capture your personal banking data. A report released by European ATM Security Team shows that in 2008, fraud related ATM crimes in Europe jumped 149% when compared with the previous year. According to the report, this increase in ATM fraud is linked primarily to a dramatic increase of skimming attacks as show in Figure 5. During 2008, a total of 10,302 skimming incidents were reported in Europe (see Figure 5).

According to the same report, the losses due to ATM fraud were significant and a total loss of almost EUR 500 million was reported in which over 4 million was due to skimming as indicated in Figure 6.

More recently, the EAST European Fraud Update report for 2010 which is based on country

Figure 5. ATM related fraud attacks by number of incidents 2008 (Source EAST & EPC)

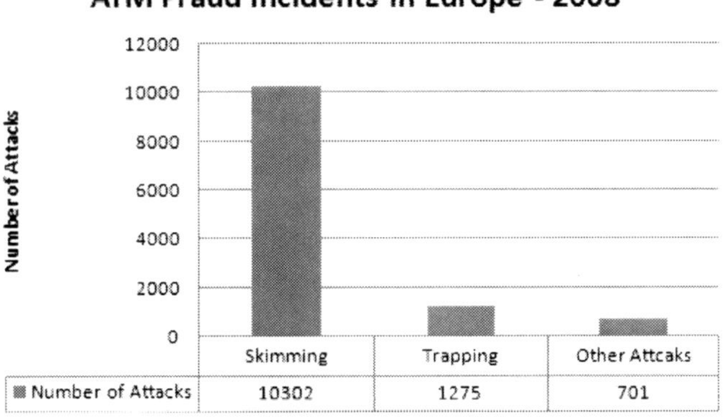

Figure 6. Losses due to ATM fraud in 2008 (Source EAST & EPC)

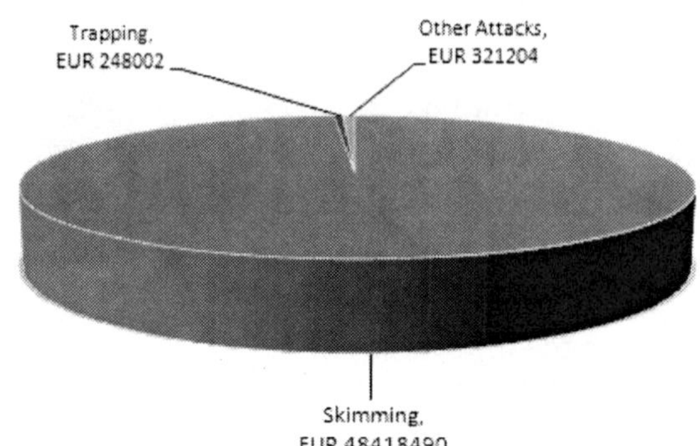

crime updates from 19 European countries, found that ATM skimming, despite the wide launch of EMV/chip-and-PIN technology, remains a primary security issue in the European Union, with repeat attacks at single ATMs continuing to take place.

Some counter measures against skimming as suggested by Diebold Incorporation are:

Jittering: Process that controls and varies the speed of movement of a card as it's swiped through a card reader, making it difficult (if not impossible) to read card data by the external device.

Alert systems: These systems monitor routine patterns of withdrawals and notify operators or financial institutions in the event of suspicious activity.

Chip-based cards: These cards house data on microchips instead of magnetic stripes, making data more difficult to steal and cards more difficult to reproduce.

Foreign object detection: ATMs equipped with this type of technology can alert owners, operators, or law enforcement in the event that a skimming device is added on the fascia of an ATM.

Card Trapping

This involves placing a device directly over or into the ATM card reader slot. In this case, a card is physically captured by the trapping device inside the ATM and the fraudster tries any method to capture the customer's PIN. When the customer leaves the ATM without their card, the card is retrieved by the thieves and used to make fraudulent cash withdrawals or to make other purchases. Typically only one card is lost in each attack. The criminals have to withdraw the whole device each time a card is trapped, although recently a card trapping device has been seen that can stay in place for a period of time and that allows removal of trapped cards without the removal of the device. The most common variant is known as the Lebanese Loop (see Figure 7). Thieves place a device fitted with a loop of tape, wire, or strong thread over an ATM card reader. This allows a card to be inserted and read by the ATM, but not returned. The criminals obtain the PIN by watching the user entering the PIN (shoulder-surfing), and retrieve the card after the victim has left the ATM under the impression

Figure 7. Lebanese Loop (trapping device)

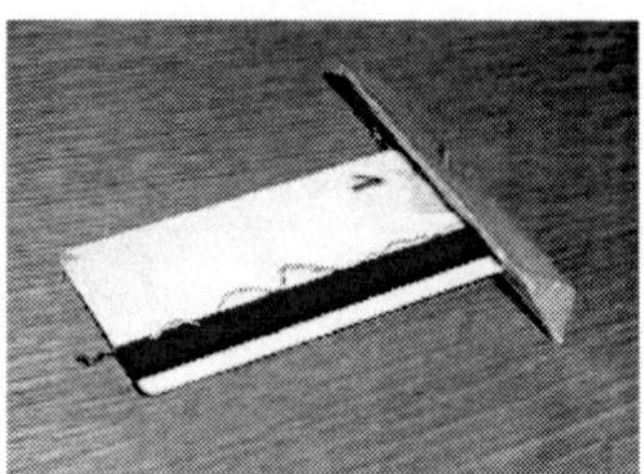

that the card has been retained by the ATM for other reasons.

There are multiple techniques used to capture the customer's PIN including the use of video cameras, offering advice and distracting the customer while they input their PIN. Another variant of card trap is known as the Algerian V.

PIN Cracking

A research paper by (Bond and Zielinski 2003) shows how a complex mathematical attack can yield a PIN in an average of 15 guesses. By design, it shouldn't be possible to guess a four-digit pin in less than an average of 5,000 attempts. The attack, documented in the paper is directed against the decimalisation tables used to translate between a card PIN and the hexadecimal value of a PIN generated when the hardware security module checks the validity of a number. The attack works by simply manipulating the contents of the decimalisation table in order to gain clues (such as which digits are or are not present in the PIN). Refining the technique, which allows a PIN to determine in an average of 24 iterations, might allow an attack to succeed in 15 guesses. In practice, the risk of attack comes from a corrupt insider, perhaps in computer operations and with access to sensitive manuals who might be able to use the attack to refine what would otherwise be a brute force attempt to guess PIN numbers. In the short term, the best way to guard against the attack is to make sure it isn't possible to change the decimalisation table without permission. As a stop gap an audit trail in ATM hardware security module will also allow the banks to spot when something suspicious occurs.

In a similar research conducted by (Berkman and Ostrovsky, 2006) explains how the processing system used by banks is open to abuse. One of the attacks targets the translate function in switches - an abuse functions that are used to allow customers to select their PINs online. In either case, the flaws create a means for an attacker to discover PIN codes, for example, those entered by customers while withdrawing cash from an ATM providing they have access to the online PIN verification facility or switching processes. A bank insider could use an existing Hardware Security Module (HSM) to reveal the encrypted PIN codes and exploit them to make fraudulent transactions, or to fabricate cards whose PIN codes are different than the PIN codes of the legitimate cards, and yet all of the cards will be valid at the same time. Even worse, an insider of a third-party Switching provider could attack a bank outside of his territory or even in another continent.

Phishing/Vishing Attack

Fraud and scams using mail communication have existed for many years. With the advent of email, cell phones and the Internet this scam has quickly spread worldwide. Phishing scams are designed to entice the user to provide the card number and PIN for their bank card. Thieves will send an email representing them as a bank and claiming that your account information is incomplete, or that the user needs to update their account information to prevent the account from being closed. The user is asked to click on a link and follow the directions provided. The link however is fraudulent and directs the user to a site set up by the thieves and designed to look like the user's bank. The site directs the user to input sensitive information such as card numbers and PINs. The information is collected by the thieves and used to create fraudulent cards, withdraw funds from the user's account and make purchases. In Nigeria, more traditional phishing e-mails encouraged the receiver to register on-line for an enhanced security plan. Commercial banks in Nigeria warned consumers of such fake phishing e-mail claiming to be from the Central Bank of Nigeria (CBN) advising that ATM cards required upgrading. Example of such phishing e-mail message is shown in Figure 8.

Figure 8. Phishing e-mail message

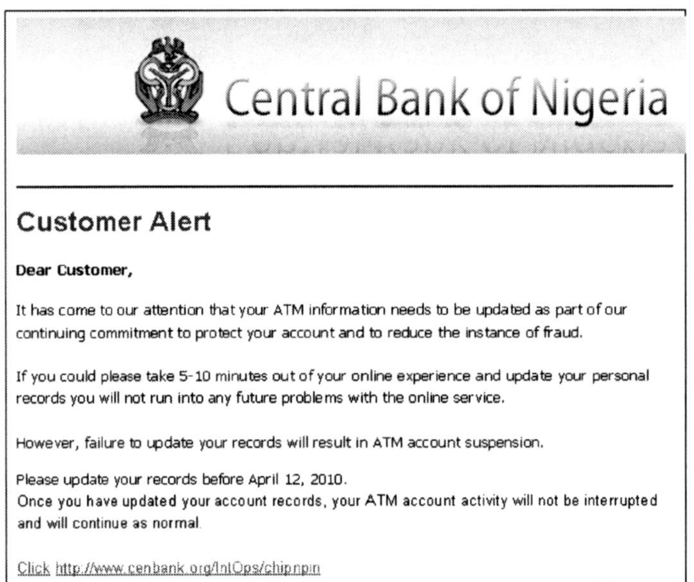

Figure 8 is an example of a phishing e-mail, disguised as an official e-mail from a fictional bank. The sender is attempting to trick the recipient into revealing confidential information about his/her ATM card. Note that although the URL of the bank's webpage appears to be legitimate, it actually links to the phisher's webpage. This can be verified by pointing the mouse at the link in which the actual website will be shown (which is usually different from what is written physically). Also one can notice that after clicking the URL will be diverted to another link. In this case, the link will divert the user to the actual URL which is http://verificationsonline100.t35.

Figure 9. Phisher's webpage

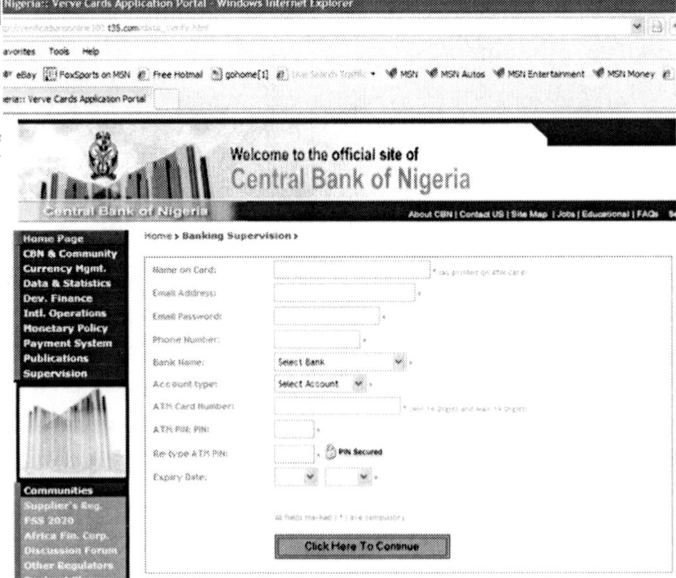

com/data_verify.html as shown in Figure 9. This looks like the actual real bank website (http://www.cenbank.org/)

In 2008, the financial services industry has seen an increase in the numbers of phishing attacks that are expected to continue into 2010, including sophisticated spear phishing and Rock Phish attacks. The Anti-Phishing Working Group (http://www.antiphishing.org/) reports that the financial services sector remains the most targeted sector being attacked, with an average of more than 90 percent of attacks being directed at financial services.

Traditionally, after a successful phishing attack, the criminal would extract the needed information and go onto the online account and remove the victim's bank funds. This has changed for some of the more sophisticated criminals in recent years were instead of looting the victim's account, they don't set up fake bill pay or take money directly from the account. Instead they go to the check image page, where they take a copy of the victim's check. Many financial institutions are now offering check images as part of their online banking services to their customers. The checks contain the victim's bank account number, signature, address, phone etc. These details are treasure for most criminals. They can either take the copy or make paper counterfeit checks to distribute, or take that information and create PayPal accounts or other online payment accounts that will leave the victim on the hook for any purchases.

Malicious Software

ATMs often now use publically available operating systems and off the shelf hardware and as a result are susceptible to being infected with viruses and other malicious software. The malicious software is injected into the ATM through network attacks, or through other infected devices. Once installed on the ATM, the malicious software will collect card information and PINs. According to a report by (Linda, 2009), some security researchers have found malware code that lets a criminal take control over ATMs.

Another report by SpiderLabs (the forensics and research arm of TrustWave), found a Trojan family of malware that infected 20 ATMs in Eastern Europe. The researchers warn that the malware may be headed toward US banks and credit unions, as well as other parts of the world. The malware lets criminals take over the ATM to steal data, PINs and cash (SpiderLabs, 2009). Trustwave's performed analysis of the malicious software and found that the malware captures magnetic stripe data and PIN codes from the private memory space of transaction-processing applications installed on a compromised ATM. The compromised ATMs ran Microsoft's Windows XP operating system. The malware is designed to allow third parties to control different aspects of the machine's operation, including the gathering of sensitive data from the magnetic stripe on the card. It is also possible to use the software to force an ATM to dispense all of the cash stored in its cassette. The malware was produced by a developer serving an organized team, according to experts from the company. It codifies roles and responsibilities with different privileges, accessed using different trigger cards, with identity data designed to specify the holder's role codified on the magnetic strip. SpiderLabs analysts do not believe the malware includes networking functionality that would allow it to send harvested data to other, remote locations via the Internet. The malware does, however, allow for the output of harvested card data via the ATM's receipt printer or by writing the data to an electronic storage device (possibly using the ATM's card reader). Analysts also discovered code indicating that the malware could eject the cash dispensing cassette. What follows is a high-level summary of the key features identified during Trustwave's in depth analysis of the malware sample. It is, however, believed that this is a relatively early version of the malware and that subsequent versions may have additions functionalities.

The malicious code, which is detected as *Troj/Skimer-A,* contained references to Diebold DLLs and appeared to be sending instructions that would assist in the stealing of PINs and information from cards entered into the machine. In addition, it appears that the malicious code is designed to skim money from accounts in Russian, Ukrainian and American currency. Figure 10 depicted the malicious code. The Trojan is believed to be attacking Diebold ATM machines. In view of this Diebold had contacted customers in January warning them about the urgent security threat to their systems.

Diebold issued an update to its ATM software, and recommended that it be installed on all of its Windows-based ATMs globally. According to the company, the update should prevent the Skimer-A Trojan horse from successfully stealing information from cash machine users.

ATM hacking

Hackers use sophisticated programming techniques to break into websites which reside on a financial institution's network. Using this access, the hackers access the bank's systems to locate the ATM database. The hackers collect card numbers, and if necessary, alter the PIN for the cards they are planning to use. The hackers then sell the cards and their data to other hackers. Those hackers create ATM cards using the stolen information, and use the cards to withdraw cash from the accounts. Though hacking should really only be used to describe attacks against the internals of the ATMs software or the ATMs systems security but is also commonly used to describe attacks against card processors and other components of the transaction processing network. Many reports have shown that US have experienced a number of high profile 'ATM hack' attacks against well known credit card and debit card processors. Some of the systems security breaches have included compromise of the PIN in addition to the card data, with subsequent fraudulent spend using cloned credit cards and cloned debit cards at ATMs.

According to ATM Market Place (http://www.atmmarketplace.com/), illegal ATM software is to blame for many recent ATM hacking attacks. In spite of reports regarding more frequent hacking of ATM software, banks and financial institutions of some countries not only do not invest in ensuring safety, but tend to install illegal and non-secured software, which increases security risk even more.

Physical Attack

The main objective of conducting ATM physical attacks is to gain access to the cash within the ATM safe or the ATM security enclosure. Some of the most common methods include ram raids (smash and grab), explosive attacks (gas and non-gas)

Figure 10. Troj/Skimer-A – Malicious Code (Source Sophos Plc)

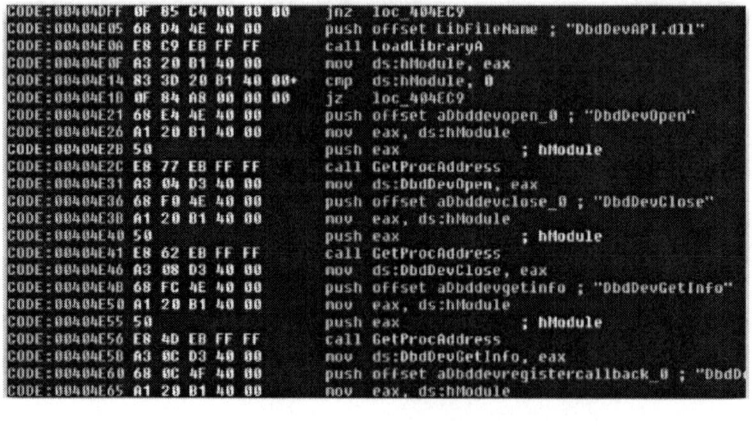

```
CODE:00404DFF 0F 85 C4 00 00 00       jnz     loc_404EC9
CODE:00404E05 68 D4 4E 40 00          push    offset LibFileName ; "DbdDevAPI.dll"
CODE:00404E0A E8 C9 EB FF FF          call    LoadLibraryA
CODE:00404E0F A3 20 B1 40 00          mov     ds:hModule, eax
CODE:00404E14 83 3D 20 B1 40 00+      cmp     ds:hModule, 0
CODE:00404E1B 0F 84 A8 00 00 00       jz      loc_404EC9
CODE:00404E21 68 E4 4E 40 00          push    offset aDbddevopen_0 ; "DbdDevOpen"
CODE:00404E26 A1 20 B1 40 00          mov     eax, ds:hModule
CODE:00404E2B 50                      push    eax             ; hModule
CODE:00404E2C E8 77 EB FF FF          call    GetProcAddress
CODE:00404E31 A3 04 D3 40 00          mov     ds:DbdDevOpen, eax
CODE:00404E36 68 F0 4E 40 00          push    offset aDbddevclose_0 ; "DbdDevClose"
CODE:00404E3B A1 20 B1 40 00          mov     eax, ds:hModule
CODE:00404E40 50                      push    eax             ; hModule
CODE:00404E41 E8 62 EB FF FF          call    GetProcAddress
CODE:00404E46 A3 08 D3 40 00          mov     ds:DbdDevClose, eax
CODE:00404E4B 68 FC 4E 40 00          push    offset aDbddevgetinfo ; "DbdDevGetInfo"
CODE:00404E50 A1 20 B1 40 00          mov     eax, ds:hModule
CODE:00404E55 50                      push    eax             ; hModule
CODE:00404E56 E8 4D EB FF FF          call    GetProcAddress
CODE:00404E5B A3 0C D3 40 00          mov     ds:DbdDevGetInfo, eax
CODE:00404E60 68 0C 4F 40 00          push    offset aDbddevregistercallback_0 ; "DbdD
CODE:00404E65 A1 20 B1 40 00          mov     eax, ds:hModule
```

and cutting (e.g. rotary saw, blow torch, thermal lance, diamond drill). Robbery can also occur when ATMs are being replenished or serviced. Staffs are either held up as they are carrying money to or from an ATM, or when the ATM safe is open and cash cassettes replaced. Sometimes, physical attacks are attempted on the safe inside the ATM. The goal is to penetrate the ATM to open the safe door or to make an opening in the safe sufficiently large to remove the cash. ATM explosive attacks or ram raid occurs globally but are most prevalent in the US, perhaps partly due to the large number of ATMs deployed in soft-target locations such as convenience stores. Incidents about ATM physical attacks from many countries are reported in (SecurityDigest, 2010). There are a variety of mechanical and physical factors that can inhibit attacks to the safe.

- The certification level of the safe (UL 291 Level 1 is recommended as a minimum for ATMs placed in unsecured, unmonitored locations)
- Alarms and sensors that will detect physical attacks on the safe
- Ink stain technologies that will ruin and make unusable any removed banknotes

SECURITY MEASURES

As technology advances, as ATM applications become more ubiquitous, as more confidential data is transmitted over the ATM system, as more sensitive transactions are conducted, as more threats breaches are reported, the challenge of securing the system becomes more urgent. Many security services in bank transactions are dependent on authenticating users such as generation of accurate audit trails, non-repudiation in communications, preserving confidentiality (Miller, 2003), and other input validation techniques such as batch totals, format checks, reasonableness checks, and transaction validation. These features only ensure that certain procedures are followed, and cannot

tell whether the person with the card and PIN is authorized to use it, they just ensure that the data transmitted follows certain guidelines or protocols that requests such as cash withdrawals are made within reasonable limits, that money is transferred to the proper account, and so forth. Therefore, it is essential to develop stronger authentication and identification measures to stop criminals from committing fraudulent act. Security measures against some of the attacks mentioned above are discussed below.

Ink-Staining

The rise in ram raids has spurred greater demand for solutions that help law enforcement track ATM thieves, or at least make ATM thefts unattractive. Ink-staining technology, which is triggered within an ATM's cash cassettes when the machine is jostled or moved, renders notes unusable. It's a technology that's been around a long time and has been used for years as a way to track down bank thieves, since the ink cannot really be washed off from bank notes or from the skin. A number of players provide services in this space. Wincor Nixdorf (a corporation providing retail and retail banking hardware, software, and services) offers an ink-staining module that resides within the cash cassette. If the cassette is handled incorrectly or opened by force, then the cash is sprayed. The purpose of the ink-staining technology is to cut down on ATM thefts, as well as internal thefts committed by cash carriers and ATM-service providers.

Global Positioning Systems

In addition to ink-staining, global positioning systems, or GPS, also are gaining some ground in the ATM world. While the technology is sometimes limited, such as when an ATM is placed in a van, where the van's metal exterior blocks a satellite's ability to continue tracking the ATM's GPS device, it has allowed financial institutions and law enforcement to recover stolen equipment, sometimes with the cash still intact.

PIN Security

The USA Department of Defense (DoD) Computer Security Center on password management guideline defines the probability of guessing a particular password as:

$$P = L \times R/S$$

Same idea can be used to determine the security of PINs. It can be used to determine the probability that a PIN can be guessed during its lifetime. The smaller that probability, the greater the security provided by the PIN. All else being equal, the longer the PIN, the greater the security it provides. The basic parameters that affect the length of the PIN needed to provide a given degree of security are:

- **L** = maximum lifetime that a PIN can be used to log into the system before it must be changed.
- **P** = probability that a PIN can be guessed within its lifetime, assuming continuous guesses for this period.
- **R** = guessing rate, i.e., number of guesses per unit of time that it is possible to make.
- **S** = PIN space, i.e., the total number of unique PINs that the PIN generation algorithm can generate. S is defined in turn as $S = A^M$, where **A** is the number of characters in the alphabet (the set of characters that may used in a PIN), and **M** is the PIN length.

To illustrate: If PINs consisting of 4 digits using an alphabet of 10 digits (e.g., 0-9) are to be generated: $S = 10^4$ that is, 10,000 unique 4-digit PINs could be generated. Likewise, to generate random 6-digit PINs from an alphabet of 10 digits: $S = 10^6 = 1,000,000$

Now, let us assume that a PIN lifetime is from 1 month up to one year, and that a PIN can be tried at a rate of 1,000 per second (a reasonable value on many of today's architectures), one can easily compute the probabilities of guessing PINs of various lengths. As we lower our estimate of **A** or increase our estimate of **R** (to account for faster processors), these probabilities only gets worse. Manipulating our equation also gives us a procedure for determining the minimum acceptable PIN length for a given system:

1. Establish an acceptable PIN lifetime **L** (a typical value might be one month).
2. Establish an acceptable probability **P** (the probability might be no more than 1 in 1,000,000).

Solve for the size of the PIN space **S**, using the equation derived from the previous one:

$$S = L \times R/P$$

Determine the length of the PIN, M, from the equation:

$$M = Log\ S/Log\ A$$

When other parameters (**L** and **R**) are not considered (i.e. setting their values to 1), it is very easy to calculate the probability as **P = 1/S**. Table 1 gives an idea about the PIN's security.

As you can see, the longer your PIN is the harder it would be to guess.

EMPLOYING BIOMETRICS: PROPOSED DESIGN

Biometric identification is utilized to verify a person's identity by measuring digitally certain human characteristics and comparing those measurements with those that have been stored in a

Table 1. Probability of Guessing a PIN based on the number of characters Used

Characters In PIN	Probability of Guessing the PIN
1	1 in 10
2	1 in 100
3	1 in 1,000
4	1 in 10,000
5	1 in 100,000
6	1 in 1,000,000
7	1 in 10,000,000
8	1 in 100,000,000

template for that same person. Templates can be stored at the biometric device, the institution's database, a user's smart card, or a Trusted Third Party (TTP) Service Provider's database. Where database storage is more economic than plastic cards, the method tends to lack public acceptance. However, (Polemi, 1997) found that TTPs can provide the confidence that this method is missing by managing the templates in a trustful way.

There are two major categories of biometric techniques: *physiological* (fingerprint verification, iris analysis, hand geometry-vein patterns, ear recognition, odor detection, DNA pattern analysis and sweat pores analysis), and *behavioral* (handwritten signature verification, keystroke analysis and speech analysis). (Deane *et al.* 1995) found that behavior based systems were perceived as less acceptable than those based on physiological characteristics. Of the physiological techniques, the most commonly utilized is that of fingerprint scanning.

In developing countries such as Nigeria, ATM fraud seem to be committed by mostly individuals linked to bank officers who are able to provide pin numbers and other relevant information required to commit such crimes. With biometrics, such fraudulent incidents can be minimized, as an added layer of authentication is now introduced that ensures that even with the correct pin information and in possession of another person's ATM card, a fraudster will not be able to withdraw

any money since the biometric features of every individual is unique.

The advantages of this may include: all attributes of the ATM cards will be maintained, counterfeiting attempts are reduced due to enrolment process that verifies identity and captures biometrics, and it will be extremely high secure and excellent user-to-card authentication. However, memory limitation in current cards may jeopardize this approach. Table 2 gives the required bytes for various biometrics. Additional information about biometric technology and standards can be found from the following organizations: The Biometric Consortium (www.biometrics.org), International Biometric Industry Association (www.ibia.org), or BioAPI Consortium (www.bioapi.com).

In general, the primary advantage of biometric authentication methods over other methods is that they use real human physiological or behavioral characteristics to authenticate users. These biometric characteristics are permanent and thus cannot easily be changed, lost, faked or forgotten. These advantages are for the benefit of users as well as system administrators because the problems and costs associated with lost, reissued or temporarily issued can be avoided, thus saving some costs of the system management.

On the other hand, the major risk posed by the use of biometric systems in an authentication process is that a malicious subject may interfere with the communication and intercept

Table 2. Required Bytes for Biometrics

Biometric	Bytes Required
Finger scan	300-1200
Finger geometry	14
Hand geometry	9
Iris recognition	512
Voice verification	1500
Face recognition	500-1000
Signature verification	500-1000
Retina recognition	96

the biometric template and use it later to obtain access (Luca et al, 2002). Likewise, an attack may be committed by generating a template from a fingerprint obtained from some surface. Further, performance of biometric systems is not ideal, as there is a trade-off between FAR (False Acceptance Rate) and FRR (False Rejection Rate), and 100% FAR/FRR is absolutely impossible. Two neutral reports on the test of some biometrics products are (Tony et al. (2001); Steven (2002)). As a negative sound, ACLU (American Civil Liberties Union) has also reported poor performance of face-recognition technology in practice (Jay & Barry, 2002). Although few biometric systems are fast and accurate (in terms of low false acceptance rate) enough to allow identification (automatically recognizing the user identity), most of current systems are suitable for the verification only, as the false acceptance rate is too high.

Our end to end ATM system simulation program will be taking a smart card, a maximum of 8 characters, numbers or mix of the both PIN and fingerprint as verification factors of the authentication process. The smart cards we used in the simulation program are the ACOS smart card; the PIN created by the user will be stored inside cards. In the verification part, the users have to submit the correct PIN DES encrypted current session key to get access to the next level. Users have 3 successful attempts to enter the correct PIN, else the cards will be locked and render it to useless.

Lastly, we use the fingerprint as the biometric identifiers as it is a unique identifier born with any human races. As we know, fingerprints are part of the DNA and no two humans in the whole world owns the same ones. We use fingerprint instead of other biometric elements, such as voice, because fingerprint is the most simple biometric identifier technique which takes shortest enrollment time and not affected by other factors such as illness. Other biometric identifier such as voice can be altered by many causes, illness, stress, background noise which made the identifying process troublesome (Christine, 2003). What worse is that users' voice can be recorded and be modified easily using a computer.

Our system integrate biometric identification into normal, traditional authentication technique use by electronic ATM machines nowadays to ensure a strong, unbreakable security and also non-repudiate transactions. In order to demonstrate the strength of our proposed authentication

Figure 11. AET60 BioCARDKey

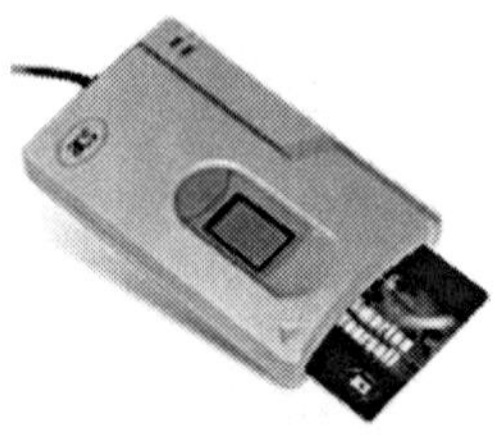

protocol using the combination of three authentication methods of card, PIN and fingerprint, we used AET60 BioCARDKey development kit manufactured by Advanced Card System Ltd as shown in the Figure 11.

The proposed design involves two phases namely enrollment phase and verification phase. Each of the phases is briefly describe below.

Enrollment - Prior to an individual being identified or verified by a biometric device, the enrollment process must be completed. The objective of this enrollment process is to create a profile of the user. The process consists of the following two steps:

1. Sample Capture: the user allows for a minimum of two or three biometric readings, for example: placing a finger in a fingerprint reader. The quality of the samples, together with the number of samples taken, will influence the level of accuracy at the time of validation. Not all samples are stored; the technology analyzes and measures various data points unique to each individual. The

number of measured data points varies in accordance to the type of device.

2. Conversion and Encryption: the individual's measurements and data points are converted to a mathematical algorithm and encrypted. These algorithms are extremely complex and cannot be reversed engineered to obtain the original image. The algorithm may then be stored as a user's template in a number of places including servers and ATM card.

A new and blank ATM card has to be enrolled with user details before it can be verified later. Enrollment system is usually operated by the admin to enter their customer details into the card. However, exception applies to the PIN entry where it should be entered by the user themselves and need to enter the PIN again to make sure they enter the correct ones.

Identification and Verification - Once the individual has been enrolled in a system, he/she can start to use biometric technology to have access to his account via the ATM machine or related system to authorize transactions.

Figure 12. Flowchart for the enrollment process

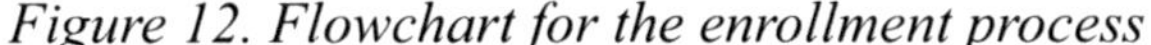

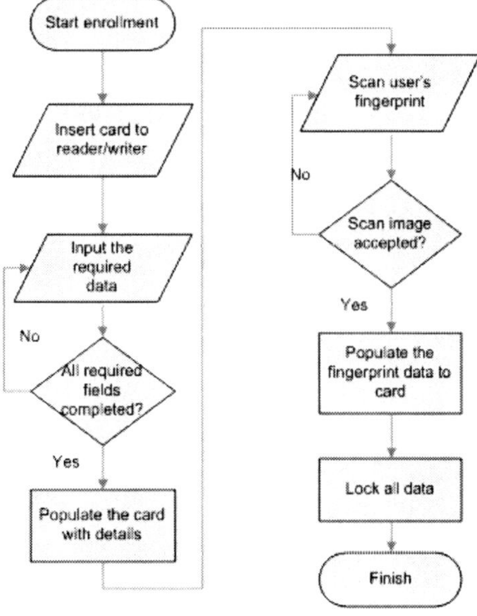

Figure 13. Implementation design for the enrollment process

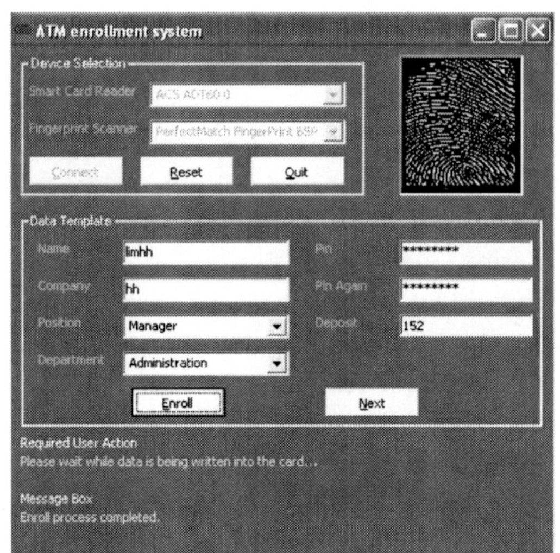

1. *Identification*: a one-to-many match. The user provides a biometric sample and the system looks at all user templates in the database. If there is a match, the user is granted access, otherwise, it is declined.
2. *Verification*: a one-to-one match requiring the user provides identification such as a PIN and valid ATM card in addition to the biometric sample. In other words, the user is establishing who he/she is and the system simply verifies if this is correct. The biometric sample with the provided identification is compared to the previously stored information in the database. If there

Figure 14. Flowchart for the verification process

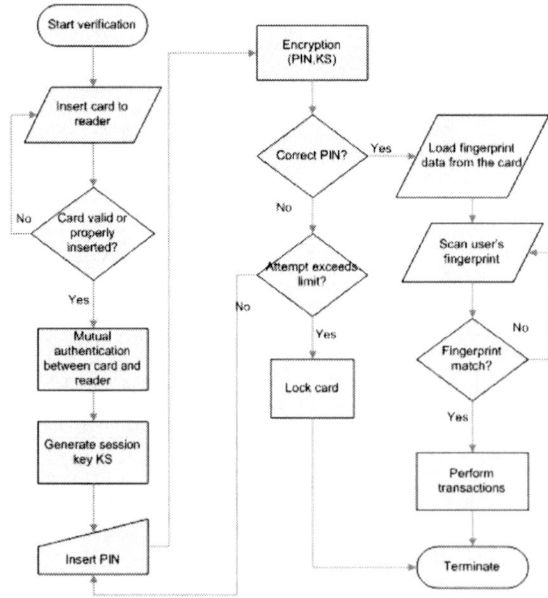

is a match, access is provided, otherwise, it is declined.

After the card has been enrolled with user data, this particular card will be the user's ID. The PIN and fingerprint sample from the user were also encrypted and save into the card. In order to get access into the ATM machine, the user has to present the card to the card reader, and then verify the PIN and lastly matched their fingerprint detail with the card. In this particular system, the ATM interface is quite a simple one just showing the simple debit and credit function, what we tried to emphasis in our project is the complex verification part which includes the MAC and PIN encryption.

ADVANTAGES AND DISADVANTAGES OF THE PROPOSED SYSTEM

As with any other technology, biometrics has its own advantages and disadvantages. The best reason why biometrics is getting more popular and widely implemented is a convenience of having authenticating mechanisms with a user. We can't forget parts of our body at home, and we can't lend it. We don't need to memorize fingerprints and then change it every 3 months as with passwords. Biometrics can last virtually forever, until something is amputated or damaged. More details can be found in literatures (Kim et. al., (2003); Lin and Lai (2004); Yoon and Yoo 2005))

On the opposite side, there is a factor of users accepting or not accepting a particular biometric technique. Some people are still hesitant to be authenticated using fingerprints, since it was associated for a long time with criminals and prisons. However, most people accept voice recognition. Retina and iris recognitions trouble some people due to the exposure to the light, which they consider to be harmful for the eyes etc. Further, a problem common to all biometric systems including fingerprint is that unauthorized use of biometric information is very easy (Bolle et. al. 2002). For example, a fingerprint can be acquired from objects touched by the person. Originally, fingerprint personal authentication was put to practical use on the precondition of a close range or face-to-face interface. Therefore, protecting the privacy of fingerprint information has not been given sufficient consideration. Some of the advantages and disadvantages of the all

Figure 15. Implementation design for the verification process

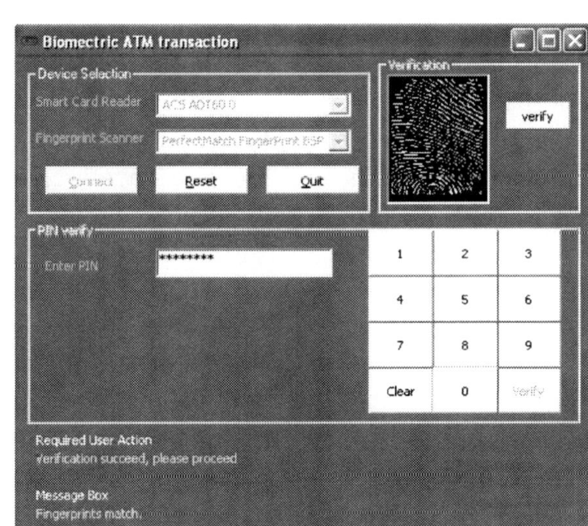

Table 3. Comparison between ATM Card and Biometrics

Technology	Advantages:	Disadvantages:
ATM Card	Two-factor authentication. Physically secure Support multiple applications and Cryptographic capabilities. Ensures user's privacy. Easy to use and wider acceptance by the public due to portability On board processing capabilities. Inexpensive and convenience	Must be with the user. Easily lost or stolen. Split-in-trust. PIN guessing and brute force attacks
Biometrics	Harder to impersonate. Not transferable/shareable. Easy and faster to use. Cannot be lost High security. Roaming; with its owner at all times	Fail To Enroll (FTR) rate Some methods are not applicable to some individuals. Privacy, anonymity, and users acceptance issues. Not very reliable due to FAR/FRR. Increases system's cost. Lack of standardize
Biometric ATM	Strongest authentication with high accuracy rate. High degree of non-repudiation. Blocks guessing, theft, cloning, lost, or forgotten, problems etc Additional layer of security: three-factor authentication.	Lack of standardization Some methods cannot be implemented due to card memory limitations. Can inherit some of threats associated with biometrics and or card. Time consuming for the customers.

three well-known authentication mechanisms are given in Table 3

CONCLUSION

Automatic Teller Machines have become a mature technology which provides financial services to an increasing segment of the population in many countries. Biometrics, and in particular fingerprint scanning, continues to gain acceptance as a reliable form of securing access through identification and verification processes. This chapter identifies a high-level model for the modification of existing ATM systems to economically incorporate fingerprint scanning; and, outlines the advantages of using such system. As Biometrics technology is becoming cheaper both in its application and usage, financial institutions need to invest in this technology as a way of securing transactions and gaining customers confidence as well as satisfaction. In addition to fingerprints, other biometric ATM technologies are emerging; Fujitsu provides a highly reliable biometric authentication system based on palm vein pattern recognition technology. Already deployed at leading financial institutions in Asia, the Fujitsu palm vein device has added a new level of security for employees and customers. The results have an extremely high degree of accuracy with a false acceptance rate of less than 0.00008%, while maintaining a false rejection rate of only 0.01%.

Considering most of the ATM frauds discussed, biometrics will certainly be a chosen security measure. There is certainly no silver bullet method or technology advocated that will guarantee a 100% eradication of ATM fraud completely (there never is), since the emergence of new technology everywhere in the world is followed closely by a subverting technique or method but can certainly go a long way in minimizing it. By integrating the biometric identifiers into the current ATM system, the access will be strongly protected by three factor authentications as well as high accuracy. Problems of cloning of the cards and the breaking of the PIN code will be tackled as well because hackers cannot easily sneak pass the most complex and final session of the authentication process, with is biometric identifiers. Besides, high degree of non-repudiation will also be guaranteed as the owners cannot deny their DNA themselves.

ACKNOWLEDGMENT

The author wishes to acknowledge King Fahd University of Petroleum and Minerals (KFUPM) Saudi Arabia and Hafr Al-Batin Community College for their support in providing the various facilities utilized in the process of producing this chapter and the book in general. This work was supported by the Deanship of Scientific Research (DSR) program of King Fahd University of Petroleum and Minerals (KFUPM), under Project Number: # **IN101001.**

REFERENCES

ATM Market Place. (2009a). *ATM scam nets Melbourne thieves $ 500,000*. Retrieved December 2, 2009, from http://www.atmmarketplace.com/article.php?id=10808

ATM Market Place. (2009b). *Australian police suspect Romanian gang behind $ 1 million ATM scam*. Retrieved November 13, 2009, from http://www.atmmarketplace.com/article.php?id=10883

Berkman, O., & Ostrovsky, O. M. (2006). *The unbearable lightness of PIN cracking*. Retrieved May 3, 2009, from http://www.arx.com/files/Documents/ The_Unbearable_Lightness_ of_ PIN_Cracking.pdf

Bolle, R., Connell, J., & Ratha, N. (2002). Biometric Perils and Patches. *Pattern Recognition, 35*, 2727–2738. doi:10.1016/S0031-3203(01)00247-3

Bond, M., & Zielinski, P. (2003). *Decimalisation table attacks for PIN Cracking*. Retrieved December 9, 2006, from http://www.cl.cam.ac.uk/techreports/UCAM-CL-TR-560.pdf

DailyNews. (2009). *ATMs on Staten Island rigged for identity theft; bandits steal $500G '*. Retrieved September 9, 2009, from http://www.nydailynews.com/news /ny_crime/2009/05/11/2009-05-11_automated_theft_bandits_steal_ 500g_by_rigging_atms_with_pinreading_gizmos.html#ixzz0J8qBVdar&D

Deane, F., Barrelle, K., Henderson, R., & Mahar, D. (1995). Perceived acceptability of biometric security systems. *Computers & Security, 14*(3), 225–231. doi:10.1016/0167-4048(95)00005-S

Diebold. (2003). *EMV White Paper*. Retrieved April 11, 2010, from www.diebold.com/solutions/a tms/opteva/emv.pdf

EMV. (2004). *Integrated circuit card specifications for payment systems*. Retrieved January 14, 2010, from https://partnernetwork.visa.com/vpn/global /category.do?userRegion=1&categoryId=61&documentId=94

Gershon, C. (2003). Biometrics Authentication & Smart Cards. *GSA/FTS Network Service Conference,* Managing the Future: Mastering the Maze. Retrieved December 9, 2009, from http://www.fts.gsa.gov/2003_network_conference/ 5-1_biometric_smartcards/

Inforsecurity. (2009). *$9m lifted in RBS Worldpay ATM heist*. Retrieved April 16, 2010, from http://www.infosecurity-us.com/ view/524/9m-lifted-i n-rbs-worldpay-atm-heist

Jay, S., & Barry, S. (2002). Drawing a blank: The failure of facial recognition technology in Tampa, Florida. *An ACLU Special Report*, Jan. 2002. Retrieved October, 9, 2009, from http://www.aclu.org/issues/ privacy/d rawing_blank.pdf

Kim, H. S., Lee, J. K., & Yoo, K. Y. (2003). ID-based password authentication scheme using smart cards and fingerprints. *ACM SIGOPS Operating Syst. Rev.*, *37*(4), 32–41. doi:10.1145/958965.958969

Lin, C. H., & Lai, Y. Y. (2004). A flexible biometrics remote user authentication scheme. *Computer Standards & Interfaces*, *27*(1), 19–23. doi:10.1016/j.csi.2004.03.003

Luca, B., Bistarelli, S., & Vaccarelli, A. (2002). Biometrics authentication with smartcard, *IIT TR-08/2002*, Retrieved October, 9, 2009, from http://www.iat.cnr.it/attivita/progetti/ parametri biomedici.html

McGlasson, L. (2009). *ATM Fraud: 7 Growing Threats to Financial Institutions*. Retrieved April 2, 2010, from http://www.bankinfosecurity.com/ articles. php?art_id=1523&opg=1

NetWorld Alliance. (2003). *Timeline: The ATM's history*. Retrieved June, 20 2009, from http://www.atm24.com/NewsSection/Industry%20 News/Timeline%20-%20The%20ATM%20History.aspx

News, B. B. C. (2009). *Shoppers are targeted in ATM scam*. Retrieved July 11, 2009, from http://news.bbc.co.uk/2/hi/uk _news/england/tees/4796002.stm

Polemi, D. (1997). *Biometric Techniques: Review and evaluation of biometric techniques for identification and authentication, INFOSEC*. Institute of Communications and Computer Systems, National Technical University of Athens.

RBR. (2010). *Global ATM Market and Forecasts to 2013*. Retrieved May 7, 2010, from www.rbrlondon.com

SecurityDigest. (2010). *ATM Fraud and Security Digest News*. Retrieved April 7, 2010, from www.atmsecurity.com/monthly-digest March 2010

Snopes. (2004). *Thieves Equip ATMs with Duplicate Card Reader and Wireless Camera*. Retrieved April 20, 2010, from http://www.snopes.com/fraud/ atm/atmcamera.asp

SpiderLabs. (2009). *ATM Malware Analysis Briefing*. Retrieved May 15, 2010, from https://www.trustwave.com/ spiderLabs-papers.php

Steven, K. (2002). Testing iris and face recognition in a personnel identification application. *In The Biometric Consortium Conference*, February 2002. Retrieved October, 21, 2009, from http://www.itl.nist.gov/div895/isi s/bc/bc2001/FINAL_BCFEB02/FINAL_1_Final%20Steve%20King.pdf

Tony, M., Gavin, K., David, C., & Jan, K. (2001). Biometric product testing final report. *Issue 1.0, CESG/BWG Biometric Test Programme*. Retrieved August 17 2009, from http://www.cesg.gov.uk/technology/ biometrics/media/Biometric% 20Test%20Report%20pt1.pdf

VISA. (2004). *Guidelines for PIN Security Requirement: Version 2.0*. Retrieved March 6, 2010, from http://partnernetwork.visa.com/st/pin/pdfs/ PCI PIN Security Requirements.pdf

Yoon, E. J., & Yoo, K. Y. (2005). A new efficient fingerprint-based remote user authentication scheme for multimedia systems, in *9th Int. Conf. Knowledge-Based & Intelligent Information & Engineering Systems (KES 2005)*, 2005, (pp. 332–338), Paper LNAI 3683.

KEY TERMS AND DEFINITIONS

ATM: A computerized device that provides the customers of a financial institution with the ability to perform financial transactions.

Biometrics: Techniques for identifying or verifying people based on their physiological or behavioral characteristics.

Shoulder Surfing: A security attack where the attacker uses observation techniques, such as looking over someone's shoulder, to get information.

Phishing Scams: A scam (usually by e-mail) that encompasses fraudulently obtaining and using an individual's personal or financial information.

Card Skimming: The illegal copying of information from the magnetic strip of a credit or ATM card.

Card Trapping: The term used to describe attacks where the user's ATM card is trapped and prevented from being return back to him/her.

Chapter 14
Network Security through Wireless Location Systems

André Peres
Federal Institute of Science and Technology – Rio Grande do Sul, IFRS, Brazil

Raul Fernando Weber
Instituto de Informática, UFRGS, Brazil

EXECUTIVE SUMMARY

The advantage of wireless local area networks, giving the mobile stations the possibility of moving freely inside the network access range comes with a security drawback. The fact that microwave signals can transpose walls and suffers with attenuation, reflections, refraction, diffraction and dispersion, depending of the obstacles, makes very difficult to define the network access range. Without the knowledge of the network boundaries, the network administrator cannot define a physical delimiter to network access. Without the user-location, it is impossible to restrict the network access based on the physical access boundaries defined by the administrator. When the wireless network operates indoor, the many obstacles and the dynamic behavior of these obstacles (some people moving around, for instance) make the micro-wave signal behavior change the range and aspect of the network. This work proposes a new approach to indoor user-location mechanism, based on the dynamic behavior of the obstacles and consequent changes on network range in IEEE 802.11 networks. Finally a new authentication system WlanAuth, based on the user location is proposed.

INTRODUCTION

When we use wireless networks, our goal is to grant network access with stations mobility and flexibility. The stations must be capable of access the network while moving freely around the access area, without losing connection, and the network physical infrastructure must support the addition of new wireless devices and the disconnection of them without any physical impact.

Because of the behavior of the signal propagation, however, when we compare wireless networks with wired ones, we identify that there are some differences in the management and security aspects that must be considered.

DOI: 10.4018/978-1-60960-015-0.ch014

In wired networks we can easily confine the physical network inside a room or building, according to the network connection points (switch ports and cables). Also, it is easy to segregate different subnets in the same building, in separate rooms or areas using routers and/or firewalls.

When we have a minimal IP address organization (subnet oriented), it is easy to determine the physical location of a station, only analyzing the IP address information.

In wireless networks, the physical coverage area is difficult to define due to the microwave signals behavior. The reflection, refraction, diffraction, scattering, attenuation and multi-path, distribute the coverage area with non-uniform patterns. The network access area is defined by the obstacles that the microwave signal encounters in the environment.

This means that the network physical access area definition is not possible in a easy way, and a wireless station can capture the network signals even outside the building.

Related to segregation, besides the fact that the WLAN (Wireless Local Area Networks) IEEE802.11 uses multiplexed channels to deliver different networks in the same environment, the responsibility of channel selection relies on the wireless station. This means that the network manager can not control the subnet in which a client tries to connect.

Because of the mobility, the wireless stations can be in any place inside the coverage area. This means that only by analyzing network data, it is not possible to locate the device. A malicious stations can be anywhere inside (or outside) the building.

In order to conceive a wireless network with the minimum of security, the IEEE presents some mechanisms to achieve device authentication and data privacy in IEEE802.11 networks. The data privacy is achieved by one of the mechanisms IEEE (1999), IEEE (2003), IEEE (2004):

- *WEP*: Wired Equivalent Privacy. It is a symmetric cryptography protocol (same key to cypher and decipher the data) base in the RC4 algorithm;
- *WPA*: Wireless Protected Access. Based in the WEP algorithm, but with temporal keys - TKIP (Temporal Key Integrity Protocol). Can be used with an initial pre-shared-key (PSK) or with 802.1x protocol;
- *WPA2*: or IEEE802.11i. It uses the AES cryptography algorithm, which is much more robust than WEP and WPA. It also can be used with a PSK or 802.1x.

WEP was proven by Fluhrer (2001) to have security vulnerabilities based on weak keys generated by the cryptography algorithm. The WPA tries to overcome this vulnerabilities through TKIP, changing the shared secret from time to time. It is possible to break WPA by capturing the authentication packets and discovering the first key (pre-shared key) through brute force Moskowitz (2003).

Because WPA2 uses AES, it is considered the more robust cryptography protocol for IEEE802.11 networks.

The authentication can be made trough the protocols Gast (2002):

- *open system*: the station submits an authentication request, and the access point always returns a success response. This means that open system is a null authentication protocol as all stations are always accepted;
- *shared key*: the station submits an authentication request. The AP (Access Point) generates a challenge (random text) e sends it to the station. The station must then cipher the challenge with the WEP algorithm, and returns the result to the AP. The AP then verifies that the station knows the shared key.
- *802.1x*: uses a RADIUS server in order to identify the user with user/password challenge. The AP manages a communication

between the station and the RADIUS server. The server indicates to the AP if the user is valid.

Using the cryptography mechanisms, and authentication protocols, it is possible for the network administrator, to avoid the malicious access to network data, and the control of in which network the device have credentials to access. It is not in the scope of this work to describe the existent security mechanisms in more detail.

Besides the existents security mechanisms, the major difference between wired and wireless network management and security remains in the impossibility of the physical location of a device in the wireless network access area.

This can be exemplified in the academic environment used in the development of the WlanAuth mechanism.

This environment takes place in the ULBRA university (campus Guaiba, Brazil) where the network is segregated with a different subnet for each classroom. Before the class hour, the teacher can specify which web sites the students can access during class in a proxy configuration specific system. The access control is then made by the network proxy, with the defined rules been applied to that specific classroom.

The problem is that with wireless access, the wireless network devices are placed in the wireless subnet, and distributed in several classrooms. Because of this physical distribution, there is no way to apply a unique proxy rule to all the devices in the wireless subnet.

Imagine that one student in classroom X is forced to obey the teacher rules if he/she is using the wired network, but if he/she is using the wireless network the access is not controlled.

With wireless device location, it is possible to define the physical location of a specific device, and with this information, we can apply the proxy rules defined to that location to the specific station IP address.

The main goal of the WlanAuth is to finds out, in which room are each wireless device, and then apply the security rules of that perimeter to each specific station.

It is important to call attention to the fact that with this kind of control, the security policy can migrate from a subnet/IP address oriented based, to a physical perimeter's base.

BACKGROUND

There are several techniques and models to determine a wireless device location. All of them need two or more known points as location references (usually the access points) and some exchange of information between the mobile device and a location server.

With the exchange of information between the device and the network, it is possible to locate the device by:

- AoA - Angle of Arrival: with information about the angle of arrival of microwave signal from the device in two known (and distinct) points of the building, it is possible to determine two lines that intersect. The intersection point is the (most likely) location of the device. Sayed (2005);

- *AmpoA*: Amplitude of Arrival: with information about the amplitude of arrival of the microwave signals from the device, it is possible to locate the device through fingerprinting (a matrix made by the network administrator with sample points of signal amplitude in the building), or through free space path loss (FSPL) calculation (the microwave attenuation in obstacle free environments), and determine the distance between the known points and the device. With the distance it is possible to triangulate the location;

- *ToA*: Time of Arrival: this technique uses the time that it takes to a signal to travel between the device and the access point and obtain the distance between them. With the distance it is possible to triangulate the location.

As some examples of AoA, we have:

- Elnahrawy (2007), where the authors use mobile directional antennas to determine the angle of arrival of microwaves signals and the signal rate.

The angle should be obtained as a line connecting the device and the AP. For this, there must be placed several directional antennas in the AP covering 360 degrees, or directional antennas capable of moving. When a device signal is received, the location server must determine which antenna received the signal with the greater signal amplitude. With this information, the location server discovers the angle between the AP and the station. With 2 APs it is possible to draw two lines, and determine the intersection point of this lines. The intersection point is the possible device's location.

Some authors that used AmpOA:

- in Bahl (2000) and Taheri (2004), the authors used fingerprint to locate the mobile devices. These two proposals determines that should be constructed a matrix with samples of signal rates between a generic device and each access point in the environment (at least three access points must be visible in all sample points). It is necessary to map each point of the environment, setting the signal rate between the point and each access point presented in the environment and insert the signal rates obtained into a matrix. Each AP has one of this sample matrixes mapping the environment. Those matrixes are stored in the location server. In order to locate a device, this device should collect the signal ampli-

tude rates (from it to each access point) and send this information to the location server. The server searches for the closest sample values in the matrixes to locate the device. The error in this case is directly associated with the quality of the samples, the number of sample points, the differences between the antennas used to do the samples and the antenna used by the device, and the dynamic obstacles in the building.

- Faria (2005), the author presents the relation between FSPL and location. It is used the Log-Distance Path Loss formula to distance calculation, and then the triangulation is made. In this technique there are no matrices, and with the amplitude information received from the device to be located is used with triangulation or trilateration in order to locate it.

The ToA approach is used in:

- Morrison (2002). The author uses special hardware (oscilloscope) attached to the wireless network interface to obtain the time between sending a datagram to the network, and receiving an ACK (acknowledgement) datagram (atomic action in 802.11 networks);
- Capkun (2008). The authors use application level software in order to obtain the time that it takes for information be exchanged between the wireless station and the location server. This time is used in order to determine the distance between them.

Because of the microwave behavior, all the cited techniques have their accuracy dependable of the environment. Our objective is to consider the environment in the construction of the location mechanism. As presented in Stoyanova (2007) and Yasar (2006), simple variations of environment can lead to precision error in the location process for all technique.

We choose AmpOA technique to develop our solution. The choose of AmpOA comes from the fact that ToA needs some kind of special hardware to do the job (the hardware is needed because of the light-speed microwave propagation, which needs nanosecond precision clock to be accurate), and the need of special antennas in AoA technique (not usual in commercial APs).

Our proposed technique uses the same fingerprint method as Bahl (2000) and Taheri (2004) with the increment of adding the dynamic obstacle identification in the location process, as in Kitasuka (2003), Pandey (2005) and Moraes (2006). The fingerprint models in Bahl (2000) and Taheri (2004) consider only the obstacles that are in the sampled environment in the moment of sampling process. This means that any change in the environment will affect directly in the location precision. The fingerprint matrix must be updated every time a mobile device is located in order to increase this precision. In Kitasuka (2003), Pandey (2005) and Moraes (2006) the dynamic obstacle identification is made, without considering the use of the location process in a security mechanism.

In addition, because of the obstacles in the environment, in some cases, the discovered location point is far from the actual physical location of the device. If the device informs the amplitude with a great degree of variation (caused by the obstacles) the fingerprint location system can locate the station in distant points on the matrix, not relative to the amplitude variation. This is not the case in triangulation/trilateration, because the circles radius variations are directly related to the amplitude variation informed by the station.

With this in mind, we suggest that the system must use a mix-technique, using fingerprint and trilateration. The trilateration (which does not consider any obstacles, fixed or dynamic) can inform a location area in the fingerprint matrix. After delimiting this area, the fingerprint matrix should be updated according with the present obstacles, and the fingerprint location technique is used.

Also, we must consider the use of the location process in a security mechanism. This means that all the devices involved in the location must be trusted.

This is not the case in Moraes (2006), Pandey (2005) and Kitasuka (2003). In those papers, the authors used client stations in order to discover the environment obstacles (as amplitude sniffers devices). This can not be used in our scenario, because of the lack of trust in the students stations and the probability of compromising those stations with malicious objectives.

In Buschmann (2007), the authors use the amplitude comparison among neighbor wireless sensor in order to obtain one sensor's location. Each sensor have a list of neighbor sensors and the expected amplitude of signals. When the system must locate a single sensor, it consults this tables and the location is determined according with the number of common neighbors.

As a similar approach, Krishnan (2005) suggests that low cost stations should be distributed in the environment in order to measure their amplitude and locate a specific wireless station.

In Kuwabara (2009), a initial map is constructed, based on few amplitude samples in the environment. Each sample is analyzed and its distance to each AP is stored. Based on these samples a fingerprint matrix is constructed. When analyzing the samples, the difference between the expected amplitude and the real signal received is used as a base to determine the obstacles in the environment. The obstacles is assumed as been in the middle point between the sample location and the AP. This information is important, because it is used as a base to construct the fingerprint matrix.

Our technique uses the fingerprint with dynamic obstacle identification in a security mechanism. This means that the informations collected to obtain the obstacle identification should be made by trusted devices, and the information collected in the user mobile device should be confirmed by the network.

The dynamic obstacle identification, and the confirmation of the signal rate informed by the user mobile device are made by the location mechanism by consulting the network access points.

WIRELESS LOCATION FOR SECURITY MECHANISMS

During the microwave signals propagations, each obstacle is capable of changing the signal direction and amplitude. The more important aspects are attenuation, reflection and refraction.

The microwave signal changes its direction, every time it encounters a metal surface. The same behavior occurs when it collides with water. Every time the microwaves changes the propagation material (when it transposes a wall, for instance) the changes in the material density changes the propagation direction. Those behaviors depends directly of the obstacles surface and material.

If we do not consider obstacles, the attenuation can be measured with the Free Space Path Loss, as shown in formula (1).

$$FSPL = 20\log\left(4\grave{A}d \ / \ \text{»}\right) \tag{1}$$

where *FSPL* is the attenuation in dB, d is the distance between transmitter and receiver in meters, and λ is the length of the microwave in meters (0.125m to 2.4Ghz).

When a transmitter sends the signal, it's strength in the receiver depends of the power of the transmitting interface *Tx* (dB), the attenuation in the cable between the interface and the antenna *Ct* (dB), the gain of the transmission antenna *Gt* (dBi), the *FSPL* attenuation *FSPL* (dB), the gain in the receptor antenna *Gr* (dBi), and the attenuation between the reception antenna and the receiver interface *Cr* (dB), as formula (2).

$$Rx = Tx - C_t + G_t - FSPL + G_r - C_r \tag{2}$$

This means that with the signal strength obtained by the device from the access point transmission, and knowing the antennas used by transmitter and receiver it is possible to discover the distance between them.

But, every time that a microwave signal is transmitted in the air, or have to transpose some obstacle, it's amplitude is attenuated. If we use the signal strength to try to locate some device, it is necessary to observe each obstacle in the way, and its attenuation ratio (a brick wall, for instance, can attenuate a microwave signal in 6 dB, and a human body in 3 dB).

This means that we must consider the dynamic attenuation caused by obstacles in the environment in order to use the signal obtained by the device in the location process. If we consider *Ad* as the dynamic attenuation, we can redefine the *Rx* formula as (3).

$$Rx = Tx - C_t + G_t - FSPL + G_r - C_r - A_d \tag{3}$$

With this information, when we collect the signal amplitude received by some wireless device, we can the discover its distance to the AP, by using FSPL and the informations about transmission power and antennas used, as formula (4) and (5).

$$FSPL = Tx - C_t + G_t + G_r - C_r - A_d - Rx \tag{4}$$

$$d = \left(10^{\left(FSPL/20\right)}\text{»}\right) / 4\grave{A} \tag{5}$$

Note that with formula (4) and (5), we can use the amplitude information obtained in the client wireless device, and discover its distance to the AP. The informations about the transmission power of the AP can be easily obtained, as the information about its cable attenuation and antenna gain. The receiver antenna gain and attenuation in the receiver, is difficult to foreseen, and a generic value must be used. The only thing that keeps incomplete is the dynamic obstacle attenuation factor in the environment, that must be obtained by the location system.

If we used the fingerprint technique, the only information we need is the received signal amplitude, in order to compare it withing the fingerprint matrix. But, if the technique used is trilateration, the distance is the more important information.

In order to locate some device with the fingerprint technique, the network administrator must first take samples in each possible location point in the environment. All the physical perimeter must be divided in location points and in each point a amplitude sample of all the APs in range and a wireless device.

This sample point are used to build a fingerprint matrix of the environment. Each AP has its own fingerprint matrix.

When a wireless device must be located, it informs the amplitude signal obtained for all APs in range. The amplitude values are then used in order to find the closest value in all matrix cells and determine the wireless device location point.

For instance, if the wireless device informs that it is receiving from AP_i the amplitude P_i, then the matrix M_i of AP_i is consulted and a new temporary matrix is constructed with the difference between P_i and the value of each cell, as can be seen in formula (6).

$$D_i[x, y] = mod\left(M_i[x, y] - P_i\right) \qquad (6)$$

This process must be repeated for each AP in station's range. And after creating one temporary matrix for each AP, those matrices are added, creating a new matrix with the sum of the amplitude differences. The cell with the smallest value is the potential device location.

If there is more then one cell with the same value, and this value is the smallest in the matrix, then the location system must distribute the location probability among those cells.

The trilateration technique does not need the initial sampling process. This technique uses only the distance between the station and at least three known APs.

With the distance d known, we can construct a circle with the AP position as center and radius equals to d.

With the three circles formed, it is possible to locate the device by identifying the intersection area among the circles. In order to find the intersection area, first we need to define the circle equations, and the intersection points between circle 1 (with center x1,y1) and 2 (with center x2, y2). The circle equation is presented in formula (7).

$$R_i^2 = \left(x - x_i\right)^2 + \left(y - y_i\right)^2 \qquad (7)$$

Putting the formula into a system, to find the intersection points we have formula (8).

$$x^2 + y^2 - 2xx_1 - 2yy_1 + x_1^2 + y_1^2 = R_1^2$$
$$-\left\{x^2 + y^2 - 2xx_2 - 2yy_2 + x_2^2 + y_2^2 = R_2^2\right\} \qquad (8)$$

$$-2xx_1 + 2xx_2 - 2yy_1 + 2yy_2 + x_1^2 + y_1^2 - x_2^2 - y_2^2 = R_1^2 - R_2^2$$

Approaching the equation, we have the formula (9).

$$\left(-2x_1 + 2x_2\right)x + \left(-2y_1 + 2y_2\right)y + x_1^2 + y_1^2 - x_2^2 - y_2^2 = R_1^2 - R_2^2 \qquad (9)$$

And isolating y, and breaking the formula into blocks we obtain the formula (10).

$$A = R_1^2 - R_2^2 - x_1^2 - y_1^2 + x_2^2 + y_2^2 \qquad (10)$$

$$B = -2x_1 + 2x_2$$

$$C = -2y_1 + 2y_2$$

$$y = \left(A - \left(xB\right)\right) / C$$

Combining the formulas, we can replace the equation and form the formula (11) and (12).

$$x^2 + \left(\left(A - xB\right)/C\right)^2 - 2xx_1 - 2y_1\left(A - \left(xB\right)/C\right) + x_1^2 + y_1^2 - R_1^2 = 0 \tag{11}$$

$$x^2 + A^2 / C^2 - 2AxB / C^2 + x^2B / C^2 - 2xx_1$$
$$-2y_{1A} / C + 2y_1Bx / C + x_1^2 + y_1^2 - R_1^2 = 0 \tag{12}$$

We form a second-degree equation, with the therms D, E and F as seen in (13).

$$D = \left(1 + B^2 / C^2\right) \tag{13}$$

$$E = \left(-2AB / C^2 - 2x + 2y_1 B / C\right)$$

$$F = \left(A^2 / C^2 - 2y_1 A / C + x_1^2 + y_1^2 - R_1^2\right)$$

$$x^2 D + xE + F = 0$$

Finally, with D, E and F defined, we can find the intersection points between the two first circles with Baskara as in formula (14) and (15).

$$x' = -E + \left(\sqrt{E^2 - 4DF}\right) / 2D \tag{14}$$

$$x'' = -E - \left(\sqrt{E^2 - 4DF}\right) / 2D$$

$$y' = \left(A - \left(x'B\right)\right) / C \tag{15}$$

$$y'' = \left(A - \left(x''B\right)\right) / C$$

Using this equations, we will find 2 intersection point to each 2 circles. If there is 3 APs in range, we find 6 points of intersection AP1 x AP2, AP1 x AP3 and AP2 x AP3. In order to achieve the identification of one unique point, we identify the 3 closest points and construct a triangle with them. The center point of the triangle is the possible station location. The identification of this point is made with formula (16).

$$x = \left(x_1 + x_2 + x_3\right) / 3 \tag{16}$$

$$y = \left(y_1 + y_2 + y_3\right) / 3$$

In WlanAuth, the trilateration technique is used in the first phase of the system. After collecting the amplitude information of the wireless station, the system delimits a area in the fingerprint matrix in which the station should be. This area is used for all the remain location process.

Dynamic Obstacle Identification

In our system, we use a dynamic obstacle identification method. The goal of the dynamic obstacle identification is to make the dynamic behavior of obstacles and microwave propagation part of the location system.

We used a 627 m² area, as presented in the Figure 1, divided in 14x7 points, forming 13x6 squares. Each square has 2m x 2m.

The access points (APs) are represents as triangles, with fixed and known location. To discover dynamic obstacles in the environment, the APs are used to measure the attenuation variations among them using the site survey feature.

Figure 1. Experiments scenario

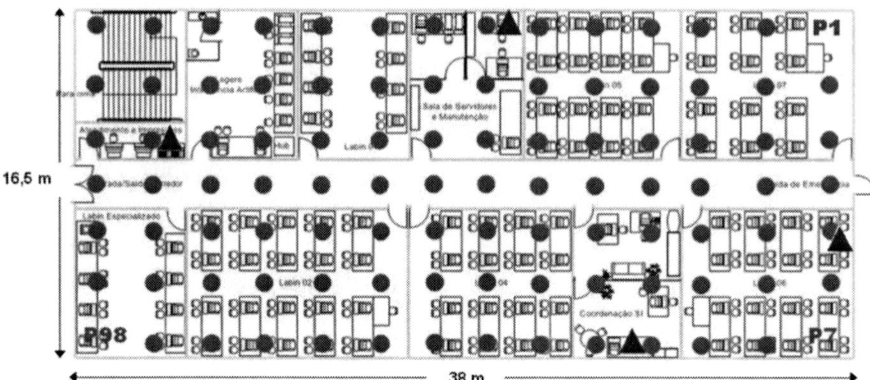

The location server collects from those devices the signal rate from time to time and uses this information to update the location system.

Each AP sends information about others APs in range, and the signal amplitude between them. If there is a new obstacle between two APs the received signal amplitude before the obstacle appears and during the appearance are shown in the two samples. The difference is used in the location system.

If a new amplitude value is obtained, it should be reflected in the fingerprint matrices of the two APs involved. As the system can not know in which cell the obstacle are, the system distributes this value in all the cells between those two APs. The way the system identifies which cells should be update is through Euclidean distance. Also, according with the distance between the APs a alpha value is used. This alpha value increases the number of cells, distributing the new value in a ellipsis area (instead of a line of cells).

The complete process is: first the system identifies the obstacle, then it update the matrix of the AP if the cell is between the APs with Euclidean distance = 1 + alpha.

As the alpha value depends of the environment, a new sample phase should be executed in order to determine the best alpha for each two APs.

To measure the impact of the obstacles in the environment, we collected the signal strength between one access points and a mobile station in an interval of 5 seconds, during 48 hours. The results can be seen in Figure 2, where is presented a 24 hour graph compiling the 48 hour data collection. As it can be seen, in the interval between 19:00h and 22:30h there are more variations in the obtained values. This can be explained by the class hour which is from 19:10h to 20:45h (with one interval from 20:45 to 21:00) and from 21:00h to 22:30h.

As the system can only locate dynamic obstacles between the APs, there is no way to know if an obstacle outside the range of the line between the APs exists.

WLANAUTH

After we defined that the use of signal amplitude and dynamic obstacle consideration was the best way to locate the devices, we defined 4 ways to validate the system:

1. *fingerprint*: we used pure fingerprint technique to serve as base of the location accuracy. Using it as reference, we can vali-

Figure 2. Dynamic obstacles signal attenuation

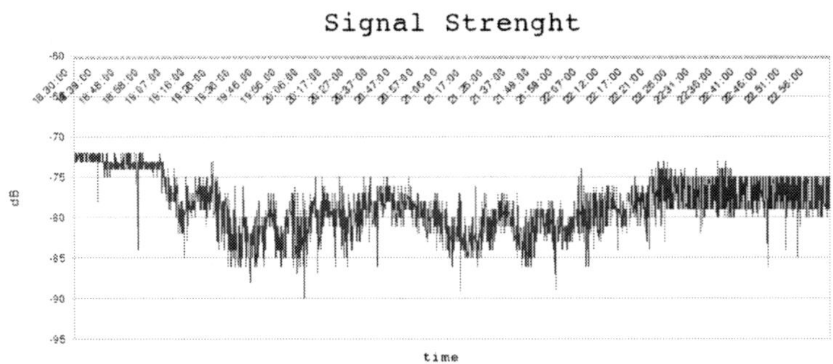

date the increase the accuracy of obstacles consideration in our technique;

2. *fingerprint with dynamic obstacle consideration*: we test the system accuracy using the obstacle identification and fingerprint updated matrices and compare it with the fingerprint technique;

3. *trilateration*: we used trilateration to locate the devices without the sampling process used in the fingerprint technique, based only in the obtained distance between the wireless station and all the APs in range (we use FSPL);

4. *trilateration with fingerprint and obstacle consideration*: in this final technique, we used the results obtained in the trilateration technique (3) to delimit the fingerprint area used in the location process (2).

Also, the security concern about the trust in the wireless device amplitude information leads the system to validate the information with the APs. This means that the system must consult the wireless devices for the amplitude information, and after that, validate the value obtained with the AP.

The security mechanism was build on top of the location system together with the security system already in use for the wired network. The mobile stations have a server software listening for connections. When a student authenticate with the wireless network, he/she have all communica-tions blocked by a captive portal software (we use the wifidog captive portal). In this captive portal, the user must authenticate with a username and password. The captive portal was modified, so that when the user enters the password, the system will connect with the mobile station server (in order to obtain the device amplitude information, a server software was developed and installed in the wireless devices) and receive the signal strength data to perform the location procedure.

When the captive portal system receives the signal strength data, it will send this information to the location server. The location server returns to the captive portal the room that was identified as the user location. The captive portal will then modify the proxy's configuration so that the mobile station IP address will receive the same security rules that the wired subnet in which the mobile station are.

In mobile based systems, there is no guarantee that the mobile station will send the correct information to the location system. A malicious user can send false signal values to the system so that its location will not be correct. In order to avoid spoofed information from the mobile client, the security protocol confirms the user data with the network infrastructure (network based location).

To achieve this control, the system must connect with the AP and request the signal strength of the mobile station it is locating. In order to obtain this information, the mobile station must be associated with the access point (as the access points only monitor signal strength to associated stations).

The system must verify the information received from the mobile station with at least three access points. The mobile station must associate with those APs during the signal strength collection phase of the protocol.

Figure 3 presents the security protocol used to impose the security policy to a mobile station. The communication occurs as follows:

1. the mobile station request authentication/association with the access point;
2. the access point grants authentication/association to the station;
3. the station access the captive portal;
4. the captive portal returns a web site requesting username/password;
5. the user in the mobile station enters with username/password;
6. the captive portal connects to the mobile station server in order to receive the signal strength data among the mobile station and all access points in range;
7. the mobile station server software returns the signal strength data to the captive portal;
8. the captive portal connects with the AP the station is associated to confirm the client information;
9. the AP returns the signal information about the mobile station;
10. the captive portal sends to the station the request to connect with another AP;
11. the mobile station must repeat the process for at least 3 times, with 3 different access points;
12. the captive portal sends the received data to the location server. The location server returns the room that the mobile station is in;
13. the captive portal modify the proxy's configuration and returns the result to the mobile station.

Figure 3. Security mechanism protocol

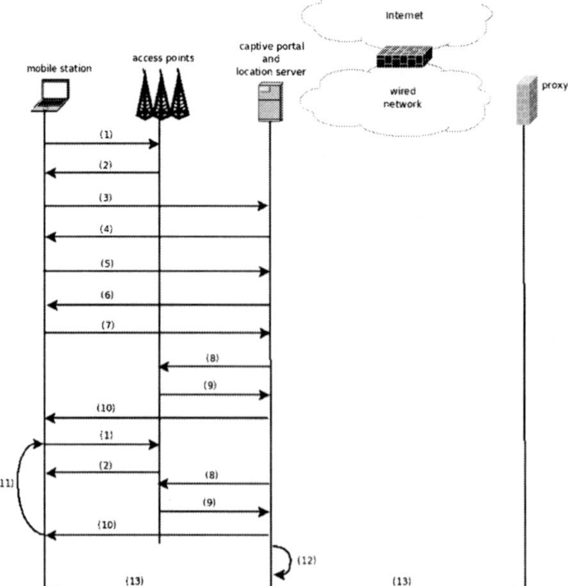

The signal strength value received by the AP is different from the value informed by the mobile station, because of the transmission power of the wireless device, as we can see in formula (2). In our experiments there is a compatibility table in order to validate this information. This compatibility is needed to verify that the station information can be trusted.

EXPERIMENTS

In order to evaluate the proposed mechanism, there was made a series of location tests. The tests was divided in three situations: 1. location with few dynamic obstacles; 2. location with inserted obstacle and; 3. location with dynamic obstacles.

The first situation was made with few personal in the building, which means that there was little impact of dynamic obstacles in the environment. The only source of interference was the fixed obstacles mapped in the sample process of fingerprint. The mobile station was placed in classroom 6.

There was made 80 location inferences and for each inference, the mobile station informs the average of 50 signal amplitude samples. The same information was used in the fingerprint location process, and the fingerprint with dynamic obstacle identification process. Figure 4 presents the location points obtained in those two techniques. We also use this situation in order to define the alpha value to be used in all the other situations. The best value of alpha was 1 between AP1 and AP2, and 3 between AP1 and AP3, as it returns the best location values.

The average error for all the variations of the techniques was:

- Fingerprint: 2.71m;
- Fingerprint with dynamic obstacle identification: 3.48m;

The dynamic obstacle identification increase the average error in this case, but not in a way of compromising the mobile station room identification.

In the second situation, the mobile station was in room 10. In this situation, there was made two different tests. One with no artificial obstacle (situation 2a), and another placing one obstacle in between the AP2 and the mobile station (situation 2b). Figure 5 shows the location points obtained in the two techniques in situation 2a. There was made 50 location inferences and for each inference, the mobile station informs the average of 50 signal amplitude samples.

Figure 4. Situation 1: location points

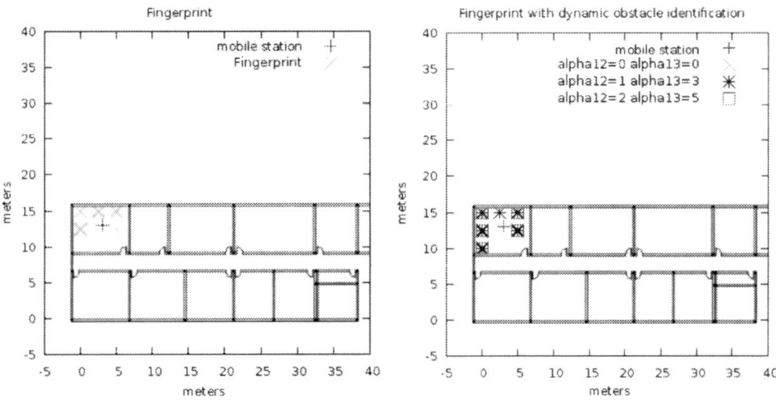

Figure 5. Situation 2a: location points

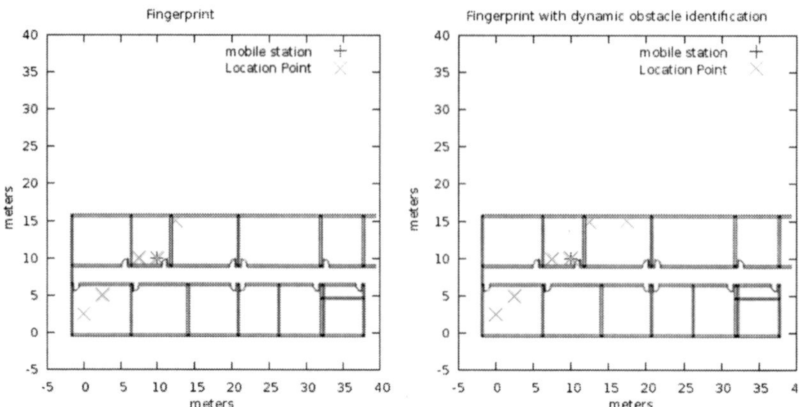

The average error for all the variations of the techniques was:

- Fingerprint: 2.71m;
- Fingerprint with dynamic obstacle identification: 3.48m;

The room location accuracy was:

- Fingerprint: 44%;
- Fingerprint with dynamic obstacle identification: 74%;

When we placed one obstacle between AP2 and the mobile station (situation 2b), the fingerprint with dynamic obstacle identification increase the number of location points for the 50 inferences, but the fingerprint technique increase the location error. Figure 6 presents the location points in this situation.

The average error for all the variations of the techniques was:

- Fingerprint: 5.7m;
- Fingerprint with dynamic obstacle identification: 2.15m;

The room location accuracy was:

- Fingerprint: 44%;

Figure 6. Situation 2b: location points

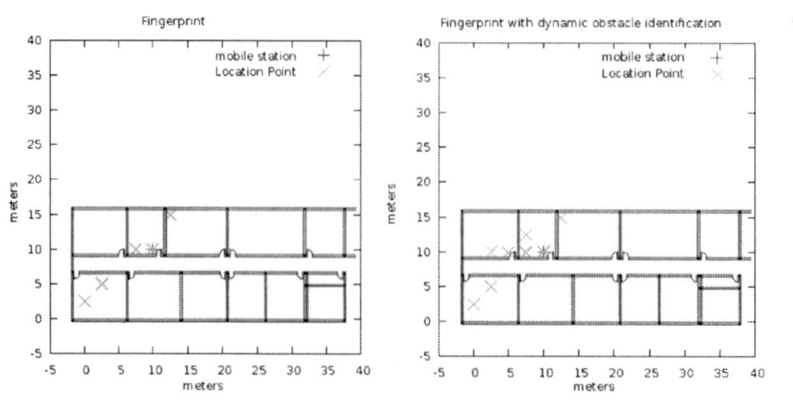

- Fingerprint with dynamic obstacle identification: 80%;

The third situation was placed during the class hour. This means that there was a great number of dynamic obstacles in the environment. The expected in this situation is the increase of the location error.

The mobile station was placed in room 5, and the location points are presented in Figure 7. As in the situation 2, some location inferences indicates the wrong room.

The average error for all the variations of the techniques was:

- Fingerprint: 2.63m;
- Fingerprint with dynamic obstacle identification: 4.55m;

The increase of the location error in meters is greater in the dynamic obstacle identification. The reason of this value is because of the inferences in which the location technique indicates the room 4 as the location point (16m from the actual station location). But this error does not reflect the increase of room identification. The room location accuracy was:

- Fingerprint: 12%;

- Fingerprint with dynamic obstacle identification: 40%;

As seen in this last experiment, the location error was greater as the number of dynamic obstacles increases. In this case, we then include the trilateration technique to delimit the location area. With this in mind, the location process was:

1. obtain the information from the wireless device;
2. after the information validation with the APs involved in the process, we execute the trilateration location process;
3. with the point obtained by the trilateration, we convert it to a location in the fingerprint matrix;
4. the point in the matrix was used as a center point in the definition of the location area of the wireless device. We used a 3 cells ratio area as parameter;
5. the fingerprint with obstacles consideration updated matrices was used to locate the device within this area.

The results obtained in the trilateration process are shown in Figure 8. This figure presents the points obtained in the 50 location inferences, and

Figure 7. Situation 3: location points

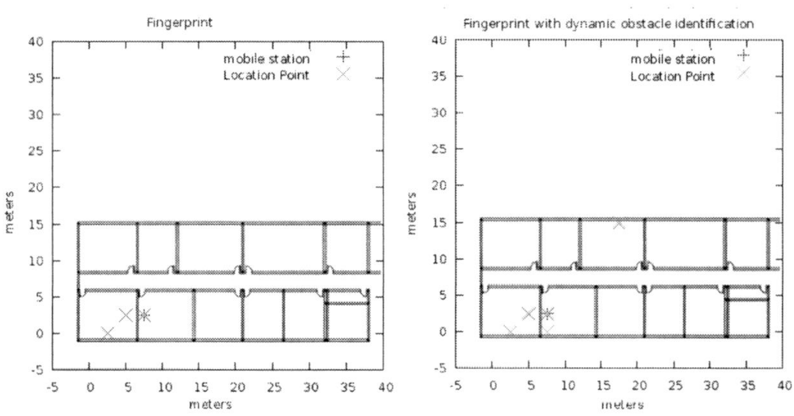

the points are used to delimit a 3x3 cells area to the fingerprint location.

Those points was obtained by the intersection points of the circles defined by the amplitude signal received from the wireless devices. The 50 circles have the smallest, medium and greatest values presented in Figure 9.

Figure 10 presents the point obtained by the fingerprint with dynamic obstacles consideration, after delimiting the matrix area. This is the WlanAuth location technique.

The new results in this case have the average error of 1.96 meters and room location accuracy of 40%. This means that the room identification accuracy was maintained, but the average error decrease significantly with the use of trilateration combined with fingerprint.

FUTURE RESEARCH DIRECTIONS

The location process is complex and involves all different aspects in the environment in order to locate a wireless device. Besides the presented need to consider the dynamic obstacles, others aspects should be used in future research, such as:

- *the antennas involved in the location process*: it is very important to note that the wireless device antenna has a big deal in the location process. A way to identify the client antenna or to create a technique to bring this information in the location process in such a way that the location system can increase his accuracy should be of great contribution to the process;

- *temperature*: the temperature variations also have great influence in the signal amplitude. Researches that bring more informations and tests in this subject should also be of great contribution to the location process;

- *more performance to the security mechanism*: one of the things that have a significant impact in the security protocol is the fact that a AP cannot returns the signal amplitude relative to a non associated device. This means that in order to verify the validation of the amplitude values received

Figure 8. Situation 3: location points obtained in trilateration

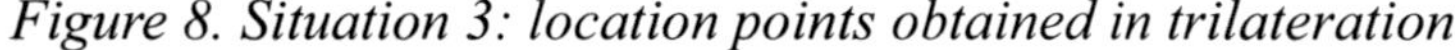

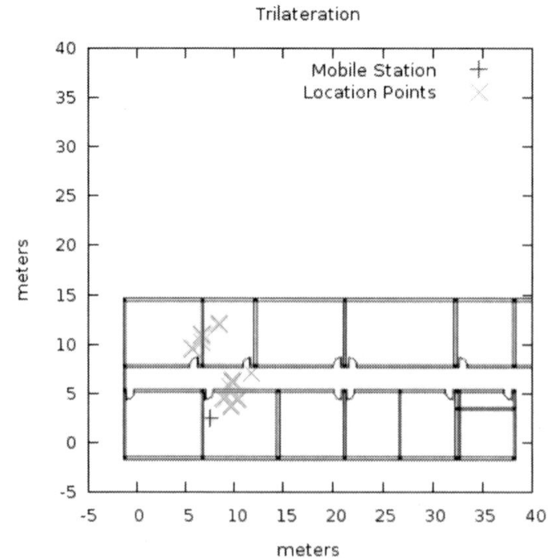

Figure 9. Situation 3: trilateration circles (lowest, medium and greatest radius)

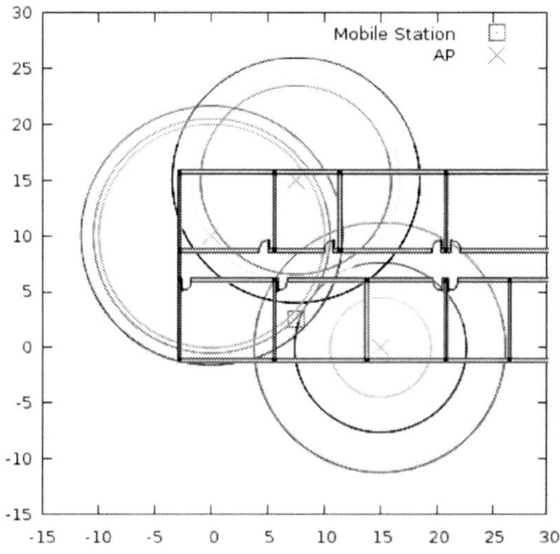

by the wireless device, it should associate with at least tree APs. This process is time consuming and new ways to deliver a more rapid validation are welcome.

Also, as the location systems available still with accuracy that can be improved, all the effort to increase the precision in the location process in indoor environments can be of great help.

Figure 10. Situation 3: location points with fingerprint and dynamic obstacles consideration, after trilateration

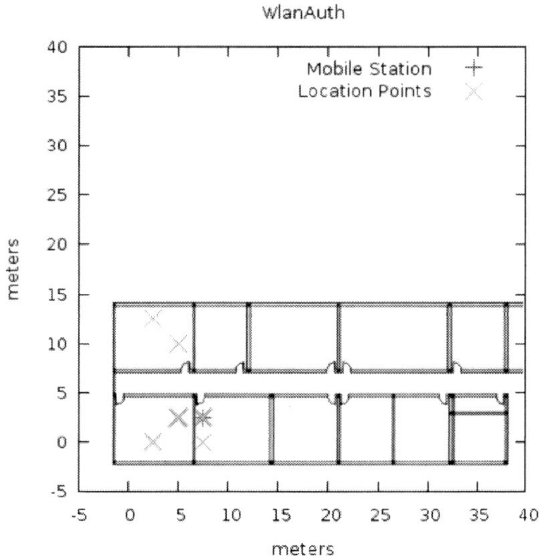

CONCLUSION

The use of wireless network in an academic scenario brings flexibility and mobility to such a dynamic and technological environment. However, the use of this network technology must respect the same rules and security of the wired one.

During the class, we must concern about the quality and restrictions imposed by the teacher to keep the students focused in the discipline's content.

This research aims to bring to the classroom this type of control through identifying the physical location of the students and applying to them the same security policy of their colleagues that use the wired network.

The concern with the location precision is justified by the need of eliminating any place in the classroom where the student can escape the security rules, or any place in the public area where some wireless network user receives restrictions incorrectly. Our security mechanism achieve its main goal of doing that, with a sufficient precision in locating a mobile station and applying the proper security policy.

As in any security mechanism, the devices used to obtain information must be trusted. We can not use a users station in this kind of task. The proposed mechanism also achieve the increase in the security role of mobile device location, using only trusted devices (the access points).

The location process proved to increase the accuracy with the inclusion of trilateration technique in order to delimit a location area, and with this area defined, the technique manage to decrease the fingerprint location error. Also the dynamic obstacles consideration in the fingerprint technique proved to increase the room identification with considerable value to the location process.

REFERENCES

Bahl, P., et al. (2000, February). *Enhancements to the RADAR User Location and Tracking System.* (Microsoft Research Technical Report), Retrieved April 2004 from: http://citeseer.ist.psu.edu/ bahl00enhancements.html

Buschmann, C., et al. (n.d.). Radio propagation-aware distance estimation based on neighborhood comparison. In *Proceedings of the European Workshop on Sensor Networks*, 2007. (pp.325–340, Springer Lecture Notes in Computer Science, v.4373).

Capkun, S., & Hubaux, J.-P. (2006). Secure Positioning in Wireless Networks. [JSAC]. *IEEE Journal on Selected Areas in Communications*, *24*(2), 221–232. doi:10.1109/JSAC.2005.861380

Elnahrawy, J., et al. (2007). *Adding angle of arrival modality to basic rss location management techniques.* Retrieved June 2008 from: http://paul.rutgers.edu/ eiman/ elnahrawy07AoA.pdf

Faria, D. B. (2005). *Modeling Signal Attenuation in IEEE 802.11 Wireless LANs - Vol. 1.* (Technical Report) TR-KP06-0118, Kiwi Project, Stanford University.

Fluhrer, S., et tal. (2001). Weaknesses in the Key Scheduling Algorithm of RC4. *Lecture Notes in Computer Science, 2259*, doi:10.1007/3-540-45537-X_1

Gast, M. (2002). *802.11 Wireless Networks: the definitive guide.* Sebastopol, CA: O'Reilly and Associates, Inc.

IEEE. (1999). *IEEE 802.11b - Part 11: wireless lan medium access control (mac) and physical layer (phy) specifications: higher-speed physical layer extension in the 2.4 ghz band.* Retrieved June 2003 from: http://standards.ieee.org/getieee802/download/802.11b-1999.pdf

IEEE. (2003). *IEEE 802.11g Part 11: wireless lan medium access control (mac) and physical layer (phy) specifications amendment 4: further higher data rate extension in the 2.4 ghz band.* Retrieved December 2003 from: http://standards.ieee.org/getieee802/ download/802.11g-2003.pdf

IEEE. (2004). *IEEE 802.11i Part 11: wireless lan medium access control (mac) and physical layer (phy) specifications amendment 6: medium access control (mac) security enhancements.* Retrieved October 2004 from: http://standards.ieee.org/ getieee802/ download/802.11i-2004.pdf

(2005)... *IEEE Signal Processing Magazine, 22*(4), 24–40. doi:10.1109/MSP.2005.1458275

Kitasuka, T., Nakanishi, T., Fukuda, A (2003). Wireless LAN Based Indoor Positioning System WiPS and Its Simulation. *Communications, Computers and signal Processing, 1*(28), 272–275.

Krishnan, P., et al. A System for LEASE: location estimation assisted by stationery emitters for indoor rf wireless networks. *Twenty-third Annual Joint Conference of the IEEE Computer and Communications Societies, v.2, n.7, p.1001–1011, 2004.* Retrieved March 2005 for: http://citeseer.ist.psu.edu/ krishnan04system.html

Kuwabara, M., & Nishio, N. (n.d.). Wi-Fi based radio map for location sensing by hypothesizing existence of barriers. In *ICUIMC '09: Proceedings of the 3rd international Conference on Ubiquitous Information Management and Communication,* 2009, New York.

Moraes, L. F. M., & de, Nunes, B. A. A (2006). *Calibration-free WLAN location system based on dynamic mapping of signal strength.* In MOBI-WAC '06 *Proceedings Of The 4th Acm International Workshop On Mobility Management And Wireless Access, 2006*, New York.

Morrison, J. D. (2002). *IEEE 802.11 wireless local area network security through location authentication.* (Masters Thesis. Naval Postgraduate School Monterey, California). Retrieved January 2003 from: http://cisr.nps.edu/downloads/ theses/02thesis_morrison.pdf

Moskowitz, R., & Fleishman, G. (2003). *Weakness in Passphrase Choice in WPA Interface.* Retrieved January 2004 from: http://wifinetnews.com/ archives/002452.html

Pandey, S., et al. (2005). Client assisted location data acquisition scheme for secure enterprise wireless networks. In *Proceedings of the ACM, 2005.. . v.2, p.1174–1179.*

Sayed, A. et al. Network-based wireless location: challenges faced in developing techniques for accurate wireless location information.

Stoyanova., et al. Evaluation of impact factors on RSS accuracy for localization and tracking applications. In MOBIWAC '07: *Proceedings of The 5th ACM International Workshop on Mobility Management and Wireless Access,* 2007.

Taheri, A., et al. *(2004).* Location fingerprinting on infrastructure 802.11 wireless local area networks (WLANs) using Locus. *In:* Anual Ieee International Conference - Local Computer Networks, *29.*

Yasat, A.-U.-H., et al. Low cost solution for location determination of mobile nodes in a wireless local area network. In ACE '06: *Proceedings Of The 2006 Acm Sigchi International Conference On Advances In Computer Entertainment Technology,* 2006, New York, NY.

Section 5
Other Application Areas

Chapter 15
EDFA and EDFL Review

Belloui Bouzid
Hafer Al-batin Community College & King Fahd University of Petroleum & Minerals, Saudi Arabia

EXECUTIVE SUMMARY

In this chapter, I propose a comprehensive study of erbium-doped fiber amplifier (EDFA) and erbium doped fiber laser (EDFL). The chapter is based on three principal levels: the first is at the atomic level, where it is evident and meaningful to give general and deep studies on erbium spectra at theoretical background angle. The important part that needs to be understood in the erbium is its energy level splitting and lasing. The second level is based on the EDFA and EDFL critical, where many research papers have been reviewed to show and clarify their strong and weak side at different views. To specify the weakness of the classical EDFA and EDFL, and to describe the future generations and its characteristics, it is very important to review the recent published papers and books. At the experimental level a full investigation is given. Vast and new designs were invented showing high-gain and low-noise-figure (NF) utilizing a new technique called double pass with filter. An efficient amplification occurs at the signal wavelength of 1550 nm when it travels along the design quadruple pass double stages with filter amplifier (QPDSF). The highest gain of 62.56 dB with a low NF of 3.98 dB was achieved for an input signal power of -50 dBm and pump powers of 10 and 165 mW in the second and first stage amplifiers respectively. This important result shows also, a large difference of 40 dB gain between the QPDSF and the single stage single pass (SPSS) EDFA configuration. This design is used to show high gain of 62.56 dB compared to SPSS which records only 20 dB. A higher power and wider spectrum of ASE is observed for the double pass compared with single pass. A comparative investigation is presented and analyzed for various configurations. At the end, a high output power EDFL configuration is reported. It incorporates a double stages linear cavity with fiber loopback and a tunable bandpass filter TBF. The configuration increases the output power by suppressing the amplified spontaneous emission and achieves a highly stable output power of more than 18 dBm at 1560 nm. A standard spectrum is attained with TBF adjustment.

DOI: 10.4018/978-1-60960-015-0.ch015

INTRODUCTION

As it is found in the vast literature review, laser and amplifier take an important part in this scientific age due to their effects in this new generation of communications and Tbps transmission [1]. The importance of EDFA and EDFL are owing to their ability to amplify the signal and revive it through millions of kms on this earth. The lasers phenomena in general, let the researchers focus on the development and enhancement of optical amplifier and give wide and deep understanding of amplification and lasing. Thousand of books and millions of papers have been published since the early discover of laser in 1960 by Theodore Maiman. The roots of the fiber amplifier began in 1964 with the first amplification experiment of Snitzer. It is an interesting task to study, illustrate, and investigate the beneath behavior of laser at specific conditions of design, and verify their performance parameters.

The laser was discovered but the modeling was followed to much the experiment results. And the base was the quantum theory based on Planck and Einstein formulas. To understand and elaborate the construction of laser phenomena, it is of great consequence to combine theory and experiment in one thinking head.

The elucidation of laser and amplifier is related to what we call the energy level or the atomic structure that emit the photon. How this photon is born? How it is constructed within the sublevel of the atomic orbits? Or what is the physical meaning of the electron jumping? How the amplification phenomena can be explained? All these questions are important to be answered to understand the laser and amplifier conceptions.

The rare earth with its puzzle of emission and absorption played latter an important role in lasing and amplifications due to the 4fn, where n varied from 1 to 14 electrons. The erbium ion is the main part in the optical amplifier and laser, this importance is owing to the overlap of lowest absorption in fiber optic and erbium emission at C and L bands.

In general, all the scientific community in the photonics fields knows, what is the real effect of optics and laser on the huge development of internet, and on the progress of terabits transmission? [1]. Laser with the stimulated emission phenomena are considered to be the main key to the future revolution of communication. Let us think internet without fiber optics or without fiber amplifier? How the narrow band of electronics can be solved? I believe this huge communication that we are living in, will be abolished without fiber optics, laser, and EDFA. At the beneath of the laser phenomena there are many promising future developments and new discoveries that can be achieved. Optical amplifier and lasers are used nearly in all the wide spectrum of science such as medicine, military, education and manufacturing.

After a decade of research in amplifier and laser, and after a deep study of EDFA and EDFL in the past and present design, a remarkable effect of configuration is observed. The simple EDFA configuration is used by splicing the WDM with the active medium EDF and with the pump power, an amplification of an input signal will occur with the generation of amplified spontaneous emission (ASE) noise. In all cases of single pass single stage (SPSS) the gain shows small increase even by changing the pumping power 980nm or 1480nm or using the co-propagating or the forward propagating or even putting the 980 and 1480 in one direction. The gain gap between the SPSS types of configurations doesn't show high difference and the saturation will occur a t low pump power.

The vast published papers of SPSS don't show a sufficient increase of gain difference. In the double passes double stages (DPDS) the circulators are used as loop-back of ASE and laser beam. It was observed a high difference between gains. It can be noticed, that the configuration structure has the most important part in the design of EDFA. This impressed result is due to the output power that can be generated after a specific change of the design parameters. The study presented in this chapter will open new window of research where, different parameters and factors of configurations are changed to make an efficient EDFA and EDFL.

The spectrum of ASE from an EDF shows a non-uniform profile and it is limited to 1520 – 1620 nm range. The NF of an EDFA improves as its population inversion increases with pumping power augmentation. Backward pumping, while having a higher noise figure, also has higher output power because the stronger pump powers at the output delays the commencement of gain saturation. Therefore, forward pumping is preferred to maintain a low NF, and backward pumping is preferred to achieve a high output power. Hybrid pumping with 980nm forward pumping and 1480 nm backward pumping, takes advantage of the high population inversion provided by 980 nm pumps and the high power. A recent and new idea shows a slightly higher gain and lower NF by putting the 980 and 1480 nm in one side.

The use of input optical isolator will prevents ASE signals from propagating in the backward direction. In another words, reflected ASE would reduce the population inversion, thereby reducing the gain and increasing the NF. The output isolator prevents light from output reflections from re-entering the EDFA, however, many researchers attempted to implement EDF without isolator. In general, lower cost design is preferred by using single 980 nm. The pump, the input signal, WDM, isolators, single stage, double stages, double passes, double stages double passes are an important factors in EDFA design.

Furthermore, the influences of the length and concentration have been intensively studied to investigate their effect on gain and NF [2-8]. The amplifiers make use of the fact that the erbium gain peak shifts to longer wavelengths as the EDF length is increases. Indeed, the EDFA gain spectrum changes with population inversion and fiber length. Non silica erbium doped fibers, such as fluoride and telluride have also been proposed as alternatives because they do not require as much

filtering to achieve a flattened spectrum. These materials widen the erbium spectra because they have lower phonon energy, which increases the lifetime of the highest stable levels, or maybe is due to the amorphous nature of glass.

In addition, a tremendous progress has been made in the development of broadband EDFA, which form the backbone of high capacity light wave communication systems. The amplifier provides high output power and low NF to support the ever-increasing capacity demand on light wave systems. In addition, various techniques have been proposed to flatten the gain and expand the amplification window.

EDFA theory is related to laser and its phenomena of interaction of matter-light-matter, where the stimulation of emission is occurred at specific conditions. Based on the lasers studies, a huge and vast number of formulas are given in different books and papers to find the exact model for lasing and amplification and to find a suitable and precise formula. But owing to the vast factors affecting the output it is very complicated to find the precise formula for output laser, gain, and NF.

In general, the basic formalism used for modeling light amplification in EDFA is based on [9, 10]:

- Classical Electromagnetism
- Quantum Mechanics
- Laser Physics

The fundamental laser parameters are:

- Er^{3+} dopent density
- Fluorescence life time
- Cross section is related to the fiber parameter.

The rate equation is to combine the following:

- Signal
- Pump
- ASE

Spectral gain ripples and non-uniformities of Silica-based erbium-doped fiber amplifiers represent a bottleneck in broadband all-optical light wave systems. This is resulting in gain and signal-to-noise ratio (SNR) discrepancies between channels. Different techniques have been used to overcome this impediment: Using fiber Grating, Acousto-Optic tunable filter, dual-core fiber, phase shifted long period fiber grating, high birefringence [11-14].

In this chapter, a focus is given to three main parts:

First is to give a brief description of atomic structure and their characteristics of lasing and amplifications, second is to give critical view regarding the laser and amplification in general, third is to show designs and their experimental results starting from single pass single stage to quadruple pass double stages for amplifier, and ring cavity and double stages linear cavity.

AT THE ATOMIC LEVEL

The relationship between the principal quantum number is organized as shown in Table 1. It is very clear that all the quantum numbers are ordered in such way that gives the specific structure of the atom. This specific structure, will affect strongly the characteristic of the atom and its interaction with light absorption or emission.

The Er atom is shown in Figure 1, following the subshells order of electrons position in atom their division is following the order 2, 8, 18, 30, 8, 2 based on $1(s^2)$, $2(s^2p^6)$, $3(s^2p^6d^{10})$, $4(s^2p^6d^{10}f^{12})$, $5(s^2p^6)$, and $6(s^2)$ see Figure 2. The sum of all electrons are 68 electron located in the erbium atom. If the erbium atom loss three electrons the atom becomes an ion Er^{+3}. In this case $6s^2$ and f^{12} will loss three electrons. The $4f^{11}$ is coved by the $5p$. Following the energy level progress and the distributions of electrons throughout the whole positions of electrons in the Er^{+3} ions three positions of electrons are not filled inside the $4f^{11}$ as can be shown in the Figure 4.

The Russel-Saunder theory is labeling the energy level with the following label: $^{2S+1}L_J$, where L is the total orbital angular momentum, S is the total spin of electrons, and j is the total angular momentum.

Following Figure 3, $S = (1/2)+(1/2)+(1/2) = 3/2$

L - the total orbital angular momentum quantum number defines the energy state for a system of electrons. These states or term letters are represented as follows:

From Figure 3 and Table 2 L = 6 and 6 is coincided with I.

The $^{2S+1}L_J$ can be calculated by the following:

Table 1. Quantum number relation ship

n, n^2, $2n^2$ Relationships			
n	Subshells	n^2	$2n^2$
1	1s	1	2
2	2s2p	4	8
3	3s3p3d	9	18
4	4s4p4d4f	16	32
5	5s5p5d5f5g	25	50
n = Principal quantum number (energy level) *n = Number of kinds of subshells at energy level n* *n^2 = Number of orbitals (total) at energy level n* *$2n^2$ = Maximum number of electrons at energy level n*			

Figure 1. Erbium atom and 68 its electrons

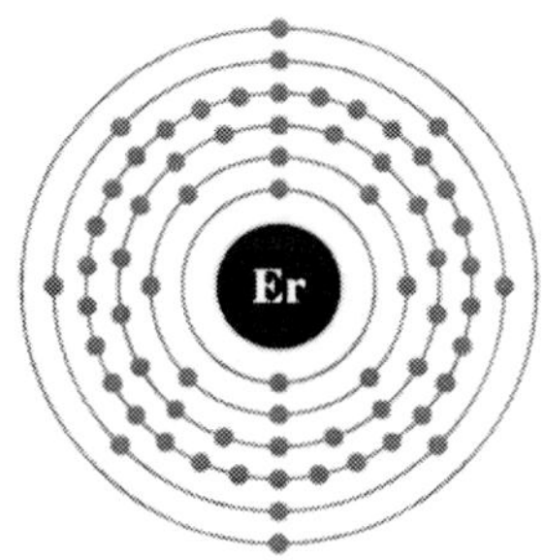

$2S+1 = 2(3/2)+1 = 4$

$L = I$

$J = L+S, L+S-1, L+S-2....L-S.$

J can be calculated as the following:

$J = 6+3/2 = 15/2$

$J = 6-1+3/2 = 13/2$

$J = 6-2+3/2 = 11/2$

$J = 6-3+3/2 = 6-3/2 = L-S = 9/2$

The number of fine manifold can be measured based on the following formula $g = (2J+1)/2$

$g1(J=15/2) = 8$, $g2 (J=13/2) = 7$, $g3 (11/2) = 6$.

The energy levels distribution of the Erbium ion can be shown in Figure 4.

AT THE CRITICAL LEVEL

- Most of the published papers and books on EDFA and EDFL are focusing on the experimental process and results with less concentration on theory and modeling. This owes to the complexity and difficulties faced during the analysis and explanations of stimulated emission. Dealing with the fiber laser, endless of factors are controlling the laser and amplifier output such

Figure 2. The approximate order of filling of atomic orbitals, following the arrows

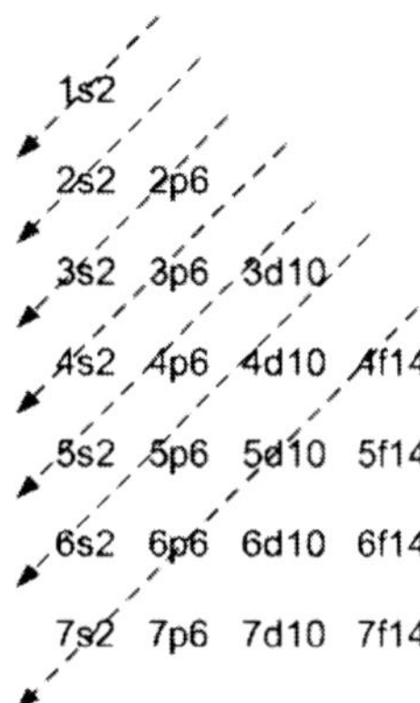

as, EDF length, erbium concentration, material host, type of optical component, type of configuration, pump signal overlap, and the filter. All these factors and parameters have their direct impact on the output laser, wavelength, flattening, gain, and NF.

- Based on this complexity, only the scientists from the physics background are able to theorize and analyze laser and amplifier. The combination of theory and experiment are necessary to understand the real phenomena and this is what is not fully shown in the published papers and books. To find an agreement between theory and experiment is a difficult task to achieve.

- Most of the experimental works are just descriptions of graphs and their trends and not physical explanation phenomena based on the formula. The vast factors and parameters used in laser and amplifier increase the ambiguity. This complexity doesn't let ex-

Table 2. Total orbital momentum

S	P	D	F	G	H	I	J	
0	1	2	3	4	5	6	7	L

Figure 3. Energy level following the electrons distribution in Erbium ion

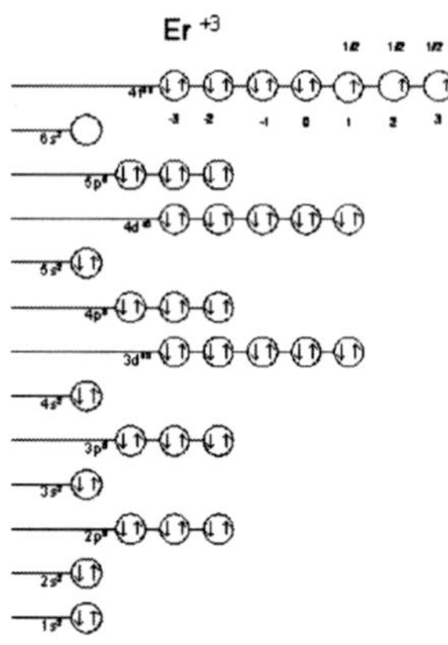

Figure 4. The energy levels distribution of the erbium atoms

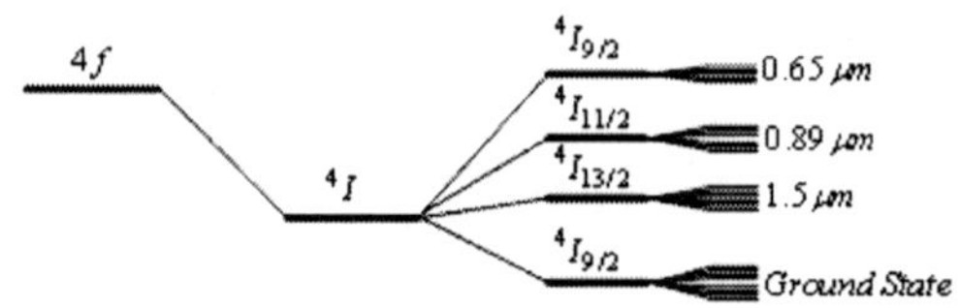

perimental scientists to fully combine between the theory and experiment. Laser in communications system and amplifier still in its early stage and this need a heavy push for the next generation laser and amplifier. I believe it is very important and necessary to find new simple formula for laser and amplifier and understand clearly what happened within the atomic subshells.

- There is a need for global simple formula to explain laser and amplifier.
- There are less published papers, studying the comparison between lasers and amplifiers at different configurations.
- Since decade the EDFA gain is not increased, and the noise generated from the amplifier is not solved.
- Flattening in EDFA gain still a major problem since the discovery of optical amplifier at the end of eightieth.
- Nano-photonics fiber laser and amplifier also still new and only few journals and labs, at the international level, are interested in this topic.
- Less interest is given to laser and amplifier for the undergraduate study level.

AT THE DESIGN LEVEL

Erbium Doped Fiber Amplifier

Design and implementation of single stage optical amplifier using EDF spliced with WDM and optical isolator is a task performed and realized successfully. The fiber used is under the following characteristics: Core: silica / germania doped with Er ion with 440 ppm (Distributed from Fibercore LtD) and the fiber diameter is 125 μm.

Figure 5(a) shows the experiment configuration of the forward pumping single stage. The input signal power generated by the tunable laser source (TLS) passing through the optical isolator then, multiplexed with 980nm pump power by the WDM. The signal will be amplified inside EDF due to the effect of stimulated and spontaneous emission then detected from the optical spectrum analyzer (OSA). The forward pumping has low NF, low gain and low pumping power saturation compared with double stages or double passes.

The second Figure 5(b) is the backward pumping power. The input signal power travels the reverse of pumping power. The backward pumping power has higher gain and higher NF compared to forward pumping configuration. The third configuration is seen in Figure 5(c) where, the pumping is generated from the two sides of EDF, and the signal is traveling reversed to pumping power. It is remarked that the bi-directional pumping configuration has higher gain and middle NF compared to forward and backward pumping configurations.

Figure 5. Forward pumping (a), backward pumping (B), and bi-directional pumping (C)

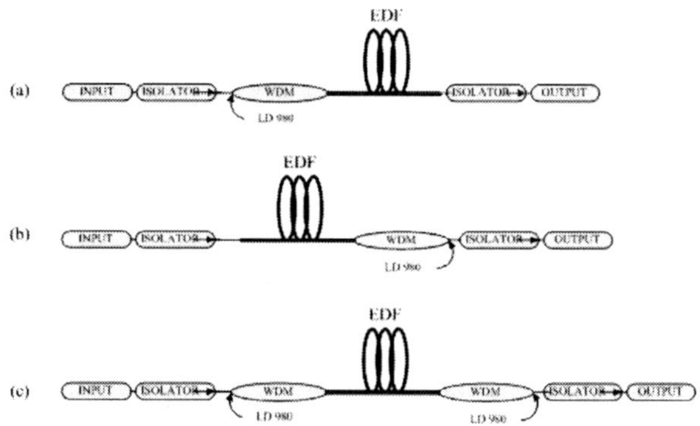

Since the first experimental demonstration of a high-gain EDFA, significant effort has been directed towards achieving a perfect amplifier with high gain and a low NF, with minimum cost. To enhance an EDFA, the main concern is to improve its performance, such as effective bandwidth, gain, noise figure, and efficiency, by optimizing parameters such as; concentration, length, position, and component used of the amplifier. These impressive efforts have been the main focus of past and current research. Recently, reported papers have defined the highest gain as between 30 and 55 dB and the lowest NF as approximately 3dB. In this chapter, a new EDFA structure, called the dual-stages quadruple pass (DSQP), is introduced; this new architecture is used to demonstrate an enhancement of gain and NF at short EDF length [15-20].

We give the details of this new architecture and we analyze the phenomenological behavior of the high gain and low NF achieved. Increasing gain gives high sensitivity for the amplifier and increases the distance between two successive optical amplifiers. In addition, the results have been interpreted to investigate the effect of this new configuration on the surprising increase in gain, giving importance to the role of the two filters included between the two ports (3 and 1) of the two circulators. Using the double passes with filter has been developed to increase the gain higher. Such an increase in gain with this technique shows that this new architecture can give better results and open original and novel ideas for a new generation of EDFAs.

It is the right time for scientists to investigate the amplification phenomena of EDFA practices and to focus on the principles of next generation EDFAs with high-quality amplifications. The standard for the next generation is to achieve the maximum possible gain and the minimum possible NF.

The configuration of the DSQP [15] with filter is shown in Figure 6. A 980 nm semiconductor laser is used as a forward pump source (maximum power of 175 mW). Figure 6 shows the new configuration structure where one circulator (CIR1) with four ports and another two circulators (CIR2 and CIR3) with three ports have been used. CIR1 was used for the input signal power (port 1) and output signal power (port 4), and the other two circulators, CIR2 and CIR3, were used for signal feedback purposes. Two tunable band pass filters (TBF1 and TBF2) were incorporated between port3 and port1 of circulators CIR2 and CIR3. The bandpass of TBF1 is 0.28 nm and TBF2 is 1 nm. The EDF1 of 8 m length and EDF2 of 7 m length were used in the first and second stage, respectively.

The amplified signal will propagate through the CIR1 from port1 to port2 then travel through

Figure 6. Experimental configuration of DSQP. TBF: tunable bandpass filter, CIR: circulator, EDF: erbium-doped Fiber, LD: laser diode, WDM: wavelength division multiplexing, TLS: tunable laser source, and OSA: optical spectrum analyzer.

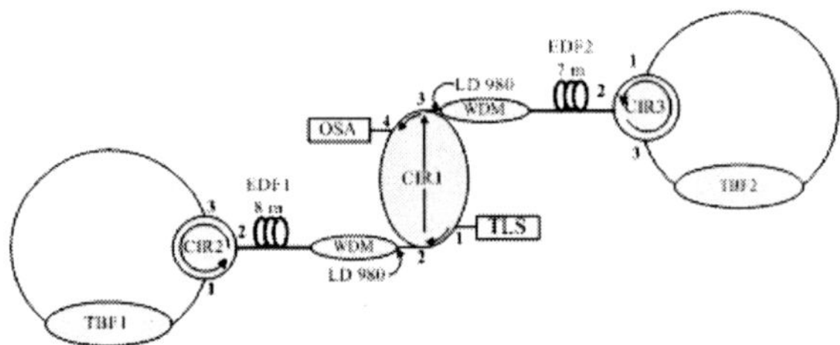

EDF1; it will be affected by the first amplification from EDF1, through port2 into port3 of CIR2, passing through the first TBF1 filter into port1 and back to port2 to be amplified during the second pass by EDF1 into port2 of CIR1, and therefore will propagate again in the second stage through EDF2, CIR3, and TBF2 for the third and fourth passes. The output signal power was displayed through the OSA from port4 of CIR1. Traveling from port1 to port4 of CIR1, the signal was affected by four amplifications during the four passes, or, as we mentioned, the new quadruple pass amplification.

Figure 7 shows gain vs. pump power and input signal power at 1550 nm signal wavelength for input signal powers from -50 to 0 dBm and pumping powers from 15 to 175 mW. The pumping power was optimized in this experiment by fixing it in the second stage at 10 mW and varying it at the first stage from 5 to 165 mW in 5 mW steps. This optimization is performed owing to instability of the signal that has been observed in the case when the two pump powers were increased together. The starting pumping power was 15 mW (pump2 = 10 mW and pump1 = 5 mW). At 15 mW pump power with 0 dBm input signal power the gain is -3 dB. At lower input signal power, which is -50 dBm, the gain value increases sharply to 38 dB. It is an attractive result when we see a very sharp shift of gain at a lower pumping power where the ratio between the gain and the pumping power is 2.5 dB/mW at -50 dBm input signal. At higher pumping power and higher gain, the ratio was decreased to 0.35 dB/mW. It is clearly observed that the increase in gain is sharp, and there is no significant evidence of gain saturation, and it is expected that the gain value can exceed 65 dB with the fifth or sixth pass at a higher pump power.

Figure 7. Experimental gain vs. pumping power and input signal power at λ = 1550 nm obtained using the DSQP

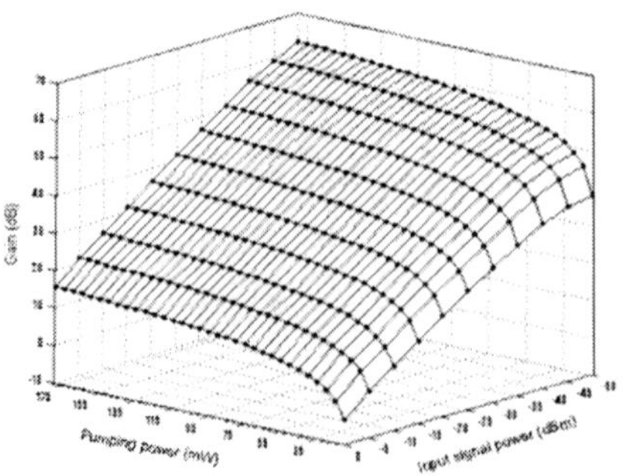

Figure 8. Experimental noise figure vs. pumping power and input signal power at λ = 1550 nm obtained using the

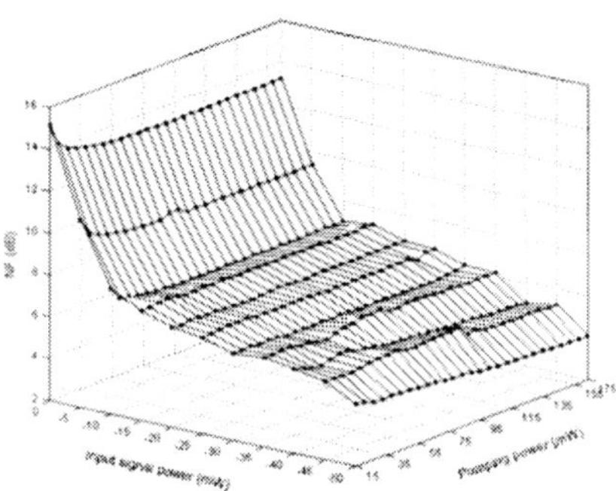

Figure 8 illustrates NF against pumping power and input signal power at 1550 nm signal wavelength. The pump power and input signal power were varied from 15 to 175 mW and from 0 to -50 dBm, respectively. In the case of NF vs. pump power, a constant behavior of NF is shown during the pumping augmentation at different input signal powers. The lowest NF is recorded at -50 dBm. During the increase in input signal power from -50 to 0 dBm, different parts of NF were characterized, the first part is at the input signal power between -50 and -10 dBm where the NF was increased from 3.98 to 7.03 dB and a minor increase in NF was recorded at this part. In the second part the NF showed a sharp increase from 7 to 14 dB. The reverse phenomenon was recorded for the NF vs. pumping power where a major change was observed for a low pumping power at 15 mW. This also may be explained on the basis of the relation between NF and the pumping power. It was observed that the filter played the role of a constant function of NF referring to the increase in pumping power.

Describing the trends of NF vs. input signal power in Figure 8, the noise showed a different behavior compared with pumping power, a sharp reduction from 14 to 7 dB of NF value was recorded between 0 and -10 dBm input signal power and a slow reduction from 7 to 4 dB of NF value was recorded between -10 and -50 dBm

input signal power. At this point, the lowest NF is recorded to be 3.98 dB. Combining all the shown figures, the highest gain of 62.56 dB was achieved with the lowest NF of 3.98 dB. This good result is considered to be the first among the current scientific research on EDFA or previously published papers.

The six configurations were shown in Figure 9 (a) SPSS: single pass single stage, (b) DPSS: double pass single stage, (c) DPSSF: double pass single stage with filter, (d) TPDS: triple pass double stage, (d) TPDSF: triple pass double stage with filter, and QPDSF: quadruple pass double stage with filter. The difference between these configurations is owing to the additions of TBF and the second stage which can be single pass or double pass. The circulators are used as loop back where port 1 and 3 are spliced and the TBF is incorporated between these ports to suppress and eliminate the unwanted ASE. The Key role of TBF in this continuous increase of gain is impressive and crucial where stimulated emission will strongly amplify the signal.

Figure 10 shows gain on dB vs. configurations and pumping power [16]. The input signal power is at 1550 nm wavelength and -50 dBm except the SPSS. From the 3D graph, all the six configurations show an increase of gain at the changing of configurations from SPSS, DPSS, DPSSF, TPDSF and QPDSF. Except for the TPDS without

Figure 9. Experimental configurations of EDFA: (a) single pass single stage (SPSS), (b) double pass single stage (DPSS), (c) double pass single stage with filter (DPSSF), (d) triple passes double stage (TPDS), (e) triple passes double stages with filter (TPDSF) and (f) quadruple passes double stages with filter (QPDSF). TBF: tunable bandpass filter, CIR: circulator, EDF: erbium-doped Fiber, LD: laser diode, and WDM: wavelength division multiplexing, INPUT: tunable laser source, and OUTPUT: optical spectrum analyzer.

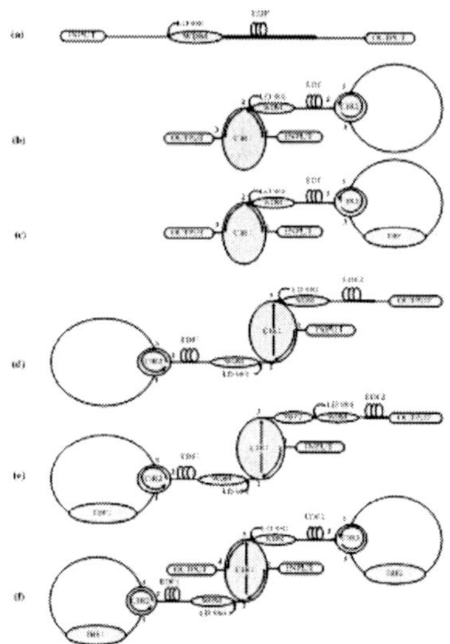

filter, which shows a lower gain compared to DPSSF and TPDSF.

It can be seen clearly, by following the variations of gain vs. configurations, at lower pump power of 10 mW, the gain is varied at different configuration where a shift between 9.65 and 45 dB is recorded for SPSS and QPDSF respectively. At higher pumping power of 90 mW the gain is shifted owing to configurations change from 20.04 to 59.49 dB. All these results are at 1550 nm input signal power and -50 dBm except the SPSS. This good result shows clearly the

Figure 10. Experimental gain vs. configurations and pumping power at 1550 nm wavelength at -50 dBm input signal power. SPSS: single pass single stage, DPSS: double passes single stage, DPSSF: double passes single stage with filter, TPDS: triple passes double stages, TPDSF: triple passes double stages with filter, and QPDSF: quadruple passes double stages with filter.

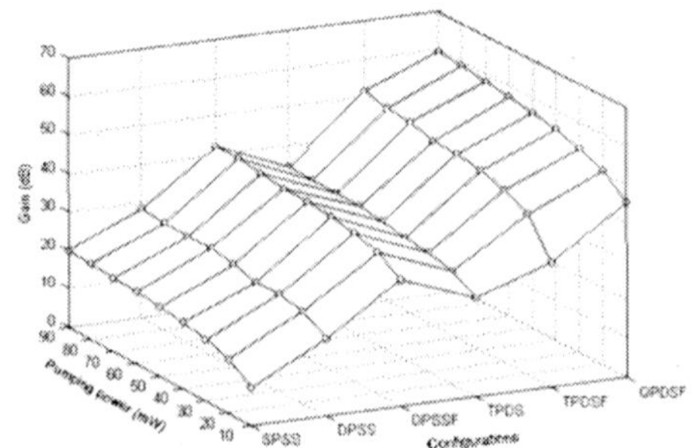

Figure 11. Experimental results of gain (dB) vs. pumping power (mW) for (•) single pass configuration and (▲) double pass dual stage configuration

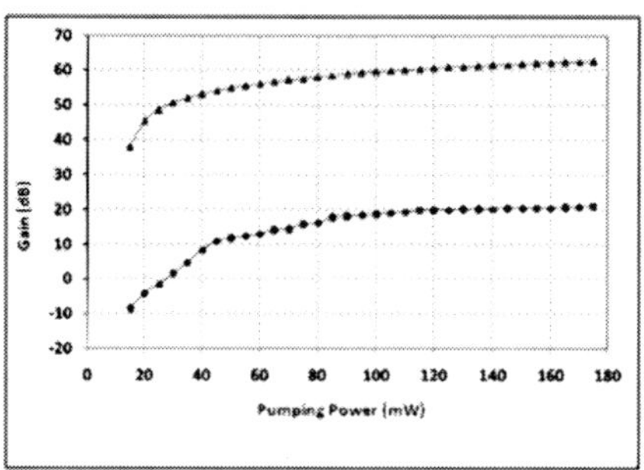

impact of the varied configurations, the filter, and the double pass on the gain value. So, with the change of configuration from SPSS to QPDSF, the gain is increased to 45 dB at low pumping power. The gain difference between the SPSS and QPDSF reach to 39.45 dB at high pump power.

The main and principal focal point was to find an idea where the gain can improve better and higher more than that, which existed in the published papers and books. The hope becomes a truth when the tunable band pass filter was positioned between the port 1 and port 3 of the circulator. This new position of the TBF increases the gain to approximately 40dB. With the same length and the same pumping power and the same wavelength the gain is jumped from 20dB single pass to 40 dB double pass with filter and this was a big achievement in that time. Adding another stage double pass to the first stage the configuration becomes dual stage double pass with filter see Figure 11 the gain reach 62.56 dB. The huge gap difference of 40 dB between the single pass configuration and the double passes dual stage shows how efficient the configuration design can control the gain value and output power.

In Figure 11 it is very clear and evident result showing the difference between dual stage double pass and single pass. By increasing the pumping power for both configurations in Figure 9(a) and Figure 9(f) the gain difference between the two

configurations is a constant value of approximately 40 dB.

Erbium Doped Fiber Laser

Tunable single-frequency lasers in the wavelength region, around 1550 nm are of much interest in a variety of applications, such as wavelength division multiplexing WDM optical communications, spectroscopy, and fiber sensors. These lasers have potential advantages because of their narrow line width and low intensity noise. They represent a natural source for fiber optical communications, since the light is already in the fiber and they can be spliced directly to the system. Other advantages include high side mode suppression ratio (SMSR), low threshold, and flat output power. These parameters are important in the design considerations for this type of lasers.

Various configurations have been proposed aimed at achieving best combination of these characteristics. They include ring cavity and linear cavity structures. The suggested tuning range in the conventional band C band and L band is reported to be 80 nm. The placement of the fused coupler for tapping the output from the system is critical due to the presence of amplified spontaneous emission ASE in the laser output. For efficient ASE filtering, the fused coupler is placed after the tunable filter. Inefficient filtering can lead to the deterioration of the SMSR value, which

Figure 12. Experimental configuration of double stage linear cavity EDFL

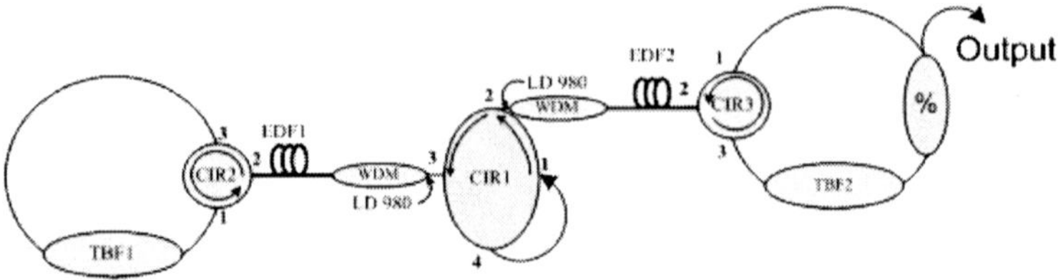

is critical for WDM transmission. We propose a new linear cavity EDFL configuration using a fiber loopback FLB embedded with tunable filters in a linear laser oscillator.

Implementing the linear cavity configuration, three circulators and two tunable bandpass filters TBFs are used. The output power of the proposed laser design is more than 18 dBm at 1560 nm. The double filtering technique enables the laser configuration to achieve higher stability as well as higher output power.

Figure 12 shows the proposed configuration of the system [17]. It consists of three circulators: CIR1 with four ports, andCIR2 and CIR3 with three ports each. They are used as loopback mirrors. The arrangement allows the insertion of the output coupler at one of the FLB mirrors. The TBF Newport is mechanically tuned with a passband of 1 nm, an insertion loss of around 1.5 dB at the center wavelength, and a tuning range limited to 40 nm from 1525 to 1565 nm. Both TBFs must be tuned and adjusted to the same wavelength in order to suppress the ASE efficiently.

The tuning process is used to stabilize the output power, to control the shape of the spectrum, and to minimize the insertion loss. The linear laser cavity consists of two portions. The first, EDF1, is a 10 m length, and the second, EDF2, is a 15 m length, both of erbium-doped fiber, with an Er^{3+} ion concentration of 440 ppm. The EDF is pumped by two 980 nm laser diodes. Each diode can provide a pump power of 220 mW at maximum. A fused coupler with 95% coupling ratio is placed after the tunable filter in one of the fiber loop mirrors to act as the output port. All connections are fusion spliced to minimize any back reflection and to achieve a low cavity loss. An optical spectrum analyzer OSA with 0.01 nm minimum resolution constituted the principal part of the measuring equipment.

The effect of pump power on the performance of the laser output was investigated by varying the power of the pump, which was provided by two 980-nm laser diodes. The power of the first pump P1 is fixed at 10 mW, and then the power of second pump P2 is varied from 10 to 220 mW in

Figure 13. Experimental results of output power (dBm) vs. pumping power at 1565 nm

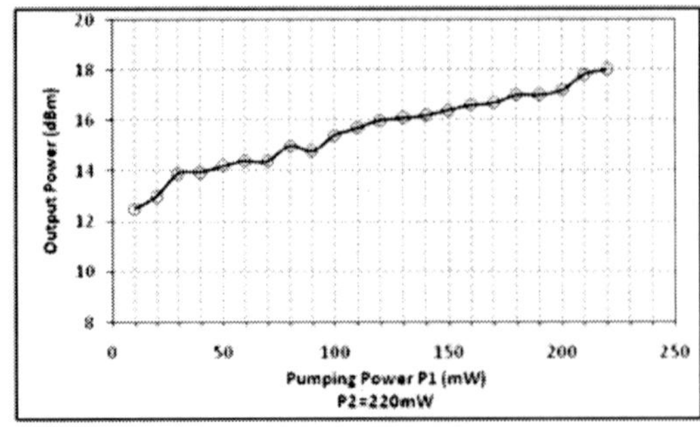

steps of 10 mW. When P2 reaches 220 mW, P1 is raised similarly in steps of 10 mW until it reaches 220 mW also. For a selected lasing wavelength of 1560 nm, the output power of the laser system is found to increase with increasing pump power until it becomes 18 dBm, with a coupling ratio of 95% as can be seen in Figure 13.

CONCLUSION

A detailed investigation was given on three principal levels first is the atomic structure where Erbium ion was investigated and interpreted. The energy levels of Erbium atom was shown calculated using the Russel-Saunder formula. The second level is the critics given to EDFA and EDFL topics where many published papers and books shows superficial and insignificant investigation concern the experiment and theory of EDFA and EDFL. The last level is the presentation of various configurations and their performance parameters related to design parameters. All these results have been published in an international conferences and journals.

ACKNOWLEDGMENT

The author wishes to acknowledge HBCC/KFUPM for their support in providing the various facilities utilized in the presentation of this paper.

REFERENCES

Ahmad, H., Harun, S. W. (2005, May). Double-pass L-band EDFA with flat-gain and improved noise figure characteristic, *3*, 75-77.

Ali, S., Khalid, A., Al-Khateeb, S., & Bouzid, B. (2008, April). A New Erbium-Doped Fiber Laser With a Double Tunable Bandpass Filter. *Optical Engineering (Redondo Beach, Calif.)*, *47*(4).

Becker, P. C., Olsson, N. A., & Simpson, J. R. (1999). *Erbium-Doped Fiber Amplifiers Fundamentals and Technology*. San Diego: Academic Press.

Bouzid, B. (in press). High-Gain and Low Noise-Figure EDFA Employing Dual Stage Quadruple Pass Technique. *Accepted in optical review Japan 2010.*

Bouzid, B. (in press). *Behavioral Variations of Gain and NF Owing to Configurations and Pumping Powers.* Submitted to PTL 2010.

Bouzid, B., Mohd. Ali, B., & Abdullah, M. K. (2003, September). A High Gain EDFA Design Using Double Pass Amplification with a Band-Pass Filter. *Photonics Technology Letters*, *15*(9), 1195–1197. doi:10.1109/LPT.2003.814901

Desurvire, E. (1994). *Erbium Doped Fiber Amplifier principle and Application*. New York: John Wiley and Sons, Inc.

Desurvire, E. *(2005). Optical communications in 2025.* Optical Communication, 2005. ECOC 2005. 31st European Conference, 1, 5-6.

Giles, C. R., & Desurvire, E. (1991, February). Modeling Erbium-Doped Fiber Amplifiers. *Journal of Lightwave Technology*, *9*(2), 271–283. doi:10.1109/50.65886

Li, S., & Chiang, K. S., & W. A. (2001, July). Gambling, Gain Flattening of an Erbium-Doped Fiber Amplifier Using a High-Birefringence Fiber Loop Mirror. *IEEE Photonics Technology Letters, 13*(9).

Lu, Y. B., & Chu, P. L. (2000, December). Gain Flattening by Using Dual-Core Fiber in Erbium-Doped Fiber Amplifier. *IEEE Photonics Technology Lrtters, 12*(12). J. R. Qian and H. F. Chen "Gain Flattening Fiber Filters Using Phaseshifted Long Period Fiber Gratings," Electronics Letters Vol. 34, No. 11, May 1998.

Masuda, H., & Takada, A. (1990). High Gain Two-Stage Amplification with Erbium-Doped Fiber Amplifier. *Electronics Letters, 26*(10), 661–662. doi:10.1049/el:19900432

Nilsson, J., Yun, S. Y., Hwang, S. T., Kim, J. M., & Kim, S. J. (1998, November). Long-Wavelength Erbium-Doped Fiber Amplifier Gain Enhanced by ASE End Reflectors. *IEEE Photonics Technology Letters, 10*(11).

Mahdi, M. A. (2004, February). *Member, IEEE,* K. A. Khairi, B. Bouzid, And M. K. Abdullah "Optimum Pumping Scheme Of Dual-Stage Triple-Pass Erbium-Doped Fiber Amplifier. *IEEE Photonics Technology Letters, 16*(2).

Sellami, A., Al-Khateeb, K., Belloui, B. (2006, May). The Influence of EDFA's Configuration on the Behavioral Trends of Gain," *vol. II, 9-11 May 2006,* Kuala Lumpur, pp 853-856.

Yun, S. H., Lee, B. W., Kim, H. K., & Kim, B. Y. Y. (2000, December). Dynamic Erbium-Doped fiber Amplifier Based on Active Gain Flattening with Fiber Acousto-optic Tunable Filters. *IEEE Photonics Technology Letters, 11*(10).

Zervas, M. N., Laming, R. I., & Payne, D. N. (1995, March). Efficient Erbium-Doped Fiber Amplifiers Incorporating an Optical Isolator. *IEEE Journal of Quantum Electronics, 31*(3). doi:10.1109/3.364402

Chapter 16
A User–Friendly Application–Based Design Aid Tool for Power Electronics Converters

Omrane Bouketir
King Fahd University of Petroleum & Minerals, Saudi Arabia

EXECUTIVE SUMMARY

Power electronics and its related subjects are well-known difficult to understand especially for students taking them for first time. This is due to nature of the subjects which involve many areas and disciplines. The introduction of general-purpose simulation package has helped the student a step further in understanding this subject. However, because of the generality of these tools and their drag-and-drop and ad-hoc features, the students still face problems in designing a converter circuit. In this section, the problem above is addressed by introducing a design aid tool that guides the student over prescribed steps to design a power electronics circuit. The tool is interfaced with Pspice and its knowledge base encompasses two types of knowledge; topologies' knowledge and switching devices' knowledge. The first step in the design procedure is the selection of an application of the desired circuit. Then few steps are to be followed to come out with the appropriate topology with the optimum switching devices and parameters. System structure, its different modules and the detailed design procedure are explained in the following paragraphs. At the end a design example is demonstrated and its results are displayed and discussed. It is aimed that this tool will enhance the understanding of the subject by introducing an interactive user friendly graphical interface that guides the user to the right topology. The complex design steps are hidden for the sake of saving the design time. However, an explanation module is included for the users who want to know how the results are drawn.

DOI: 10.4018/978-1-60960-015-0.ch016

INTRODUCTION

Different simulation software are being widely used to design and simulate electrical and electronic circuits. These software require the user to be proficient in designing the circuits and need deep training to be familiar with. Moreover, the design is based on trial and error, till the user reaches the required outputs. Indeed, these packages have facilitated the task of the design engineer by providing a virtual way to check the reliability of the circuit without the need of its hardware realization. However, an approach to overcome the drawbacks of these packages and augment their functionality is to introduce the expert system techniques along with these packages. In this sense, in literature only few considerable researches could be found. An earlier work (Cumbi et al., 1996) was the development of PECT tool. This tool is a knowledge-based system developed using object-oriented technique. The drawback of this tool is the need of many packages to develop and to operate such as HUMBLES expert system shell, HSPICE, semiconductor library and the Smalltalk-80TM system. In (Fezzani et al., 1997) an automatic design process for UPS was presented as an attempt to develop an expert system tool for computer-aided design of static converters. It was interfaced with SUCCESS simulation software and was developed using SMECI expert system shell. (Wang and Lee, 1996) proposed an expert system for designing, analyzing and optimizing power converters. Fuzzy logic was introduced to select the optimum topology; Pspice was used as a simulator and the MATSPICE tool as an optimizer. A computer algorithm (Amaya, 1998) was introduced for synthesis of switching power converters (dc choppers for instance). Although, this algorithm was not based on artificial intelligence techniques, it can be considered as an advanced stage in automating the design process. Other works in this area can be found as in (Masatoshi, 1997), (Debebe and Rajagopalan, 1995), (Fezzani, 1998) and (Bouketir et al., 2002 and 2003),

In the present tool; power electronic design aid system (PEDAS) (omrane et al., 2005) a different approach is introduced to overcome the difficulties faced in the literature in order to come out with a fully-automated tool specifically for designing power electronics converters. The tool is interfaced with *Pspice* simulator and establishes an interaction with the user starting from the selection of a specific application until arriving to the optimum topology with all parameter values and switches suggested. The topologies are stored in the knowledge base as schematic files, allowing the *Pspice Schematic* to be able to display the resulted circuit. Here, PEDAS general outlook and its graphical user interface (GUI) are illustrated. Then, the various and attractive controls and tools used to build a smooth and flexible interaction medium with the user are stated in details. The topologies knowledge base representation and implementation methods are described. This includes both types of this knowledge; type-based topologies and application-based topologies. The access paths to this knowledge and its manipulation procedures are explained when the inference engine module is elucidated. Instances of the explanation and help module are given. Lastly, the devices library module, its significance and its considerable features and functions are thoroughly explained and demonstrated.

PEDAS LAYOUT (GUI)

The general layout or the system outlook or the graphical user interface (GUI) is of great importance. It gives the user the first impression about the tool. Hence, this outlook must be designed carefully and cautiously. Fortunately, the programming tool selected for the system development makes this task easy to accomplish. *Visual Basic* programming language, one of its famous features is the ability to provide pre-designed graphical controls (e.g. text boxes, command buttons, and list boxes), dialog boxes and flexible menu development tool. Each control has its own set of properties, methods, and events. This is to provide the user with a standard way to make selections, carry out commands, and perform input and output tasks. The programmer needs only to choose the appropriate controls and place them to the required position on his layout form and then write his own code of task the control to perform. Furthermore, *Visual Basic* –in its professional edition- is equipped by a mean that allows the programmer to create his own control to fit his specific needs. This mean is called *ActiveX technology* which is an extension to the *Visual Basic Toolbox*. The controls designed by using this technology can be added to the application even though they were developed by a different programmer in different locations. This is one of the features that make *Visual Basic* flexible and widely acceptable. Obviously, it's not possible to explore all the features and characteristics of *Visual Basic* that have been employed to build PEDAS GUI, but they will be imperceptibly revealed throughout this paper. Figure 1 shows some useful controls and menus that make up PEDAS layout.

SYSTEM'S KNOWLEDGE CODING

Using *Class Builder* utility offered in the *Visual Basic Add-ins* a total of sixteen (16) classes and subclasses (objects) were built. Fifteen (15) of them represent the topologies knowledge base. One class represent the interfacing module between *PEDAS* and *PSpice*. Among the first fifteen classes, fourteen (14) are application-based knowledge, while one class encompasses the type-based knowledge. The switching devices' knowledge is represented by a database object. The hierarchy of these classes is shown in Figure 2. It is worth to note that one can build his objects without the assistance of the *Class Builder* utility, but because this utility is meant to help build class and collection hierarchy it's better to exploit it for the sake of time saving. Furthermore, the *Class Builder* utility keeps track of the hierarchy of the built classes and collections and generates the framework code necessary to implement them including their interface (i.e. properties, methods and events).

In the figure only the interface (properties and methods) of the *Single_Phase* subclass is shown.

Figure 1. An instance of PEDAS general layout (GUI)

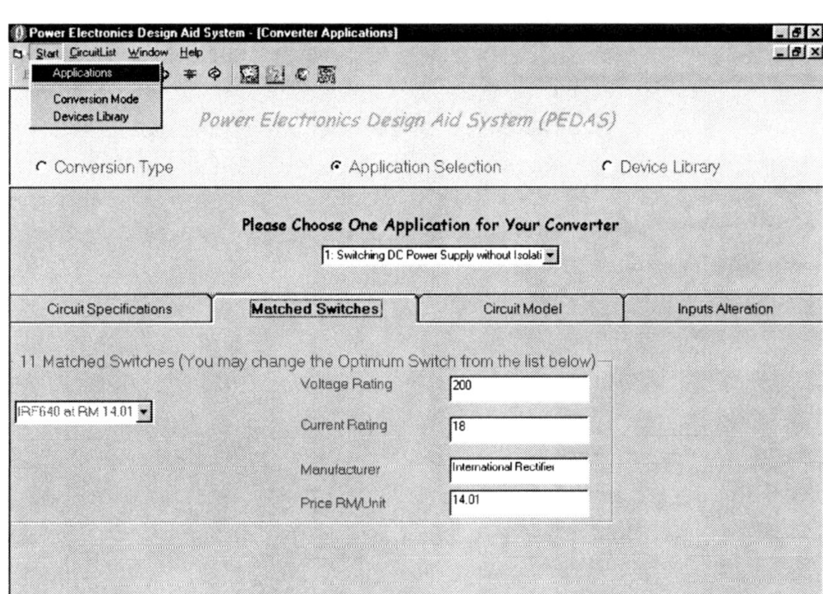

Figure 2. Class builder utility and classes' hierarchy

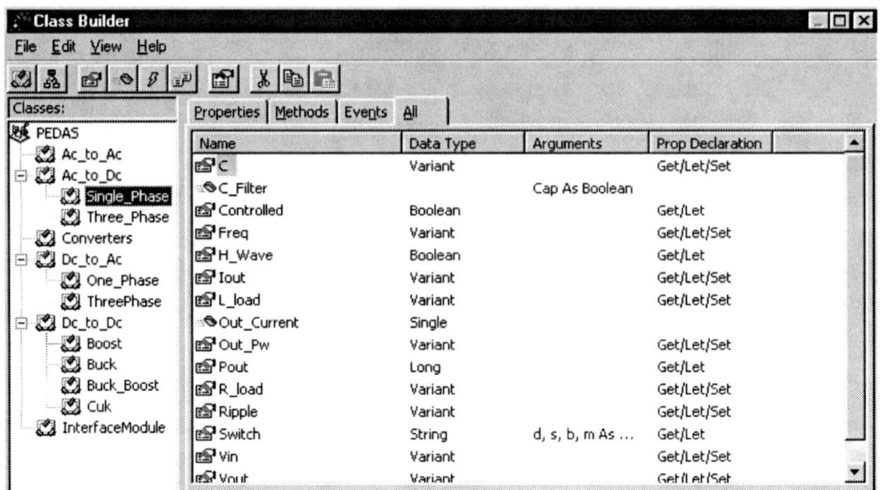

The *Converters* class is the one that represents the type-based topologies. This class and the *InterfaceModule* class were created separately from the remaining ones. We didn't use the class builder for they don't have the hierarchy as the other class do. Nevertheless, the basic ideas are the same in terms of implementation and accessibility through their interfaces.

A. Type-Based Knowledge

This part of knowledge encompasses eleven types of converter organised under the four basic types of conversions (DC-to-DC, AC-to-DC, AC-to-AC and DC-to-AC). Figures below show how these different converters appear to the user. The basic schematic and brief information about the converter are provided within this illustration. These converters are as follows:

- Buck converter (as shown in Figure 3), Boost converter, Buck-Boost converter, Cuk converter, Single-phase full wave rectifier (Uncontrolled), Three-phase rectifier (Uncontrolled), Single-phase AC controller, Three-phase AC controller (wye-connected), Three-phase AC controller (delta-connected), Square-wave inverter, PWM Inverter.

This type of knowledge is coded under only one class (object) as mentioned earlier. This class is named *Converters*, where each of its methods represents one topology among the above. All operations concerning one topology are accomplished within this method. These operations vary from requesting the user's entries to circuit parameters calculation including the guidance of the user through the process and the suggestion further steps if the inference engine fails to come out with the required circuit. Below is a segment of listing code shows the implementation of the *SinglePhaseRectifier* method, which corresponds to the single-phase uncontrolled rectifier shown above.

```
Public Function SinglePhaseRecti-
fier()
 On Error Resume Next
frst:      vinput = InputBox("Please
Enter The Input Voltage (Volt)")
         If Val(vinput) <= 0 Then
```

Figure 3. Buck converter layout in PEDAS environment

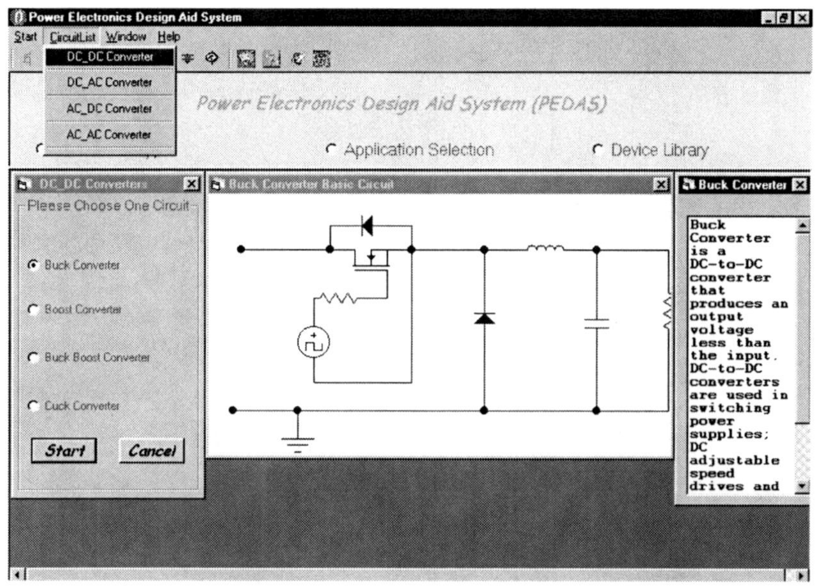


```
 res = MsgBox("The Input Voltage Must
be greater than zero", 1, "PEDAS")
         If res = vbCancel Then
Exit Sub
        GoTo frst
     End If
      vinput = 1.41 * vinput
frth:  Freq = InputBox("Please Enter
The Operating Frequency (Hz)")
        If Val(Freq) <= 0 Then
 res = MsgBox("The frequency Value
Must be greater than zero", 1, "PED-
AS")
      If res = vbCancel Then Exit Sub
          GoTo frth
     End If
fith:  RLoad = InputBox("Please Enter
The Load value (Ohm)")
       If Val(RLoad) <= 0 Then
     res = MsgBox("The Load Value
Must be greater than zero", 1, "PED-
AS")
       If res = vbCancel Then Exit Sub
          GoTo fith
        End If

capc:  Rf = InputBox("What'is the
Maxminum Ripple Factor for Vout (%)")
        If Val(Rf) <= 0 Then
     res = MsgBox("The Ripple Factor
Must be greater than zero", 1, "PED-
AS")
If res = vbCancel Then Exit Sub
         GoTo capc
       End If
    Rf = Rf / 100
    Cap = (1 / Rf)
    Cap = Cap / (2 * Freq * RLoad)
    Cap = Cap * 1000000
    Cap = Format(Cap, "##.##")
Open "c:\msim53\1phrect.sch" For In-
put As #10
 Open "c:\outp.sch" For Output As #20
    Dim srg As String
    Dim Leng As Integer
    Input #10, srg
    Close #10
    choice = 1
   Leng = Len(srg)
   For i = 1 To Len(srg)
      wrotc = False
```

```
    If Left(srg, 1) = "&" Then
    Select Case choice
    Case 1
        k = vinput
    Case 2
        k = Freq
    Case 3
        k = RLoad
    Case 4
       k = Cap
    End Select
    choice = choice + 1
    Print #20, k;
    wrote = True
 End If
 If wrote = False Then
     Print #20, Left(srg, 1);
End If
If i < Leng Then
 srg = Right(srg, Len(srg) - 1)
             Else
 srg = srg
         End If
     Next i
Close #20
SchInterface ("psched.exe c:\outp.
sch")
SendKeys "{F11}", True
End Function
```

B. Application-Based Knowledge

This knowledge constitutes the kernel of the knowledge base. It encompasses more than twenty-five (25) topologies organised under fourteen (14) objects (classes and subclasses) with their own interfaces. This is a very different knowledge from the above one. Although they may share some same topologies, the ways of representation are totally dissimilar.

This part of knowledge is arranged in such a way that the user has the access to a specific topology only through its application (see Figure 4). Nevertheless, the user can choose the type of

conversion of the circuit if he/she knows it in order to narrow the list of applications offered by PEDAS. Likewise, the internal implementation of this knowledge is based on its type of conversion following its way of representation. This implementation permits to exploit the usefulness of the inheritance feature of OOP between the class and subclass and hence reduce the development code and time drastically.

The following sections show samples of the Dc_to_Dc, Dc_to_Ac) classes and their interface implementation. Buck subclass also is dealt here with some details.

1.   Dc_to_Dc Class

This class as from its name covers all dc chopper topologies. The main applications of this type of converters are in switching dc power supplies and dc drives. They are widely used for traction motor control in electric automobiles, trolley cars, marine hoists, forklift trucks and mine haulers. They provide smooth acceleration control, high efficiency, and fast dynamic response. They can be used also in conjunction with an inductor to generate a dc current source especially for the current source inverter (Daniel, 1997).

To efficiently synthesize these converters, four basic topologies are encoded here. They are the buck, boost, buck-boost and Cuk topologies. However, other topologies such as flyback, forward, push-pull and full-bridge converters can be added to enlarge this knowledge. One should examine each of these topologies thoroughly in order to determine its necessary interface (properties and methods). Once the interface is completely determined, they can be implemented the same way as the first four were. Here only segments and passages from the source code listings are given to show the implementation of this class as it is impracticable to include the entire code.

```
Private Sub Class_Initialize()
    Set mvarBuck = New Buck
```

Figure 4. Application-based knowledge (all applications)

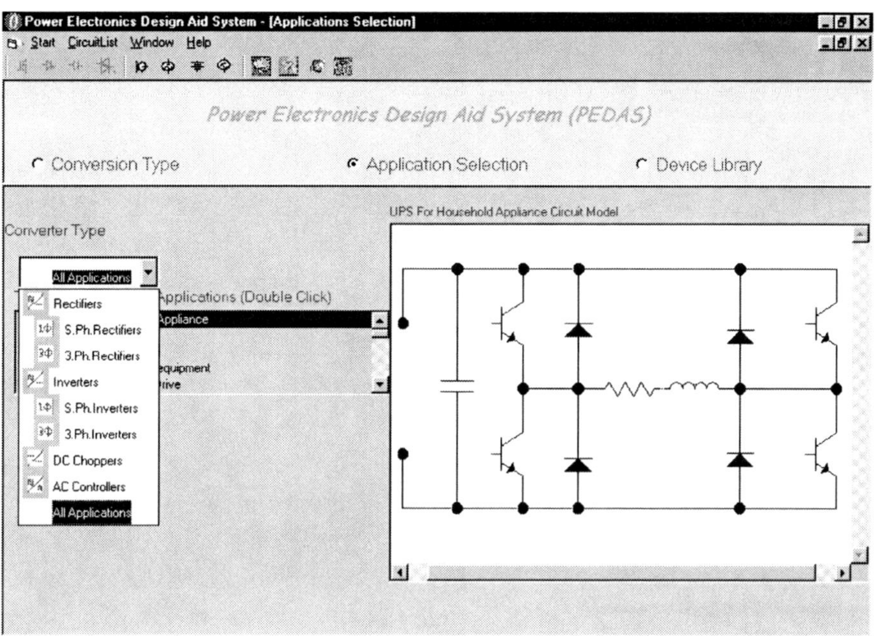

```
    Set mvarBoost = New Boost
    Set mvarBuck_Boost = New Buck_Boost
    Set mvarCuk = New Cuk
End Sub
Private Sub Class_Terminate()
    Set mvarCuk = Nothing
    Set mvarBuck_Boost = Nothing
    Set mvarBoost = Nothing
    Set mvarBuck = Nothing
End Sub
```

The first sub is to create the subclasses' instances whenever an instance of parent class is created. The second sub is to destroy the created objects and free the memory when the parent object is terminated. The following segments illustrate how to get the input voltage and output voltage values from the user. This is achieved by setting *Vin* and *Vout* properties in the parent class instead in the subclasses, this is because in all topologies these values must be set by the user. Hence these two properties are common between the four subclasses.

```
Public Property Get Vin() As Variant
        mvarVin = Val(Frm1.Text10)
        Vin = mvarVin
        mvarBoost.Vin = mvarVin
        mvarBuck.Vin = mvarVin
        mvarBuck_Boost.Vin= mvarVin
        mvarCuk.Vin= mvarVin
End Property
Public Property Get Vout() As Variant
        mvarVout = Val(Frm1.Text9)
        Vout = mvarVout
        mvarBoost.Vout = mvarVout
        mvarBuck.Vout = mvarVout
        mvarBuck_Boost.Vout= mvarVout
        mvarCuk.Vout= mvarVout
End Property
```

2.   Class Ac_to_Dc

This is a parent class to cover rectifier topologies ranging from single phase uncontrolled rectifiers to three-phase controlled rectifiers. Rectifiers are used to change the ac input to a fixed (uncontrolled rectifiers) or to a controlled (thyristor rectifiers) dc output. They are used mainly for unregulated dc power supplies and variable-speed dc drives especially in high power applications benefiting from the high ratings of SCRs. This class has two subclasses *Single_Phase* and *Three_phase* based on the type of the input source available. The initialisation and termination procedures of this class are accomplished the same way for *Dc_to_Dc* class.

Samples of some properties and methods of this class are given in the listings below.

```
Public Sub C_Filter(Cap As Boolean)
 H = mvarRipple / 100
 If Cap Then
  mvarC = 1 / (2 * mvarFreq * mvarR_
load * H)
  mvarC = 1000000 * mvarC
  mvarC = Round(mvarC)
 End If
End Sub
Public Property Get Vout() As Variant
If Not mvarControlled Then
    If mvarH_Wave Then
        mvarVout = (mvarVin * Sqr(2))
/ (3.14159)
        Vout = mvarVout
    Else
        mvarVout = (2 * mvarVin *
Sqr(2)) / (3.14159)
        Vout = mvarVout
    End If
 Else
OutVoltage:
   mvarVout = Val(InputBox("What's
your Machine Operating Voltage,
(Volt)"))
    If mvarVout <= 0 Then Exit Sub
    If mvarVout >= 0.9 * mvarVin Then
        Vin30 = MsgBox("Your Source
is Unable to Provide this Voltage,
Please Change Either the Input or the
Output Volage", vbCritical + vbAbor-
tRetryIgnore)
```

```
        If Vin30 = 3 Then Exit Sub
        GoTo OutVoltage
    Exit Sub
   End If
  Vout = mvarVout
 End If
End If
End Property
```

The first passage is to calculate the output filter value that corresponds to the desired output voltage ripple entered by the user. The last segment is to obtain the output voltage (Vout property). Here two ways to get this value; if the application selected by the user needs a controlled rectifier then this value is obtained from him by soliciting procedure. In case of uncontrolled rectifier, the output voltage value has to be calculated for that the user has no control on it once the source voltage is specified. Note that in the controlled case, the user is prompted to change the desired output voltage if the source is unable to meet it.

3.   Buck Subclass

This is only to give an example of how the subclasses are implemented as child classes of the parent classes. The Buck subclass is to cover all dc step-down converter instances. The basic topology and its parameter calculation were collected from various textbooks (8 and 9). Figure 5 shows an instance of a basic circuit of the step down converter with resistive load and square wave control scheme. Table 1 illustrates the properties and methods that were extracted by analysing this topology to build the interface of the subclass. It gives also brief description of each property and method.

The following listing passages illustrate how some methods and properties were implemented.

```
Public Sub Filter(Cfilter As Boolean)
d = mvarVout / mvarVin
If Cfilter Then
mvarC = (1 - d) / (8 * mvarL * (mvar-
```

Table 1. Buck subclass properties and methods

Name	Type	Description
C	Property	To hold the capacitor filter value (calculated from method)
Current	Method	To calculate the average output current
Filter	Method	To calculate the filters' values (L and C)
Iout	Property	To hold the output current value (calculated from method)
L	Property	To hold the inductor filter value (calculated from method)
Ripple	Property	To hold the desired ripple factor (from the user)
R_Load	Property	To hold the user's load value (from the user)
Sw_Freq	Property	To hold the suitable switching frequency (Suggested by the System)
Switch	Property	To hold the selected switching device (Selected by the System)
Vin	Property	To hold the input voltage value (from the user)
Vout	Property	To hold the desired output voltage value (from the user)

```
Ripple) * mvarSw_Freq ^ 2)
        If mvarC > 10000 Then
            res = MsgBox("The Capaci-
tor is Too Large, " & Str(mvarC) & "
Please Increase the Input Voltage "
& mvarVin & " or Decrease the Output
One" & mvarVout, vbOKCancel)
            If res = vbCancel Then
Exit Sub
            pass = False
            End If
Else
    mvarL = (1 - d) * mvarRLoad / (2
* mvarSw_Freq)
```

```
End If
End Sub
```

It is seen from the source code segment that this method serves to calculate both of the filter values (i.e. C and L). Which one is to be calculated depends on the setting of the argument (*Cfilter*) upon calling the method. If the argument is set to *True* then the capacitance will be calculated, otherwise the inductance is to be calculated and returned as a function value. The argument is set by the inference engine outside the interface, it set through the interaction module as it will be detailed later.

```
Public Property Get Switch() As Variant
```

Figure 5. An instance of basic step-down Dc chopper with resistive load

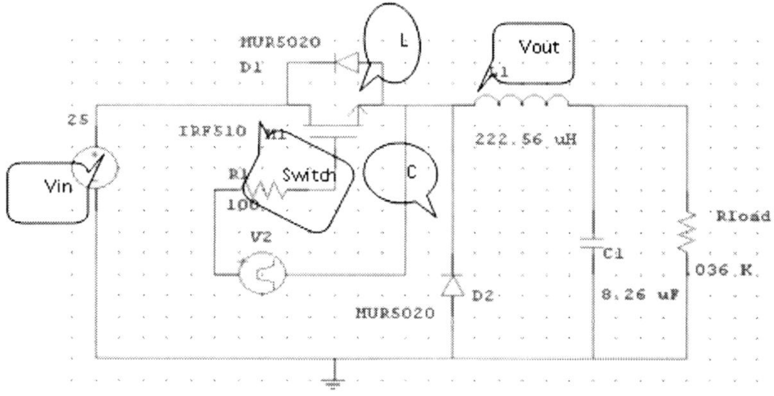

```
        mvarSwitch = Libfrm3.
SearchResult2("MOSFET", mvarVin,
mvarIout)
        Switch = mvarSwitch
End Property
```

The switch here is extracted from the database using *SerachResult2* function which is called from the devices library module where it is developed. Here the type switch selected "MOSFET" as a rule of thumb. Upon calling this function, the ratings (i.e. voltage and current ratings) are required. This means that it can not be called only after getting these two values which correspond to Vin and Iout properties respectively. This vital function was developed using structured query language (SQL) procedures and statements embedded in Visual Basic. Once the search is initiated and the ratings are within the stored values, the function doesn't only return one switch, but it returns all the devices that satisfy its arguments (i.e. the ratings). Yet it suggests and recommends the cheapest device among the resulted switches meanwhile the user is given the hand to change this device if his concern is more on other parameters (the manufacturer par example) than on the price as shown in Figure 6.

C. Inference Engine

The inference engine operates on the knowledge base in its search of solutions. It matches the facts asserted from the user inputs against the stored facts in the system's knowledge base in order to come out with results or new facts. The inference engine accesses the knowledge base through the class interfaces. Once the user selects his application or type of converter through the interaction module, the inference engine invokes the class methods and properties whenever needed to infer conclusions or assert facts. A sketch of the inference engine process flow is illustrated in figure 7.

The steps shown above are general steps to be followed in order to reach the final result. The first step is to know what type of knowledge the user wants to access in order to invoke the right class module as a response to the user action. Then, through the interaction module the user is required to insert his inputs and specification which will be used by the inference engine to assert new facts and finalise the results through the invoked class interface. Once the results are finalised, they are to be sent for displaying through the interaction and interface modules. Sample of the source code to show how to access the Boost subclass is shown below.

```
Private Sub BoostCon()
Set con = New Dc_to_Dc
Vout = con.Vout
        If Vout <= 0 Then
            res = MsgBox("The Output
Voltage Must be Greater Than Zero",
vbOKCancel)
            Exit Sub
        End If
RLoad = con.RLoad
        If RLoad <= 0 Then
            res = MsgBox("The Load
Must be Greater Than Zero", vbOKCan-
cel)
            Exit Sub
        End If
        Rload1 = RLoad / 1000 ' con-
vert to kOhm
Ripple = con.Boost.Ripple
        If Ripple <= 0 Then
            ms = "The Ripple Value Must
be Greater than Zero"
            res = MsgBox(ms, vbOKCan-
cel)
            Exit Sub
        End If
Vin = con.Vin
        If Vin >= Vout Or Vin <= 0 Then
            res = MsgBox("The Input Voltage
must be Less than the Output One" &
Str(Vout), vbOKCancel)
            Exit Sub
```

Figure 6. The returned results of the optimum switches

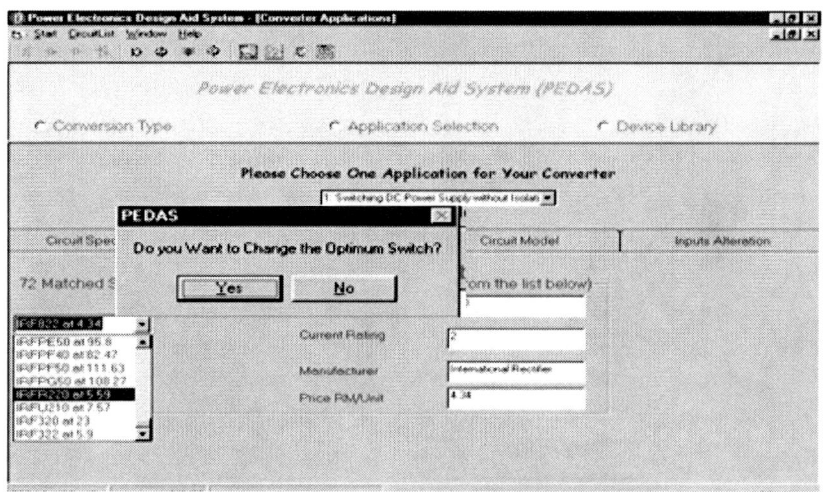

Figure 7. Ordinary steps of the inference engine flow

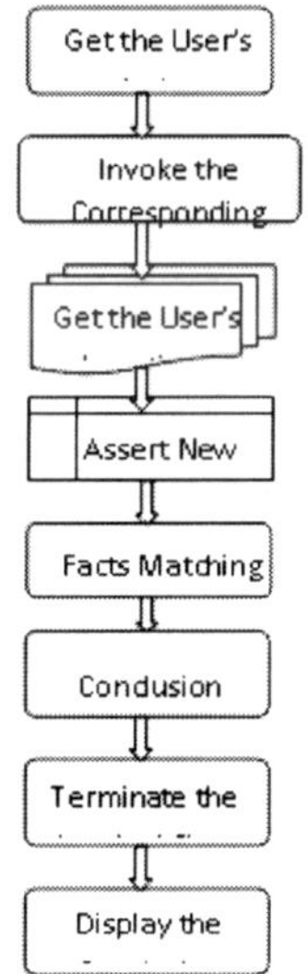


```
        End If
d = (1 - (Vin / Vout))
f = con.Boost.Sw_Freq `
Lmin = con.Boost.L
Imax = con.Boost.Iout * Lmin * f)))
C = con.Boost.C
C = Format(C, ".00")
Lmin = Format(Lmin, ".000")
```

```
Imax = Format(Imax, ".000")
swtch = con.Boost.Switch
k = 0
For i = 0 To Combo1(0).ListCount - 1
ReDim Preserve swtype(k), price(k),
VoltR(k), CurrR(k), IDa(k),
manfact(k)
price(k) = Combo1(3).List(i)
VoltR(k) = Combo1(0).List(i)
CurrR(k) = Combo1(1).List(i)
manfact(k) = Combo1(2).List(i)
IDa(K) = Combo1(5).List(i)
k = k + 1
Next i
If swtch <> Empty Then
 minp = Libfrm3.CheapPrice
 VoltageR = Libfrm3.voltagerating
 CurrRating = Libfrm3.currentrating
 manufac = Libfrm3.manufac
 Combo2.Text = swtch + "    at RM " +
Str(minp)
 Frame3.Visible = False
 If Combo2.ListCount > 1 Then
  Frame1.Caption = Str(k) + " Matched
Switches (You may change the Optimum
Switch
   from   the list below)"
```

```
Else
   Frame1.Caption = "Only One Switch
Matches Your Specifications"
End If
 Output ' call the output subroutine
to display the output results
End If
End Sub
The first step to access this segment
of the knowledge base is by creating
a new instance of the Dc_to_Dc class,
using the Set and New keywords. This
automatically will create an in-
stance of the Boost subclass in the
Class_Initialize sub as was shown in
the precedent section. After gain-
ing access to the Boost subclass, the
inference engine starts asserting the
facts and concluding results through
the subclass interface before it fi-
nalises the results and send them to
be displayed.
```

D. Interface Module

This module is the intermediate channel between PEDAS and the simulation package (PSpice). It serves in displaying the resulted circuit, its simulation process and results in PEDAS environment. After the inference engine decision is made, it sends relevant data and information (files *.sch, *.net and *.cir) to this module in order to call the simulation package to display and simulate the circuit. The connection process was achieved by using *Application Programming Interface* (API) technique. This technique is a complicated set of functions, messages, and structures allowing programmers in all types of programming languages to build applications that run on the Windows and Windows NT operating systems (Noel and Eric, 1996). PEDAS uses this set to request and carry out lower-level services performed by a computer's operating system. The following listing shows how this technique is exploited in the *InterfaceModule* class. All functions preceded by the keywords *Private Declare Function* (e.g. *GetParent* function) are API functions called by PEDAS in incoming procedures. An instance of displaying the resulted circuit within PEDAS environment is shown Figure 8.

```
Private mvarPid As Long 'local copy
Private mvarInterfProg As String
'local copy
Private Declare Function FindWindow
Lib "user32" Alias "FindWindowA"
(ByVal lpClassName As Long, ByVal
lpWindowName As Long) As Long
Private Declare Function GetParent
Lib "user32" (ByVal hwnd As Long) As
Long
Private Declare Function SetParent
Lib "user32" (ByVal hWndChild As
Long, ByVal hWndNewParent As Long) As
Long
Private Declare Function GetWin-
dowThreadProcessId Lib "user32"
(ByVal hwnd As Long, lpdwProcessId As
Long) As Long
Private Declare Function GetWindow
Lib "user32" (ByVal hwnd As Long,
ByVal wCmd As Long) As Long
Private Declare Function DestroyWin-
dow Lib "user32" (ByVal hwnd As Long)
As Long
Private Declare Function Putfocus Lib
"user32" Alias "SetFocus" (ByVal hwnd
As Long) As Long
Public Function ProgrInstance(ByVal
Target_pid As Long) As Long
Dim test_hwnd As Long, test_pid As
Long, test_thread_id As Long
    'Find the first window
    test_hwnd = FindWindow(ByVal 0&,
ByVal 0&)
    Do While test_hwnd <> 0
        'Check if the window isn't a
child
```

```
        If GetParent(test_hwnd) = 0
Then
            'Get the window's thread
            test_thread_id =
GetWindowThreadProcessId(test_hwnd,
test_pid)
            If test_pid = Target_pid
Then
                ProgrInstance =
test_hwnd
                Exit Do
            End If
        End If
        'retrieve the next window
        test_hwnd = GetWindow(test_
hwnd, 2)
    Loop
End Function
Public Property Let InterfProg(ByVal
vData As String)
'used when assigning a value to the
property, on the left side of an
assignment.
'Syntax: X.InterfProg = 5
    mvarInterfProg = vData
End Property
Public Property Get InterfProg() As
String
'used when retrieving value of a
property, on the right side of an
assignment.
'Syntax: Debug.Print X.InterfProg
    InterfProg = mvarInterfProg
End Property
Public Property Let Pid(ByVal vData
As Long)
'used when assigning a value to the
property, on the left side of an
assignment.
'Syntax: X.Pid = 5
    mvarPid = vData
End Property
Public Property Get Pid() As Long
'used when retrieving value of a
property, on the right side of an
assignment.
'Syntax: Debug.Print X.Pid
    Pid = mvarPid
End Property
```

E. Explanation Module

The explanation facility allows the system to explain its reasoning to the user in language that he/

Figure 8. Displaying the resulted circuit within PEDAS environment

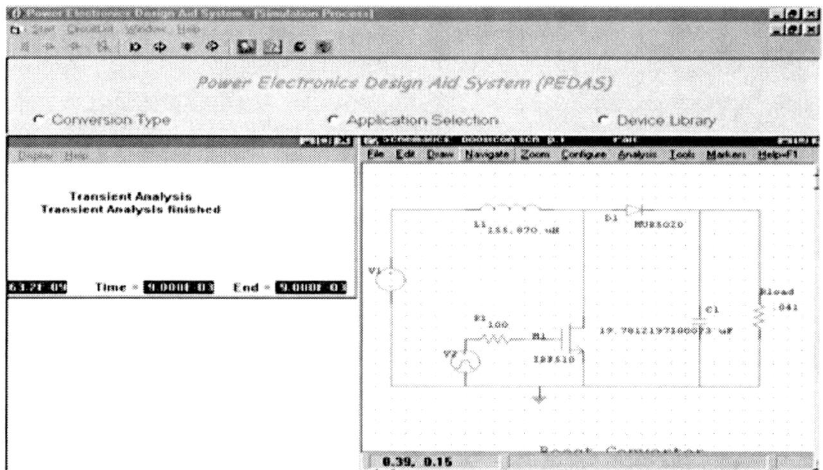

she can understand through a user interface. These explanations include justification for the system's conclusions (the know how), and the explanation why the system needs a particular data (the why query). In some systems, a tutorial explanations or deeper theoretical justifications of program's action are granted. For instance, in PEDAS this module is designed to guide and help the user:

- to find out how the results have been achieved and
- to provide general information about the circuit topologies and switching devices and
- to enhance the understanding of the converter operation by providing a tutorial-like facility.

In fact, the first point is inclusive in the interaction module. From the communication process, the user can know how certain results have been reached. A help module was developed to accomplish the second purpose. This module gathers basic information, formulas and topologies for each type of conversion. Relevant information has to be gathered and collected from various books and articles and then coded into this module. An auxiliary component to this module is developed to provide a simulation-like demo of basic converters based on their ideal parameters (see figure 9). This component can be considered as a learning aid system for students to get a comprehensive understanding of power electronics converters operations. Various parameters are made available for the user to change and see their impacts on the converter performance through its waveforms.

F. Devices Library Module

This module is a part of the knowledge base module described above. It contains power electronics switching devices along with their relevant necessary information such as type, current and voltage ratings. Figure10 gives a general view of this module. Such module encompasses huge data and allows the user to add more data during the lifetime of the system. This requires the use of a database to provide efficient handling and management of the data. Visual Basic offers a special engine called JET (Joint Engine Technology) to ease the dealing with databases. JET allows the programmer to use the methods and properties of *Data Access Objects* (DAOs) to access and manipulate database information. These methods and properties allow the user to retrieve data, modify the data and change the presentation order of the data. The programmer could even modify the structure of the database by creating, modifying, and deleting fields, tables and indexes.

Visual Basic 6 provides two controls to work with database files; the data control (with its associated bound controls) and data access objects. The two controls are not mutually exclusive, they can be used together to take advantage of each.

The first step in gaining access to information in a database is to open the database itself. "*OpenDatabase*" is a method of the "*Workspace*" object used to open the database. This module is enhanced by several functions that can be seen clearly from the main menu (or toolbar). Here only few of them are discussed in details.

1.   Search Function

Its icon is in most left side of the toolbar. It can be accessed also form the *Search* submenu under the *File* menu (Ctrl + S). As shown in Figure 11 it provides several criteria for searching a specific record. These criteria can be set all together as well as, the user has the advantage to set only some (at least one) of them for fast searching.

Note that for this function, the *Recordset* is opened as snapshot since there is no need to change the data inside the database.

2.   Update Function

Figure 9. An instance of PEDAS simulation-like Demo

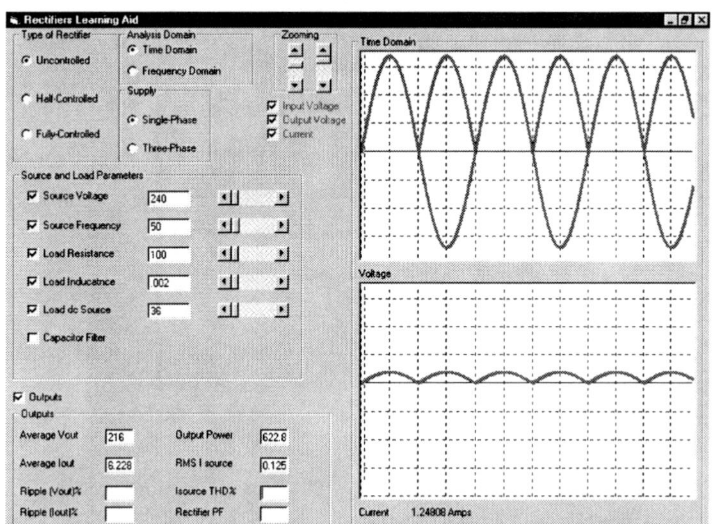

This function is to update the data in the opened *Recordset* firstly and then in the database. The *Edit* method is used to copy the new information entered by the user to the data buffer. Then the new data are assigned to fields of the *Recordset* and the *Update* method (not function) is called to write (physically) the record's changes and store them. This function is accessible from the *Update* submenu under the *File* main menu. It's also accessible from the toolbar or shortcut key "Ctrl U".

A listing of code source below shows a segment of Update function and its dialogue box is given in Figure 12.

```
Set dbsPowerDevice =
OpenDatabase(Filename, dbDriverCom-
pleteRequired, False, DatabaseCon-
nect)
    Set rstSCR = dbsPowerDevice.
OpenRecordset("SELECT * FROM " &
```

Figure 10. PEDAS switching devices' library

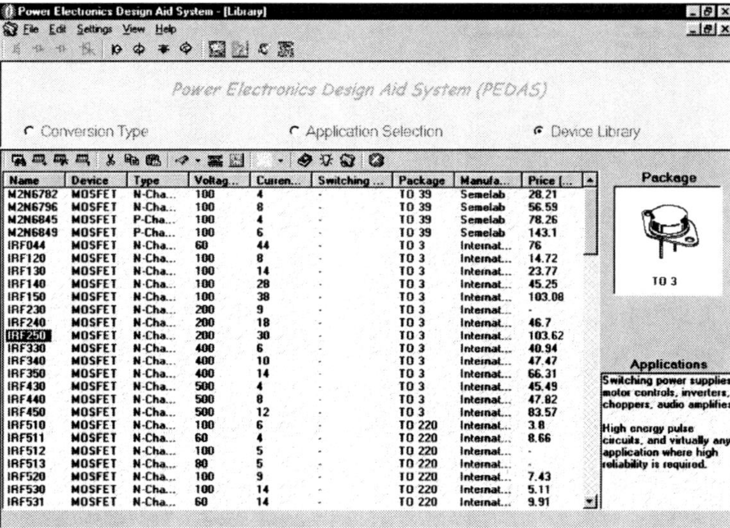

Figure 11. Search function dialog box and its search fields

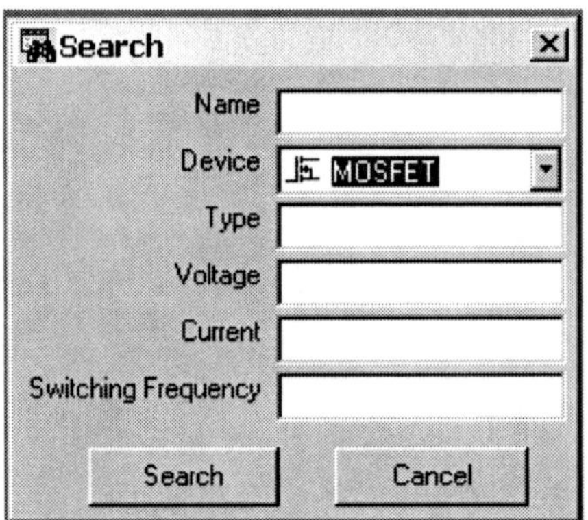


```
Devicetxt, dbOpenDynaset)
With rstSCR
!Manufacture = Manftxt
rstSCR!price = Pricetxt
.Update
.Bookmark = .LastModified
.Edit
!Name = strName
!Type = strType
End With
```

Only two fields can be modified and hence updated, these are the manufacturer and the price of the device. The *Enable* property of other fields is set to "*False*" so the user has no access to them.

3. Add Function

The Add function is to enable user to add in new components when they are introduced into the market. By this way, the user will be able to keep the program updated as and when new products are released by the manufacturers. The code below shows how the addition operation is performed.

```
Set dbsPowerDevice =
OpenDatabase(Filename, dbDriverCom-
pleteRequired, False, DatabaseCon-
nect)
    Set rstSCR = dbsPowerDevice.
OpenRecordset("SELECT * FROM " & Im-
```

Figure 12. Update function dialog box

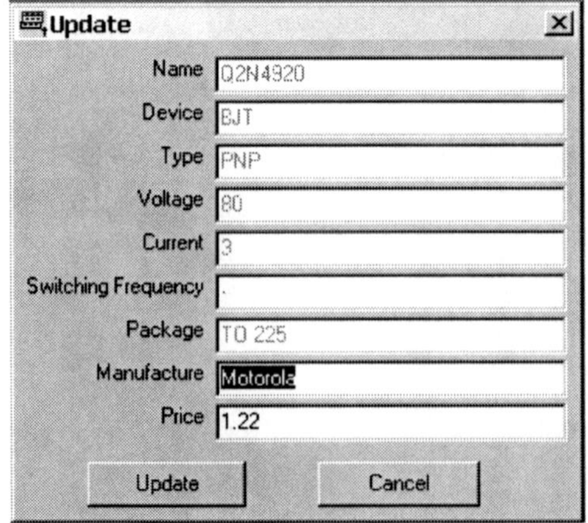

```
ageCombo1.Text, dbOpenDynaset)
   strName = NameAdd
   strDevice = ImageCombo1.Text
   strType = TypeAdd
   .........
  If strName <> "" And strDevice <>
"" And strType <> " Then
   rstSCR.AddNew
   rstSCR!Name = strName
   rstSCR!Device = strDevice
   rstSCR!Type = strType
   rstSCR.Update
   rstSCR.Bookmark = rstSCR.LastModi-
fied
   Set AItem = Form1.ListView1.List-
Items.Add()
   'To visualize the new added record
   AItem.Text = strName
   AItem.SubItems(1) = strDevice
   AItem.SubItems(2) = strType
   MsgBox ("The component is stored
into Database."),, "Add"
End if
```

There are three fields that must be specified by the user before a component can be added into the database. The compulsory fields are *'Name'*, *'Voltage'* and *'Current.'* After these ratings are entered, the component will be added to the database. User will be prompted that the component has been added.

This function is accessible by *'Add Data'* Sub-menu under *'File'* menu or by the shortcut key is 'Ctrl + A'. It can also be called upon by clicking on its corresponding icon on the toolbar menu. An instance of this function is shown in Figure 13.

4.   Delete Function

The *'DELETE'* function is to enable the user to delete a component when it is no longer exists in the market. This keeps the database alive and managed efficiently.

To delete a particular component, first select the component by highlighting it. Then, click the 'DELETE' icon on the toolbar menu a 'Delete' dialog box will appear and prompt for confirmation whether the component is to be deleted. Click 'Yes' to delete the component from the database. To cancel the process, click 'No'. The deleting process will be stopped.

Note that the component will be permanently deleted from the database by this process. If the user wishes to have the component back into the database, he needs to use the *'ADD'* function.

There are other functions provided in this module, such as the characteristic curves of certain

Figure 13. Add Function Layout

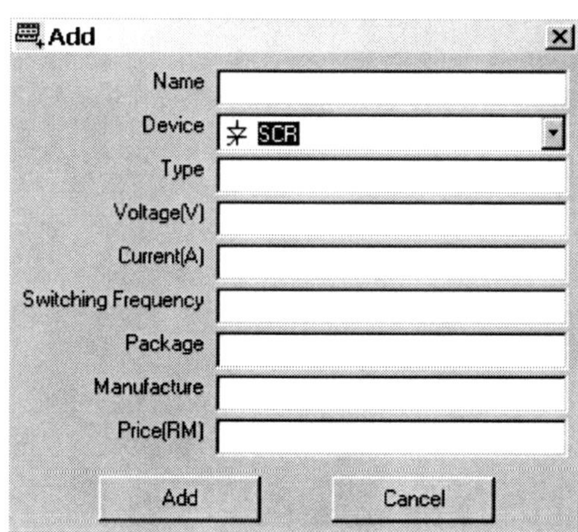

devices, their data-sheets and package numbers. This is shown in Figure 14 and Figure 15.

DEMONSTRATION EXAMPLE (FOUR-QUADRANT DC DRIVE)

This particular chopper is one type of dc-dc converters. It is mainly used in dc drives applications where the reversal of both speed and torque is needed over the period of operation. PEDAS knowledge base incorporates this converter under the application *"DC Motor Drives (4 Quadrant)"* in the dc chopper applications. This is shown in Figure 16 as well as the needed parameters (inputs) from the user. As seen, the required data from the user are:

- The operating mode of the motor
- The emf (or torque) constant.
- The required running speed
- The required developed torque
- The armature inductance
- The armature resistance and
- The input voltage which the user will be prompted for after clicking the *Next* button

The outputs of this example are shown in Figure 17 to Figure 21. It is seen that the main outputs are:

- The suitable circuit topology for the selected application; here since the application needs a reversal of the motor's speed and torque, the most appropriate circuit is the full bridge dc chopper. Both the motor's terminal voltage and the armature current can be positive or negative to meet the mode of operation selected by the user. This is achieved by computing the proper duty ratio of the switches. The motor's emf is represented by a dc voltage source with its steady-state voltage value calculated from the speed and the speed relationship (V3 in Figure 20).

The circuit switching devices (MOSFET and diode for instance); these are the main devices in the circuit to accomplish the required task. They are obtained —as discussed in chapter four- from the devices library. The calculated current and voltage multiplied by safety factors (2 and 1.2 for voltage and current respectively) are compared with the ratings of the library devices; and which-

Figure 14. Output characteristics of D1N4001 in PEDAS

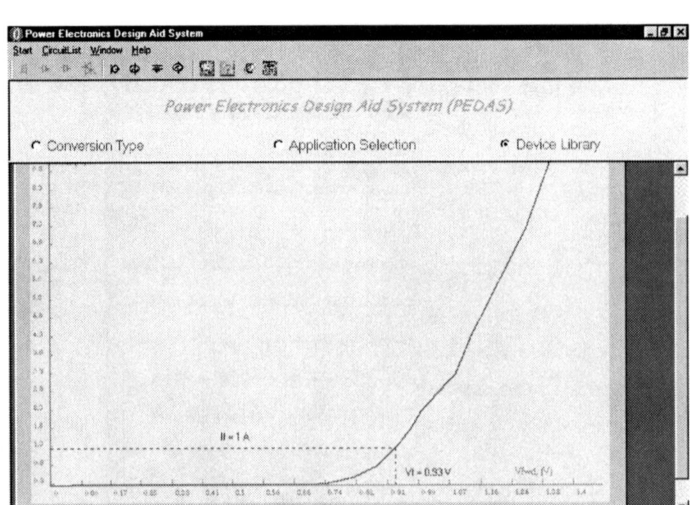

Figure 15. An instance of 'Help module' within the Devices' Library

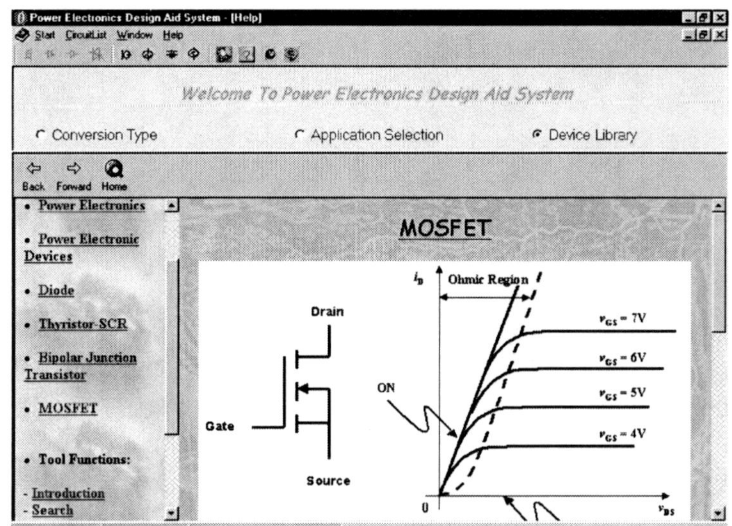

ever device satisfies this condition is selected. If more than one diode and more than MOSFET satisfy the conditions –as in this case- the cheapest devices will be suggested. However, the user is given all the devices that satisfy the ratings conditions and is allowed to choose his/her own devices. This is shown in Figure 18.

The output voltage and current. These are calculated using the user input data and the stored rules in the knowledge base. The results are shown to the user in a list along with other parameters like the suggested switching frequency and the capacitor size –see Figure 17-. However, the output voltage and current have to be confirmed by simulation upon calling *Pspice* simulation package through the interfacing module as in Figure 21. Here from Figure 17 the output voltage is found to be 75V and after simulation is shown

Figure 16. Four quadrant DC drive example

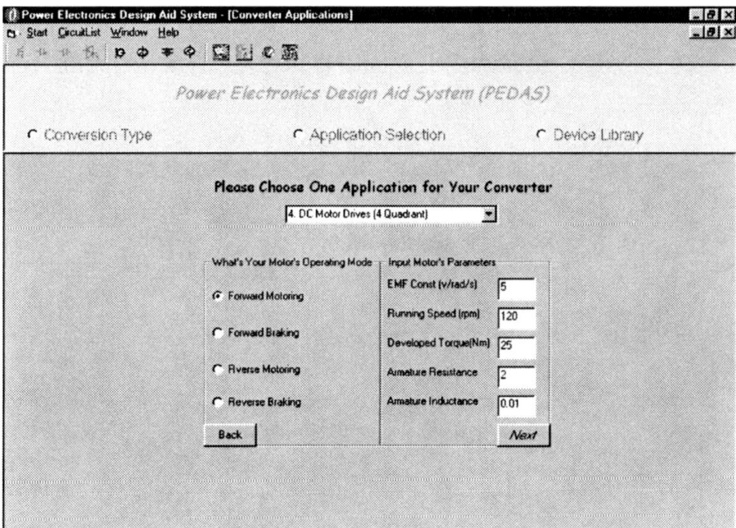

Figure 17. PEDAS results of the 4-qudrant example

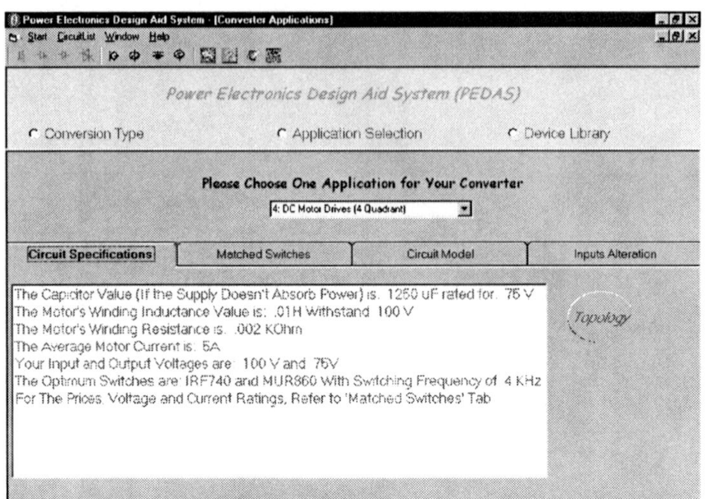

to be 68.5V. The output current is 5A while after simulation is 4.5 A. The small differences in the output values are due to the nature of the simulation which takes in account the stray parameters of the switching devices, such as the parasitic capacitances. However, the values are very close and the differences can be omitted. Anyway, if the differences are such cannot be ignored and as the simulation package is an authentic part of PEDAS architecture the outputs after the simulation are to be considered. More outputs for various different inputs are given in Table 2.

All units are as shown in Figure16.

CONCLUSION

PEDAS is academic software was developed to push the design of power electronics converters one step forward. It aimed to improve the design procedure in terms of simplicity, flexibility and

Figure 18. Suggested switches with their relevant ratings

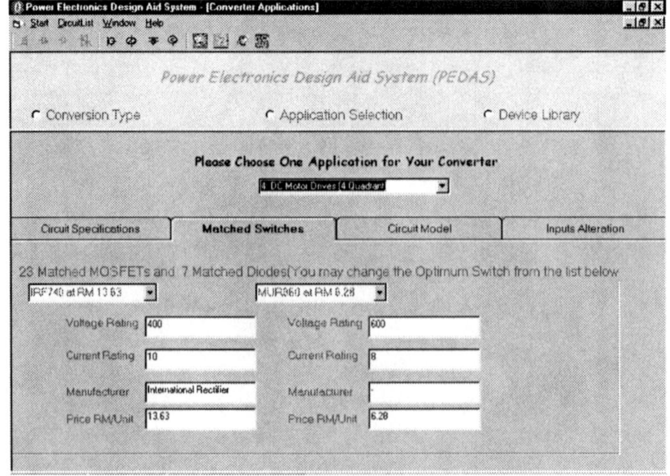

smoothness as well as time-consumption. This is successfully achieved by introducing knowledge-based techniques and object oriented paradigm. The proposed system architecture assures a flexible interaction between the user and the tool as well as among the various modules constituting the system itself. The knowledge base containing topologies and switching devices was represented using object-oriented paradigm. It is the role of the inference engine to find the suitable topology that matches the user entries. Benefiting from the object oriented programming and the design visibility features of Visual Basic programming language; an attractive user interface was developed to assure the interaction of the user with the system. Furthermore, a library module enhanced by several vital functions was developed. This library makes the developed tool independent in its devices from that of the simulation package. A help module that explains how to use the developed tool and gathers information about power electronics converters was built and linked to the tool. This was enhanced by a flexible demo for further strengthen the understanding of converters operation. A four quadrant dc drive example was designed using PEDAS and the results were analyzed and discussed. The demonstrating example showed the simplicity of using PEDAS as well as its functionality and efficiency.

REFERENCES

Amaya, L. E. (1998). *Computer Synthesis of Switching Power Converters*. (Ph.D. diss.), Dept. of Electrical and Computer Engineering Illinois Univ. at Urbana-Champaign

Bouketir, O., Norman, M., Ishak, A., Senan, M. B., & Soib, T. (2002). Expert System-Based Approach to Automate the Design Process of Power Electronics Converters. In *Proceedings of the International Conference "IEEE/PES T&D Asian Pacific*. Yokohama, Japan, 1943-1946.

Bouketir, O., Norman, M., Ishak, A., Senan, M. B., & Soib, T. (2003). Computer Aided Design Tool for Power Electronic Converters. In *Proceedings of the International Conference ROVISP, Penang Malaysia*, 709-716

Figure 19. Most appropriate topology given by PEDAS

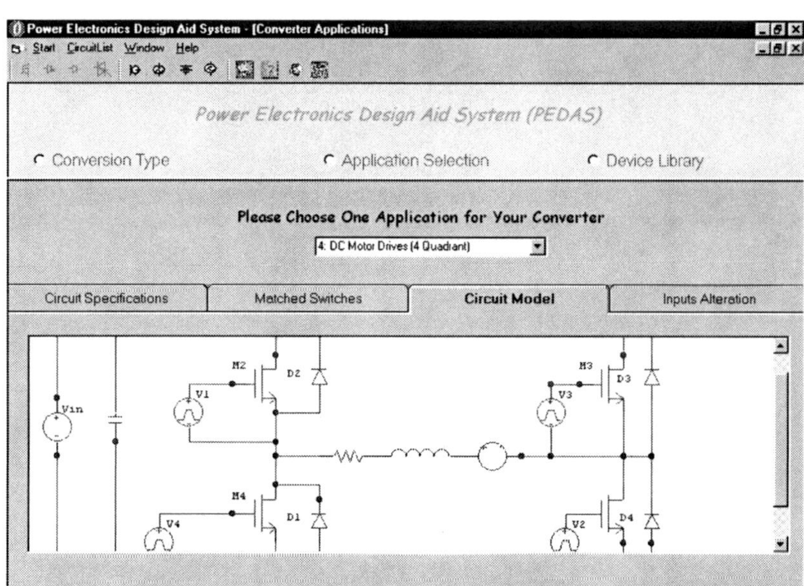

Table 2. Outputs of Four-Quadrant Example for Various Different Inputs

Mode of Operation	Inputs	Outputs	Simulation
Forward Motoring	k=2 n=75 τ=12 Ra=1 La=0.0015 Vin=30	Diode: MUR820 MOSFET: IRF530 Vt=22 Ia=6 f=13k	Vt=20 Ia=5.9
Forward Braking	k=6 n=45 τ=20 Ra=3 La=0.002 Vin=45	Diode:MUR420 MOSFET: IRF510 Vt=20.1 Ia=-3.3 f=30k	Vt=21.8 Ia=-2.4
Reverse Motoring	k=5.7 n=80 τ=32 Ra=2.4 La=0.003 Vin=70	Diode: MOSFET: Vt=-59 Ia=-5.6 f=4.8k	Vt=-58.4 Ia=-4.13
Reverse Braking	k=3.4 n=60 τ=15 Ra=4 La=0.005 Vin=12	Diode:MBR1035 MOSFET:IRF510 Vt=-2.8 Ia=4.4 f=16k	Vt=-5.1 Ia=3.95

Cumbi, M. J. N., Shepherd, D. W., & Hulley, L. N. (1996). Development of an Object-Oriented Knowledge-Based system for Power Electronic Circuit Design. *IEEE Transactions on Power Electronics*, *11*(3), 393–404. doi:10.1109/63.491632

Figure 20. Real circuit topology in Pspice displayed in PEDAS environment

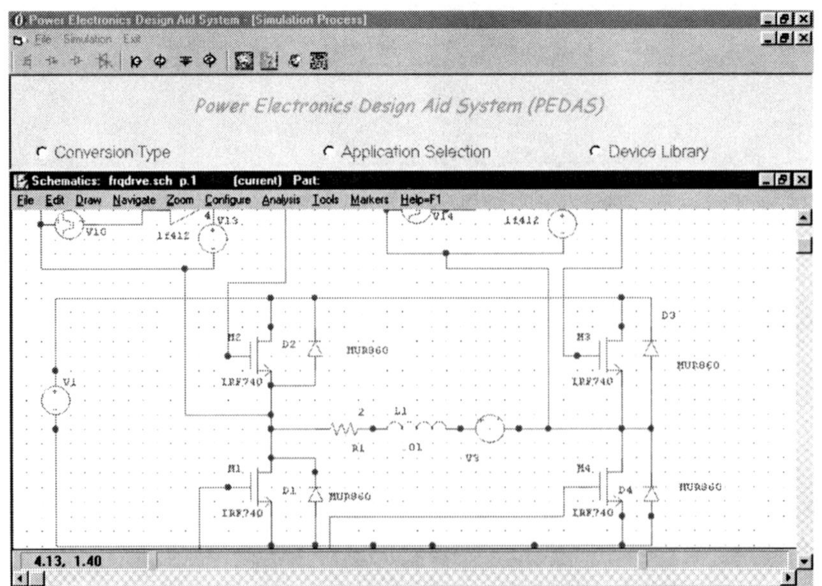

Figure 21. Simulated output current and output voltage

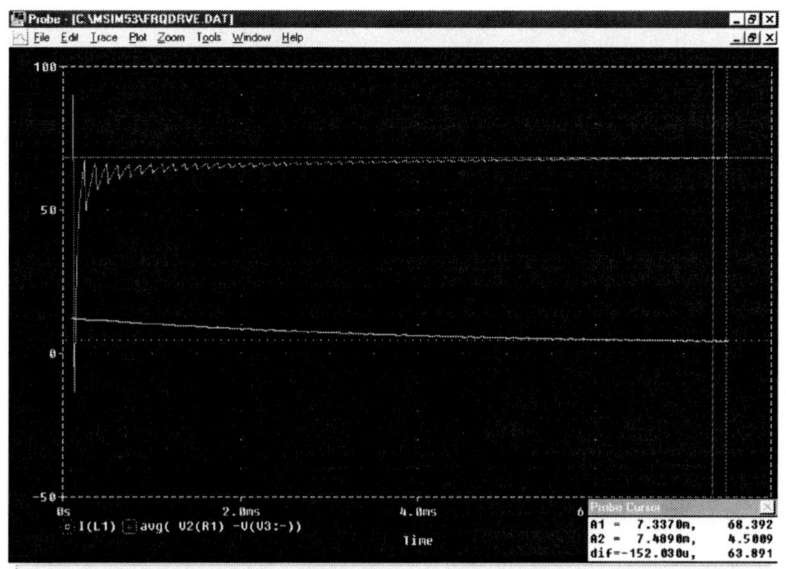

Daniel, W. H. (1997). *Introduction to Power Electronics*. Upper Saddle River, NJ: Prentice-Hall International, Inc.

Debebe, K., & Rajagopalan, V. (1995). A Learning Aid for Power Electronics with Knowledge-Based Components. *IEEE Transactions on Education*, *38*(2), 171–176. doi:10.1109/13.387220

Fezzani, D., Piquet, H., & Foch, H. (1997). Expert System for the CAD in Power Electronics – Application to UPS. *IEEE Transactions on Power Electronics*, *12*(3), 578–587. doi:10.1109/63.575685

Fezzani, D., Piquet, H., Foch, H., & Nogaret, Ph. (1998). A Few Discussions on Expert System Development for Electrical Power Systems-Optimization of Inverter-Motor of a Railway Traction Chain. *European Physics Journal*, *4*, 53–64.

Masatoshi, N. (1997). A Fast Computer Algorithm for Switching Converters. *IEEE Transactions on Power Electronics*, *12*(1), 180–186. doi:10.1109/63.554184

Noel, J., & Eric, B. (1996). *The definitive guide to using the Win32 API with visual basic 4*. Los Angeles, CA: Waite Group Press.

Omrane, B., Norman, M., Senan, M., Ishak, A., & Taib, S. (2003). CAD System for Power Electronic Converters. *Journal of Engineering Transaction*, *6*, 97–105.

Omrane, B., Norman, M., Senan, M., Ishak, A., & Taib, S. (2005). A Learning Aid Tool for Power Electronics Converters. *Journal of Electrical Systems*, *1*(2), 35–62.

Omrane, B., Norman, M., Senan, M., Ishak, A., & Taib, S. (2005). Knowledge-based design aid tool for power electronic converters, Engineering Computations. *International Journal for Computer-Aided Engineering. Emerald*, *22*(1), 5–14.

Wang, S. J., & Lee, Y. S. (1996). Development of an Expert System for Designing, Analysing and Optimising Power Converters. In *Proc. of the Nineteenth Convention of Electrical and Electronics Engineers*, 359-362

KEY TERMS AND DEFINITIONS

Converter: A circuit that converts electric power from one type to another (dc-to-ac, ac-to-dc) or a voltage from one level to another within the same type of power (dc/dc or ac/ac).

Graphical User Interface (GUI): The general layout of the system and its functions which interact between the user and the system.

Four-Quadrant Chopper: A dc to dc converter that is used mainly for dc drive and able to operate in four quadrants ($\pm$speed, $\pm$torque).

Inference Engine: An algorithm that operates on the knowledge base looking for the best solutions according to the user specifications.

Switching Device: Refers to the solid state component (diode, transistor or thyristor) that is used as switch by the converter circuit.

Compilation of References

Abdullatif, I. A., & Philip, J. K. (2009). Rethinking Models of Technology Adoption for Internet Banking: The role of Website Features. *Journal of Financial Services Marketing, 14*(1), 56–69. doi:10.1057/fsm.2009.4

Abuhaiba, I. S. I. (2007). Offline signature verification using graph matching. *Turk Journal of Electronic Engineering, 15*(1), 89–104.

Adedokun, N. A. S. (2008). *Integration of ICT into Instruction of Science and Mathematics: A Case Study of Sekolah Menengah Kebangsaan Gombak Setia, Malaysia.* (M.ed Thesis – copyright International Islamic University, Malaysia.)

Adedokun, N. A. S., & Hashim, R. (2008). Integration of Information and Communication Technology (ICT) in the Teaching and Learning of Science: Teachers' and Students' Perception. In *Proceedings of the Conference of Asian Science Education* (CASE 2008) http://case2008.nknu.edu.tw/

Advances in Cryptology - EUROCRYPT2005: Vol. 3494. LNCS (pp. 457–473). Heidelberg, Germany: Springer.

Ahlan, A. R., & Shittu, A. J. K. (2006). Issues in Information Technology Outsourcing: Case study of PETRO-NAS Bhd. In *Proceeding ICT4M 2006.* Kuala Lumpur. Malaysia.

Ahmad, H., Harun, S. W. (2005, May). Double-pass L-band EDFA with flat-gain and improved noise figure characteristic, *3*, 75-77.

Ahsan, S., & Shah, A. (2008). A Framework for Agile Methodologies for Development of Bioinformatics. *The Journal of American Science, 4*, 15–21.

Ahsan, S., & Shah, A. (2008). *Quality Metrics For Evaluating Data Provenance, Designing Software Intensive Systems-Methods and Principles* (pp. 455–473). Hershey, PA: IGI Global.

Ali, S., & Xiang, Y. (2007). Spam Classification Using Adaptive Boosting Algorithm, *6th IEEE/ACIS International Conference on Computer and Information Science* (pp.972 – 976). Australia: IEEE Computer Society.

Alkan, S., & Cagiltay, K. (2007). Studying computer game learning experience through eye tracking. *British Journal of Educational Technology, 38*(3), 538–542. doi:10.1111/j.1467-8535.2007.00721.x

Allan, R., & Ed, S. Lein. (2007). Genome-wide atlas of gene expression in the adult mouse brain. *Nature, 445*, 168–176.

Amaya, L. E. (1998). *Computer Synthesis of Switching Power Converters.* (Ph.D. diss.), Dept. of Electrical and Computer Engineering Illinois Univ. at Urbana-Champaign

Anand, V. (2007). A study of time management: The correlation between video game usage and academic performance markers. *Cyberpsychology & Behavior, 10*(4), 552–559. doi:10.1089/cpb.2007.9991

Anderson, E., & Trinkle, Bob. (2005). *Outsourcing Sales Function: The Cost of Field Sales.* Thomson, OH.

Andersson, P., & Fejes, A. (2005). Recognition Of Prior Learning As A Technique For Fabricating The Adult Learner: A genealogical analysis on Swedish adult education policy. *Journal of Education Policy, 20*(5), 595–613. doi:10.1080/02680930500222436

Androutsopoulos, I., Koutsias, J., Chandrinos, K. V., Paliouras, G., & Spyropoulos, C. D. (2000). An Evaluation of Naive Bayesian Anti-Spam Filtering. *Workshop on Machine Learning in the New Information Age, 11th European Conference on Machine Learning* (pp. 9-17). Spain: LNCS Springer.

Androutsopoulos, I., Paliouras, G., Karkaletsis, V., Sakkis, G., Spyropoulos, C., & Stamatopoulos, P. (2000). Learning to filter spam e-mail: A comparison of a naive bayesian and a memory-based approach, *4ᵗʰ PKDD's Workshop on Machine Learning and Textual Information Access*. France: LNCS Springer.

Annesley, C. (2005). *Outsourcing works better when based on trust*. Retrieved June 17, 2008 from. http://www.computerweekly.com/ Articles/2005/11/24/213137/outsourcing-works-better-when-based- on-trust-survey.htm

Antonopoulos, C., & Sakellaris, P. (2009). The Contribution of Information and Communication Technology Investments to Greek Economic Growth: An Analytical Growth Accounting Framework. *Information Economics and Policy, 21,* 171–191. doi:10.1016/j.infoecopol.2008.12.001

Argyris, C., & Schön, D. A. (1978). *Organizational Learning: A Theory of Action Perspective*. Reading, MA: Addison-Wesley.

Argyris, C., & Schön, D. A. (1996). *Organizational Learning II: Theory, Method and Practice*. Reading, MA: Addison-Wesley.

Arh, T., Dimovski, V., & Jerman-Blažič, B. (2008). *Model of impact of technology-enhanced organizational learning on business performance. V P. Cunningham, M. Cunningham (ur.), Collaboration and the knowledge economy: issues, applications, case studies, (str. 1521–1528).* Netherlands: IOS Press.

Arh, T., Pipan, M., Jerman-Blažič, B. (2006). Virtual learning environment for the support of life-long learning initiative. *WSEAS transactions on advances in engineering education*, 4(4), str. 737–743.

Astrid, D., Mitra, A., & David, M. (2008). The Role of Perceived Enjoyment and social Norm in the Adoption of Technology with Network Externalities. *European Journal of Information Systems, 17,* 4–11. doi:10.1057/palgrave.ejis.3000726

Atallah, M. J., Frikken, K. B., Goodrich, M. T., & Tamassia, R. (2005). Secure biometric authentication for weak computational devices. In A.S. Patrick, M. Yung (Ed.), *FC 2005: Vol. 3570. LNCS* (pp. 357–371). Heidelberg, Germany: Springer.

Ateniese, G., & Gasti, P. (2009). Universally anonymous IBE based on the quadratic residuosity assumption. *CT-RSA'09: Vol. 5473. LNCS* (pp. 32–47). Heidelberg, Germany: Springer.

ATM Market Place. (2009a). *ATM scam nets Melbourne thieves $ 500,000*. Retrieved December 2, 2009, from http://www.atmmarketplace.com/ article.php?id=10808

ATM Market Place. (2009b). *Australian police suspect Romanian gang behind $ 1 million ATM scam*. Retrieved November 13, 2009, from http://www.atmmarketplace.com /article.php?id=10883

Aubert, B. A., Patry, M., & Rivard, S. (1998). Assessing the Risk of IT Outsourcing, In *Proceedings of the 31ˢᵗ Annual Hawaii International Conference on System Science*, Hawaii, 685-692.

Azleen, I., Mohd Zulkeflee, A. R., & Mohd Rushdan, Y. (2009). Taxpayers' Attitude In Using E-Filing System: Is There Any Significant Difference Among Demographic Factors? *Journal of Internet Banking and Commerce, 14*(1), 2–13.

Bada, M., Stevens, R., Goble, C., Gil, Y., Ashburner, M., & Blake, J. (2004). *A Short Study on the Success of Gene Ontology*. Accepted for Publication in Journal of Web Semantics.

Baek, J., Susilo, W., & Zhou, J. (2007). New constructions of fuzzy identitybased encryption. *ACM Symposium on Information, Computer and Communications Security - ASIACCS'07* (pp. 368–370). New York: ACM.

Bahl, P., et al. (2000, February). *Enhancements to the RADAR User Location and Tracking System.* (Microsoft Research Technical Report), Retrieved April 2004 from: http://citeseer.ist.psu.edu/ bahl00enhancements.html

Bailly-Baillire, E., Bengio, S., Bimbot, F., Hamouz, M., Kitler, J., Marithoz, J., et al. (2003). The BANCA database and evaluation protocol. *Proceedings of International Conference on Audio – and Video-Based Biometric Person Authentication* (pp. 625 – 638).

Balakumar, M., & Vaidehi, V. (2008). Ontology based classification and categorization of email, *Conference on Signal Processing, Communications and Networking* (pp.199-202). USA: IEE Computer Society.

Balanskat, A., Blamire, R., & Kefala, S. (2006). *The ICT impact report: A review of studies of ICT impact on schools in Europe.* n.p.: European Schoolnet. Retrieved September 7, 2009, from http://ec.europa.eu/education / pdf/doc254_en.pdf

Balcytiene, A. (1999). Exploring individual processes of knowledge construction with hypertext. *Instructional Science, 27,* 303–328. doi:10.1007/BF00897324

Banister, F., & Remenyi, D. (2000). Acts of faith: instinct, value and IT investments. *Journal of Information Technology, 15*(3), 231–241. doi:10.1080/02683960050153183

Banister, F., & Remenyi, D. (2004). Value Perception in IT Investment Decisions. Retrieved May 7, 2005 from http://ejise.com/volume-2/volume 2-issue2/issue2-art1.htm

Banister, F., & Remenyi, D. (2005). The Social Value of ICT: First Steps towards an Evaluation Framework. Retrieved May 27, 2006 from http://www.ejise.com/volume6-issue2 /issue2-art21.htm

Barnett, J. A. (1981). Computational methods for a mathematical theory of evidence. Proceedings of *International Conference on Artificial Intelligence* (pp. 868-875).

Barracuda Networks. (2004). *An Overview of Spam Blocking Techniques,* White paper.

Barrar, P., & Gervais, R. (2006). *Global Outsourcing Strategies: An International Reference on Effective Outsourcing Relationships.* Gower Publishing.

Barthelemy, J. (2003). The Hard and Soft Sides of IT Outsourcing Management. *European Management Journal, 21*(5), 539–548. doi:10.1016/S0263-2373(03)00103-8

Barthelemy, J., & Geyer, D. (2004). The Determinants of Total IT Outsourcing: An Empirical Investigation of French and German Firms. *Journal of Computer Information Systems, 44*(3), 91–97.

Bauer, M. (1996). Approximation algorithms and decision-making in the dempster-shafer theory of evidence—An empirical study. *International Journal of Approximate Reasoning, 17,* 217–237. doi:10.1016/S0888-613X(97)00013-3

Beaver, G., & Prince, C. (2004). Management, strategy, and policy in the UK small business sector: a critical review. *Journal of Small Business and Enterprise Development, 11*(1), 34–49. doi:10.1108/14626000410519083

Beaver, K. (2003). *Healthcare Information Systems, Best Practices Series* (2nd ed.). Boca Raton, FL: CRC Presss, Auerbach Publications.

Becker, P. C., Olsson, N. A., & Simpson, J. R. (1999). *Erbium-Doped Fiber Amplifiers Fundamentals and Technology.* San Diego: Academic Press.

Becta (2003). *Using ICT to Enhance Home-school Links – an Evaluation of Current Practice in England,* Becta, UK. http://partners.becta.org.uk/index. php?section=rh&&catcode =&rid=13639- 2006, *The Becta Review 2006: Evidence on the Progress of ICT in Education,* Becta, UK. http://becta.org.uk/corporate/ publications/ documents/The_Becta_Review_2006.pdf 2007, *What Is a Learning Platform?* http://schools.becta. org.uk/index .php?section=re&&catcode =&rid=12887

Beldarrain, Y. (2006). Distance education trends: Integrating new technologies to foster student interaction and collaboration. *Distance Education, 27*(2), 139–153. doi:10.1080/01587910600789498

Benamati, J., & Lederer, L. (1999). An empirical study of IT management and rapid IT change, In *Proceedings of the SIGCPR conference on Computer personnel research, Communication of the ACM*, pp.144-153, New Orleans: Louisiana.

Benjamin, R. J., & Blunt, J. (1992). Critical IT issues: The next ten years. *Sloan Management Review, 33*(4), 7–19.

Bennett, S., Maton, K., & Kervin, L. (2008). The 'digital natives' debate: A critical review of the evidence. *British Journal of Educational Technology, 39*(5), 775–786. doi:10.1111/j.1467-8535.2007.00793.x

Berkman, O., & Ostrovsky, O. M. (2006). *The unbearable lightness of PIN cracking*. Retrieved May 3, 2009, from http://www.arx.com/files/Documents/The_Unbearable_Lightness_of_PIN_Cracking.pdf

Beulen, E., & Ribbers, P. (2002). "*Lessons learned: Managing an IT-partnership in Asia:* Theme Study: The relationship between a global outsourcing company and their suppliers." In *Proceedings of Hawaii International Conference on Systems Sciences.*

Bias, R. G., & Mayhew, D. J. (Eds.). (1994). *Cost-Justifying Usability*. Boston, MA: Academic Press.

Bicego, M., Lagorio, A., Grosso, E., & Tistarelli, M. (2006). On the use of SIFT features for face authentication. *Proceedings of IEEE International Workshop on Biometrics, in association with CVPR.*

Blaikie, N. W. H. (2003). *Analyzing quantitative data.* London: Sage Publications Ltd.

Boardman, A. E., & Hewitt, E. S. (2004). Problems With Contracting Out Government Services: Lessons From Orderly Services at SCGH. *Industrial and Corporate Change, 13*(6), 917–929. doi:10.1093/icc/dth034

Bodenreider, O., & Stevens, R. (2006). *Bio-ontologies: current trends and future directions, Briefings in Bioinformatics Advance Access.* Oxford, UK: Oxford University Journals.

Bolle, R., Connell, J., & Ratha, N. (2002). Biometric Perils and Patches. *Pattern Recognition, 35,* 2727–2738. doi:10.1016/S0031-3203(01)00247-3

Bollen, K. A. (1989). *Structural equations with latent variables.* New York: Wiley.

Bond, M., & Zielinski, P. (2003). *Decimalisation table attacks for PIN Cracking.* Retrieved December 9, 2006, from http://www.cl.cam.ac.uk/ techreports/UCAM-CL-TR-560.pdf

Boneh, D., & Franklin, M. K. (2003). Identity-Based Encryption from the Weil Pairing. *SIAM Journal on Computing, 32*(3), 586–615. doi:10.1137/S0097539701398521

Boucaut, R. (2001). Understanding workplace bullying: a practical application of Giddens' Structurational Theory. *International Education Journal, 2*(4).

Bouketir, O., Norman, M., Ishak, A., Senan, M. B., & Soib, T. (2002). Expert System-Based Approach to Automate the Design Process of Power Electronics Converters. In *Proceedings of the International Conference "IEEE/PES T&D Asian Pacific.* Yokohama, Japan, 1943-1946.

Bouketir, O., Norman, M., Ishak, A., Senan, M. B., & Soib, T. (2003). Computer Aided Design Tool for Power Electronic Converters. In *Proceedings of the International Conference ROVISP, Penang Malaysia,* 709-716

Bouzid, B., Mohd. Ali, B., & Abdullah, M. K. (2003, September). A High Gain EDFA Design Using Double Pass Amplification with a Band-Pass Filter. *Photonics Technology Letters, 15*(9), 1195–1197. doi:10.1109/LPT.2003.814901

Bransford, J., Darling-Hammond, L., & LePage, P. (2005). Introduction. In Bransford, J., & Darling-Hammond, L. (Eds.), *Preparing teachers for a changing world: What teachers should learn and be able to do* (pp. 1–39). San Francisco: Jossey-Bass.

Bringer, J., & Chabanne, H. (2008). An Authentication Protocol with Encrypted Biometric Data. *AFRICACRYPT'08: Vol. 5023. LNCS* (pp. 109–124). Heidelberg, Germany: Springer.

Bringer, J., Chabanne, H., Cohen, G., Kindarji, B., & Zemor, G. (2007a). Optimal Iris Fuzzy Sketches. [IEEE Computer Society.]. *BTAS, 07*, 1–6.

Bringer, J., Chabanne, H., Izabach`ene, M., Pointcheval, D., Tang, Q., & Zimmer, S. (2007b). *An Application of the Goldwasser-Micali Cryptosystem to Biometric Authentication. ACISP'07, 4586. LNCS* (pp. 96–106). Heidelberg, Germany: Springer.

Buchanan, D., Boddy, D., & McCalman, J. (1988). Getting in, getting on, getting out, and getting back. In Bryman, D. (Ed.), *Doing research in organisations* (pp. 53–67). London: Sage Publications.

Burmahl, B. (2001). Making the Choice: The Pros and Cons of Outsourcing. *Health Facilities Management, 14*(6), 16–22.

Burnett, A., Byrne, F., Dowling, T., & Duffy, A. (2007). A Biometric Identity Based Signature Scheme. *International Journal of Network Security, 5*(3), 317–326.

Burns, S. (2006). IT Industry Spends $66bn in Taiwan, VNU Business Publications, VNUNet.com.

Buschmann, C., et al. (n.d.). Radio propagation-aware distance estimation based on neighborhood comparison. In *Proceedings of the European Workshop on Sensor Networks*, 2007. (pp.325–340, Springer Lecture Notes in Computer Science, v.4373).

ButlerGroup. (2007). *SOA Platforms – Software Infrastructure Requirements for Successful SOA Deployments.* Ferensway Hull, UK: Butler Direct Ltd.

Cabral, L., Domingue, J., Motta, E., Payne, T., & Hakimpour, F. (2004). *Approaches to Semantic Web Services: An Overview and Comparisons.* Berlin/Heidelberg, Germany: Springer.

Cannta, N., et al. (2008). A semantic web for bioinformatics: goals, tools, systems and applications, BMC Bioinformatics. In *Proceedings of the Seventh International Workshop on Network Tools and Applications in Biology*, Pisa, Italy

Capkun, S., & Hubaux, J.-P. (2006). Secure Positioning in Wireless Networks. [JSAC]. *IEEE Journal on Selected Areas in Communications, 24*(2), 221–232. doi:10.1109/JSAC.2005.861380

Carr, N. G. (2003). IT doesn't matter. *Harvard Business Review, 81*(5), 41.

CGD. (2006). *When Will We Ever Learn? Improving Lives Through Impact Evaluation.* Washington, DC: Center for Global Development.

Chan, K. J., & Poon, J. (2004). Co-training with a single natural feature set applied to email classification, *IEEE International Conference on Web Intelligenc.* China: IEEE Computer Society.

Chang, Ai-Mei, & Kannan, P.K. (2002). *Preparing for Wireless and Mobile Technologies in Government.* IBM Center for the Business of Government.

ChanLin, L-J. (2009). Applying Motivational Analysis in a Web-based Course. *Innovations in Education and Teaching International, 46*(1), 91–103. doi:10.1080/14703290802646123

Chini, I. (2008). ICT Policy as A Governable Domain: The Theme of Greece and the European Commission. in IFIP International Federation for Information Processing: *Vol. 282. Social Dimensions of Information and Communication Technology Policy; Chrisanthi Avgerou, Matthew L. Smith, Peter van den Besselaar* (pp. 45–62). New York: Springer.

Chiu, Y., Chen, C., Jeng, B., & Lin, H. (2007). An Alliance-based Anti-Spam Approach, *Third International Conference on Natural Computation* (pp.203-207). China: IEEE Computer Society.

Chou, C., Condron, L., & Belland, J. C. (2005). A review of the research on Internet addiction. *Educational Psychology Review, 17*(4), 363–388. doi:10.1007/s10648-005-8138-1

Colardyn, D., & Bjornavold, J. (2004). Validation of Formal, Non-Formal and Informal Learning: Policy and practices in EU Member States. *European Journal of Education, 39*(1), 69–89. doi:10.1111/j.0141-8211.2004.00167.x

Collins, C. J., & Smith, K. G. (2006). Knowledge exchange and combination: the role of human resource practices in the performance of high-technology firms. *Academy of Management Journal*, *49*(3), 544–560.

Collins, A., & Halverson, R. (2009). *Rethinking Education in the Age of Technology*. New York: Teachers College Press.

Computer Economics. (2006). *IT Spending, Staffing, and Technology Trends 2006/2007 Study*. Computer Economics Inc.

Conford, T., & Smithson, S. (1996). *Project Research in Information Systems: A student's guide*. London: Macmillan Press Ltd.

Conte, D., Foggia, P., Sansone, C., & Vente, M. (2003). Graph matching applications in pattern recognition and image processing, *Proceedings of International Conference on Image Processing*.

Cook, T. A. (2007). *Global Sourcing Logistics: How to Manage Risk and Gain Competitive Advantage in a Worldwide Marketplace. American Management Association*. New York: AMACOM.

Coppola, E. M. (2004). *Powering up: Learning to teach well with technology*. New York: Teachers College Press.

Creswell, J. W. (1994). *Research design, qualitative & quantitative approaches*. Newbury Park, CA: Sage Publications Inc.

Cronin, F. J., & Motluk, S. A. (2007). Flawed Competition Policies: Designing 'Markets' with Biased Costs and Efficiency Benchmarks Published online: 24 August 2007. New York: Springer Science+Business Media, LLC 2007.

Crossan, M., Lane, H. W., & White, R. E. (1999). An organizational learning framework: from intuition to institution. *Academy of Management Review*, *24*(3), 522–537. doi:10.2307/259140

Cruz, S. M. S. D. (2005). Mining and Visualization of Logs of Bioinformatics Web Services in silico Experiments. In *Proceedings of the Brazilian Symposium on Computer Graphics and Image Processing*.

Cullen, S., & Willcocks, P. (2005). *Intelligent IT Outsourcing: Eight Building Blocks to Success*. Oxford, UK: Elsevier Butterworth-Heinemann.

Cumbi, M. J. N., Shepherd, D. W., & Hulley, L. N. (1996). Development of an Object-Oriented Knowledge-Based system for Power Electronic Circuit Design. *IEEE Transactions on Power Electronics*, *11*(3), 393–404. doi:10.1109/63.491632

Cummings, R. (2003). *Equivalent assessment: Achievable reality or pipedream*. Paper presented at ATN Education and Assessment Conference. Retrieved May 11, 2008, as Word Document from http://www.unisa.edu.au/.

Cunningham, D. J., Duffy, T. M., & Knuth, R. A. (1993). The textbook of the future. In McKnight, C., Dillon, A., & Richardson, J. (Eds.), *Hypertext: A psychological perspective* (pp. 19–49). New York: Ellis Horwood.

Currie, W. L. (1998). Using Multiple Suppliers to Mitigate the Risk of IT Outsourcing at ICI and Wessex Water. *Journal of Information Technology*, *13*, 169–180. doi:10.1080/026839698344819

DailyNews. (2009). *ATMs on Staten Island rigged for identity theft; bandits steal $500G'*. Retrieved September 9, 2009, from http://www.nydailynews.com/news / ny_crime/2009/05/11/2009-05-11_automated_theft_bandits_steal_500g_by_rigging_atms_with_pinreading_gizmos.html#ixzz0J8qBVdar&D

Daniel, W. H. (1997). *Introduction to Power Electronics*. Upper Saddle River, NJ: Prentice-Hall International, Inc.

Daugman, J. (1993). High confidence visual recognition of persons by a test of statistical independence. *IEEE Transactions on Pattern Analysis and Machine Intelligence*, *15*(11), 1148–1161. doi:10.1109/34.244676

Davenport, T. H., De Long, D. W., & Beers, M. C. (1998). Successful knowledge management projects. *Sloan Management Review*, *39*(2), 43–57.

David, Y. K. T. (2008). A Study of e-Recruitment Technology Adoption in Malaysia. *Industrial Management & Data Systems*, *109*(2), 281–300.

Davidson, R. M., Wagner, C., & Ma, L. C. K. (2005). From government to e-government: A transitional Model. *Information Technology & People*, *18*(3), 280–299. doi:10.1108/09593840510615888

Davidson, E. J. (2002). Technology Frames and Framing: A Social-cognitive Investigation of Requirements Determination. *Management Information Systems Quarterly*, *26*(4), 329–358. doi:10.2307/4132312

Deane, F., Barrelle, K., Henderson, R., & Mahar, D. (1995). Perceived acceptability of biometric security systems. *Computers & Security*, *14*(3), 225–231. doi:10.1016/0167-4048(95)00005-S

Debebe, K., & Rajagopalan, V. (1995). A Learning Aid for Power Electronics with Knowledge-Based Components. *IEEE Transactions on Education*, *38*(2), 171–176. doi:10.1109/13.387220

Denzin, N. K., & Lincoln, Y. S. (1994). Introduction: Entering the field of Qualitative Research. In Denzin, N. K., & Lincoln, Y. S. (Eds.), *Handbook of qualitative research* (pp. 1–17). Newbury Park, CA: Sage Publications.

Desurvire, E. (1994). *Erbium Doped Fiber Amplifier principle and Application*. New York: John Wiley and Sons, Inc.

Desurvire, E. *(2005). Optical communications in 2025*. Optical Communication, 2005. ECOC 2005. 31st European Conference, 1, 5-6.

Devadoss, P. R., Pan, S. L., & Huang, J. C. (2002). Structural analysis of e-government initiatives: a case study of SCO. *Decision Support Systems*, *34*, 253–269. doi:10.1016/S0167-9236(02)00120-3

Dewan, S., & Kraemer, K. L. (1998). International dimensions of the productivity paradox. *Communications of the ACM*, *41*(8), 56–62. doi:10.1145/280324.280333

Dhinakaran, C. Lee J. K., & Nagamalai, D. (2007). An Empirical Study of Spam and Spam Vulnerable email Accounts, *Conference on Future generation communication and networking* (pp.408-413). Korea: IEEE Computer Society. E-mail spam (na). *Wikipedia article*, Retrieved January 20, 2010, from http://en.wikipedia.org/wiki/Anti_spam_filter

Diamantopoulos, A., & Siguaw, J. A. (2000). *Introducing LISREL*. London: SAGE Publications.

Diana, M. L. (2009). (in press). Exploring Information Systems Outsourcing in US Hospital-based Health Care Delivery Systems. *Health Care Management Science*. doi:10.1007/s10729-009-9100-4

Dibbern, J., Goles, T., Hirschheim, R., & Jayatilaka, B. (2004). Information systems outsourcing: A survey and analysis of the literature. *The Data Base for Advances in Information Systems*, *35*(4), 6–102.

DiBella, J. A., & Nevis, E. C. (1998). *How Organizations Learn – An Integrated Strategy for Building Learning Capability*. San Francisco, CA: Jossey-Bass.

Diebold. (2003). *EMV White Paper*. Retrieved April 11, 2010, from www.diebold.com/solutions/a tms/opteva/emv.pdf

Dimovski, V., & Colnar, T. (1999). Organizacijsko učenje. *Teorija in Praksa*, *5*(36), 701–722.

Dimovski, V. (1994). *Organisational learning and competitive advantage*. Unpublished doctoral dissertation, Cleveland State University.

Dinevski, D., & Plenković, M. (2002). Modern University and e-learning. *Media, culture and public relations*, *2*, 137–146.

Dodgson, M. (1993). Organizational learning: a review of some literatures. *Organization Studies*, *14*(3), 375–394. doi:10.1177/017084069301400303

Dodis, Y., Reyzin, L., & Smith, A. (2004). Fuzzy Extractors: How to Generate Strong Keys from Biometrics and Other Noisy Data. *Advances in Cryptology - EURO-CRYPT'04: Vol. 3027. LNCS* (pp. 523–540). Heidelberg, Germany: Springer.

Doelz, R. (1994). Hierarchical Access System for Sequence Libraries in Europe (HASSEL): A Tool to Access Sequence Database Remotely. *Computer Applications in the Biosciences, 10*, 31–34.

Donegan, M. (2000). The m-commerce challenge. *Telecommunications, 34*(1), 58.

Donnerstein, E. (2002). The Internet. In Strasburger, V. C., & Wilson, B. J. (Eds.), *Children, adolescents & the media* (pp. 301–321). Thousand Oaks, CA: Sage.

Dumas, J. S., & Redish, J. C. (1994). *A Practical Guide to Usability Testing*. Norwood, NJ: Ablex.

Dwight, J., & Garrison, J. (2003). A manifesto for instructional technology: Hyperpedagogy. *Teachers College Record, 105*(5), 699–728. doi:10.1111/1467-9620.00265

Easton, J. (2002). *Going Wireless: transform your business with wireless mobile technology*. USA: HarperCollins.

Economic Planning Unit (EPU). *The Mid Term Review of the Ninth Malaysian Plan*: 2006-2010.

Ehrlich, K., & Rohn, J. (1994). Cost-justification of usability engineering: A vendor's perspective. In Bias, R. G., & Mayhew, D. J. (Eds.), *Cost-Justifying Usability*. Boston, MA: Academic Press.

Eijkman, H. (2009). The Epistemology War: Wikipedia, Web 2.0, The Academy, And The Battle Over The Nature And Authority Of Knowledge. Ken Fernstrom (Ed.), *Readings in Technology and Education: Proceedings of ICICTE 2009* (pp. 516-529). Abbotsford B.C., Canada: UCFV Press.

Eisenhardt, K. M. (1989). Building Theories from Case Study Research. *Academy of Management Review, 14*(4), 532–550. doi:10.2307/258557

Elnahrawy, J., et al. (2007). *Adding angle of arrival modality to basic rss location management techniques.* Retrieved June 2008 from: http://paul.rutgers.edu/ eiman/ elnahrawy07AoA.pdf

EMV. (2004). *Integrated circuit card specifications for payment systems.* Retrieved January 14, 2010, from https://partnernetwork.visa.com/vpn/global /category. do?userRegion=1&catego ryId=61&documentId=94

Eraut, M. (2000). Non-Formal Learning, Implicit Learning and Tacit Knowledge in Professional Work. In Coffield, F. (Ed.), *The Necessity of Informal Learning* (pp. 12–31). Bristol, UK: Policy Press.

ESCWA. (2005). *Regional profile of the information society in western Asia.* New York: United Nations.

Etzold, T., & Argos, P. (1993). SRS – An Indexing and Retrieval Tool for Flat-File Data Libraries. *Computer Applications in the Biosciences, 9*, 49–57.

Eurostat News Release 146/2006, 1-3. Nearly half of individuals in the EU25 used the internet at least once a week in 2006. Luxembourg: Eurostat Press Office.

Fan, K.-C., Liu, C.-W., & Wang, Y.-K. (1998). A fuzzy bipartite weighted graph matching approach to fingerprint verification, *IEEE International Conference on Systems, Man and Cybernetics* (pp. 4363-4368).

Farhoomand, A. F. (1992). Scientific Progress of Management Information Systems, Information Systems Research: Issues, Methods and Practical Guidelines. In Galliers, R. (Ed.), (pp. 93–111). Oxford, UK: Blackwell Scientific Publications.

Faria, D. B. (2005). *Modeling Signal Attenuation in IEEE 802.11 Wireless LANs - Vol. 1.* (Technical Report) TR-KP06-0118, Kiwi Project, Stanford University.

Fazi-Ersi, E., Zelek, J. S., & Tsotsos, J. K. (2007). Robust face recognition through local graph matching. *Journal of Computers, 2*(5), 31–37.

Fezzani, D., Piquet, H., & Foch, H. (1997). Expert System for the CAD in Power Electronics – Application to UPS. *IEEE Transactions on Power Electronics, 12*(3), 578–587. doi:10.1109/63.575685

Fezzani, D., Piquet, H., Foch, H., & Nogaret, Ph. (1998). A Few Discussions on Expert System Development for Electrical Power Systems-Optimization of Inverter-Motor of a Railway Traction Chain. *European Physics Journal, 4*, 53–64.

Figueiredo, P. N. (2003). Learning processes features: How do they influence inter-firm differences in techno-logical capability - Accumulation paths and operational performance improvement? *International Journal of Technology Management, 26*(7), 655–689. doi:10.1504/IJTM.2003.003451

Fiol, C. M., & Lyles, M. A. (1985). Organizational learn-ing. *Academy of Management Review, 10*(4), 803–813. doi:10.2307/258048

Fishman, B., & Davis, E. (2006). Teacher learning re-search and the learning sciences. In Sawyer, R. K. (Ed.), *Cambridge Handbook of the Learning Sciences* (pp. 535–550). Cambridge, UK: Cambridge University Press.

Fluhrer, S., et tal. (2001). Weaknesses in the Key Schedul-ing Algorithm of RC4. *Lecture Notes in Computer Science, 2259*, doi:10.1007/3-540-45537-X_1

Freeman, E. R. (1984). *Strategic Management – A Stake-holder Approach*. London: Pitman.

Freeman, E. R. (1994). Politics of Stakeholder Theory: Some Future Directions. *Business Ethics Quarterly, 4*, 409–422. doi:10.2307/3857340

Frost and Sullivan. (2006) Reports European Healthcare IT Outsourcing market to offer lucrative opportunities. *Hospital Business Week, 37*.

Fu, J. R., Farn, C. K., & Chao, W. P. (2006). Acceptance of electronic tax filing: A study of taxpayers' intention. *Information & Management, 43*, 109–126. doi:10.1016/j.im.2005.04.001

Gaggi, S. (1997). *From text to hypertext: Decentering the subject in fiction, film, the visual arts, and electronic media*. Philadelphia, PA: University of Pennsylvania Press.

Gail, J., & Hannafin, M. (1994). A framework for the study of hypertext. *Instructional Science, 22*(3), 207–232. doi:10.1007/BF00892243

Galliers, R. D. (1991). Choosing Information Systems Research Approaches. In Nissen, H. E., Klein, H. K., & Hirschheim, R. (Eds.), *Information Systems Research: Contemporary Approaches and Emergent Traditions*. Amsterdam: North-Holland.

Gandon, F., & Sadeh, N. (2004). Semantic Web Tech-nologies to Reconcile Privacy and Context Awareness, Proceedings of the 1st French-Speaking Conference on Mobility and Ubiquity Computing, CD-Format, New York, USA.

Gao, Y., Yang, M., Zhao, X., Pardo, B., Pappas, Y. W., & Choudhary, T. N. (2008). Image spam hunter, *IEEE International Conference on Acoustics, Speech and Signal Processing* (pp.1765-1768). USA: IEEE.

Gast, M. (2002). *802.11 Wireless Networks: the definitive guide*. Sebastopol, CA: O'Reilly and Associates, Inc.

Gee, J. P. (2003). *What video games have to teach us about learning and literacy*. New York: Palgrave Macmillan.

Gerbing, D. W., & Anderson, J. C. (1988). An updated paradigm for scale development incorporating unidi-mensionality and measurement error. *JMR, Journal of Marketing Research, 25*, 186–192. doi:10.2307/3172650

Gershon, C. (2003). Biometrics Authentication & Smart Cards. *GSA/FTS Network Service Conference,* Managing the Future: Mastering the Maze. Retrieved December 9, 2009, from http://www.fts.gsa.gov/2003_ network_con-ference/ 5-1_biometric_smartcards/

Ghyasi, A., & Kushchu, I. (2004). Uses of Mobile Govern-ment in Developing Countries. Retrieved June 18, 2005 from mGovLab, http://www.mgovlab.org

Giles, C. R., & Desurvire, E. (1991, February). Modeling Erbium-Doped Fiber Amplifiers. *Journal of Lightwave Technology, 9*(2), 271–283. doi:10.1109/50.65886

Goh, S., & Richards, G. (1997). Benchmarking the learning capability of organizations. *European Management Journal, 15*(5), 575–583. doi:10.1016/S0263-2373(97)00036-4

Goldstuck, A. (2004). *Government Unplugged: Mobile and wireless technologies in the public service.* Center for public services innovation, South Africa.

Good, B., & Wilkinson, M. (2006). The Life Sciences Semantic Web is Full of Creeps! *Briefings in Bioinformatics, 7*(3), 275–286.

Gorard, S., Fevre, R., & Rees, G. (1999). The apparent decline of informal learning. *Oxford Review of Education, 15*(4), 437–454. doi:10.1080/030549899103919

Gould, J. D., & Lewis, C. (1985). Designing for usability: Key principles and what designers think. *Communications of the ACM, 28*(3), 300–311. doi:10.1145/3166.3170

Gourier, N., James, D. H., & Crowley, L. (2004). Estimating face orientation from robust detection of salient facial structures. *FG Net Workshop on Visual Observation of Deictic Gestures.*

Graff, G. (2005). Differences in concept mapping, hypertext architecture, and the analyst–intuition dimension of cognitive style. *Educational Psychology, 25*(4), 409–422. doi:10.1080/01443410500041813

Graham, M., & Scarborough, H. (1997). Information Technology Outsourcing by State Governments in Australia. *Australian Journal of Public Administration, 56*(3), 30–39. doi:10.1111/j.1467-8500.1997.tb01263.x

Graham, P. (2003). *Better Bayesian Filtering.* Retrieved May 25, 2006 from http://www.paulgraham.com/ better. html

Greenberg, A. D. (2004). *Navigating the sea of research on videoconferencing-based distance education: A platform for understanding research into technology's effectiveness and value.* Retrieved from http://www.wainhouse.com/ files /papers/wr-navseadistedu.pdf

Greenfield, D. N. (1999). *Virtual addiction: Help for netheads, cyberfreaks, and those who love them.* Oakland, CA: New Harbinger Publications.

Greenfield, P. M., deWinstanley, P., Kilpatrick, H., & Kaye, D. (1994). Action video games and informal education: Effects on strategies for dividing visual attention. *Journal of Applied Developmental Psychology, 15*, 105–123. doi:10.1016/0193-3973(94)90008-6

Gross, J. L., & Yellen, J. (2005). *Graph theory and its applications.* Boca Raton, FL: Chapman & Hall/CRC.

Grossman, G. M., & Helpman, E. (2005). Outsourcing in a Global Economy. *The Review of Economic Studies, 72*(1), 135. doi:10.1111/0034-6527.00327

Guy, R. A., & Hill, J. R. (2007). 10 Outsourcing Myths That Raise Your Risk: Hospitals Should Be Wary Of Common Myths That Can Cause Them To Make Missteps In Developing Clinical Service Outsourcing Arrangements. *Healthcare Financial Management, 61*(6), 66–72.

Haley, D. (2004). A Case for Outsourcing Medical Device Reprocessing. *AORN Journal, 79*, 806–808. doi:10.1016/S0001-2092(06)60821-1

Hargreaves, J. (2006). *Recognition of Prior Learning: At a glance.* Adelaide, Australia: National Centre for Vocational Education Research.

Harris, E. (2004). The Next Step in the Spam Control War: Greylisting, Retrieved February 25, 2009 from http:// projects.puremagic.com/ greylisting/whitepaper. htm

Hashim, M. K. (2007). *SMEs in Malaysia: A Brief Handbook.* Petaling Jaya, Malaysia: August Publishing Sdn. Bhd.

Hashmi, N., et al. (2004). Abstracting Workflows: Unifying Bioinformatics Task Conceptualization and Specification through Semantic Web Services. In *Proceedings of the W3C Workshop on Semantic Web for Life Sciences*, Cambridge, MA.

Head, M., & Yuan, Y. (2001). Privacy Protection in Electronic Commerce – a Theoretical Framework. *Human Systems Management, 20*, 149–160.

Heeks, R. (2002). *Reinventing Government in the Information Age: international practice in IT-enabled Public Sector Reform, Routledge, Research in Information Technology and Society*. London: Routledge.

Heeks, R. (2003). Causes of e-government success and failure. Retrieved October 12, 2004 from http://www.e-devexchange.org /eGov/causefactor.htm

Heeks, R., & Lallana, E. C. (2004). M-Government Benefits and Challenges. Retrieved May 15, 2005 from http://www.e-devexchange.org/ eGov/mgovprocom.

Henriquez, A., & Riconscente, M. (1999). *Rhode Island Teachers and Technology Initiative: Program evaluation final report*. New York: Education Development Center, Center for Children and Technology.

Henry, P (2001). E-learning technology, content and services. *Education + Training, 43*(4), 251–259.

Herther, N. K. (2009). The Changing Language of Search Part 1.Nu Speak. *Searcher, 17*(1), 36–41.

Hesson, M., & Al-Ameed, H. (2007). Online security evaluation process for new e-services. *Journal of Business Process Management, 13*(2), 223–245. doi:10.1108/14637150710740473

Higgins, C. (2005). Primary school students' perceptions of interactive whiteboards'. *Journal of Computer Assisted Learning, 21*.

Higgins, C., Falzon, C., Hall, I., Moseley, D., Smith, F., Smith, H., & Wall, K. (2005). *Embedding ICT in the Literacy and Numeracy Strategies: Final Report*. UK: University of Newcastle.

Hirschheim, R., & Klein, H. (1989). Four Paradigms of Information Systems Development. *Communications of the ACM, 32*(10), 1199–1215. doi:10.1145/67933.67937

Hirschheim, R., & Lacity, M. (2006). Four stories of information systems insourcing. In Hirschheim, R. Heinzl A. & Dibbern J. (Ed.), *Information Systems Outsourcing: Enduring Themes, New Perspectives and Global Challenges*. Berlin, Germany: Springer-Verlag (pp. 303-346).

Hofer, L. (2003). *Critical issues in evaluating the effectiveness of technology. Critical Review CET 720*. New York: Springer.

Hollands, M. (2004). *Status of Offshore Outsourcing in Australia: A Qualitative Study*. AIIA Report, Australian Information Industry Association.

Hongxun, J. et al. (2006). Research on IT Outsourcing based on IT Systems Management. ICEC 06, Fredericton, Canada, *Journal of ACM 1-59593-392-1*. 533-537.

Hsiao, C., Pai, J., & Chiu, H. (2009). The Study on the Outsourcing of Taiwan's Hospitals: A Questionnaire Survey Research. *BMC Health Services Research, 9*, 78. doi:10.1186/1472-6963-9-78

Huang, Y., Lin, C., & Lin, H. (2005). Techno-economic Effect of R&D Outsourcing Strategy for Small and Medium-sized Enterprises: A Resource-Based Viewpoint. *International Journal of Innovation and Incubation, 2*(1), 1–22.

Huber, G. P. (1991). Organizational Learning: The Contributing Processes and the Literatures. *Organization Science, 2*(1), 88–115. doi:10.1287/orsc.2.1.88

Hutchinson, D. (2007). Video games and the pedagogy of place. *Social Studies, 98*(1), 35–40. doi:10.3200/TSSS.98.1.35-40

IBM SOA. (n.d.). *IBM - Service-Oriented Architecture (SOA)*. Retrieved September 15, 2008, from http://www-01.ibm.com/ software/solutions/soa/

IEEE. (1999). *IEEE 802.11b - Part 11: wireless lan medium access control (mac) and physical layer (phy) specifications: higher-speed physical layer extension in the 2.4 ghz band.* Retrieved June 2003 from: http://standards.ieee.org/getieee802/ download/802.11b-1999.pdf

IEEE. (2003). *IEEE 802.11g Part 11: wireless lan medium access control (mac) and physical layer (phy) specifications amendment 4: further higher data rate extension in the 2.4 ghz band.* Retrieved December 2003 from: http://standards.ieee.org/getieee802/ download/802.11g-2003.pdf

IEEE. (2004). *IEEE 802.11i Part 11: wireless lan medium access control (mac) and physical layer (phy) specifications amendment 6: medium access control (mac) security enhancements.* Retrieved October 2004 from: http://standards.ieee.org/getieee802/ download/802.11i-2004.pdf

IEG. (2006). *Impact Evaluation Experience of the Independent Evaluation Group of the World Bank.* Washington, DC: World Bank.

Inforsecurity. (2009). *$9m lifted in RBS Worldpay ATM heist.* Retrieved April 16, 2010, from http://www.infosecurity-us.com/ view/524/9m-lifted-i n-rbs-worldpay-atm-heist

Inkpen, A., & Crossan, M. M. (1995). Believing is seeing: Organizational learning in joint ventures. *Journal of Management Studies, 32*(5), 595–618. doi:10.1111/j.1467-6486.1995.tb00790.x

Irani, Z., Dwivedi, Y. K., & Williams, M. D. (2008). Understanding Consumer Adoption of Broadband: An Extension of the Technology Acceptance Model. *The Journal of the Operational Research Society*, 1–13.

IRB. (2001). *Annual Report 2001.* Malaysia: Inland Revenue Board.

IRB. (2006). *Annual Report 2006.* Malaysia: Inland Revenue Board.

Issac, B., & Raman, V. (2006). Implementation of Spam Detection on Regular and Image based Emails - A Case Study using Spam Corpus, *MMU International Symposium on Information and Communication Technologies* (pp.431-436). Malaysia: Multimedia University.

Ives, B., & Learmonth, G. P. (1984). The Information System as a Competitive Weapon. *Communications of the ACM, 27*(12), 1193–1201. doi:10.1145/2135.2137

Jae-Nam, L., Huynh, M. Q., & Hirschheim, R. (2008). An integrative model of trust on IT outsourcing: Examining a bilateral perspective. *Information Systems Frontiers, 10,* 145–163. doi:10.1007/s10796-008-9066-7

Jain, A. K., Flynn, P., & Ross, A. (2007). *Handbook of biometrics.* New York: Springer.

Jain, A. K., & Ross, A. (2004). Multibiometric systems. *Communications of the ACM, 47*(1), 34–40. doi:10.1145/962081.962102

Jain, A. K., Ross, A., & Pankanti, S. (2006). Biometrics: A tool for information security. *IEEE Transactions on Information Forensics and Security, 1*(2), 125–143. doi:10.1109/TIFS.2006.873653

Jain, A. K., Ross, A., & Prabhakar, S. (2004). An introduction to biometric recognition. *IEEE Transactions on Circuits and Systems for Video Technology, Special Issue on Image- and Video-Based Biometrics, 14*(1), 4-20.

Jalava, J., & Pohjola, M. (2002). Economic Growth in the New Economy: evidence from advanced economies. *Information Economics and Policy, 14,* 189–210. doi:10.1016/S0167-6245(01)00066-X

Jalava, J., & Pohjola, M. (2007). The Role of Electricity and ICT in Economic Growth: Case Finland. *Explorations in Economic History, 45,* 270–287. doi:10.1016/j.eeh.2007.11.001

Jay, S., & Barry, S. (2002). Drawing a blank: The failure of facial recognition technology in Tampa, Florida. *An ACLU Special Report,* Jan. 2002. Retrieved October, 9, 2009, from http://www.aclu.org/issues/ privacy/d rawing_blank.pdf

JBoss SOA. (n.d.). *JBoss – SOA Resource Center*. Retrieved September 5, 2008, from http://www.jboss.com/resources/soa

Jones, G. R. (2000). *Organizational Theory* (3rd ed.). New York: Prentice Hall.

Jones, R. (2003). Local and national ICT policies. In R. Kozma (Ed.) *Technology, innovation, and educational change: A global perspective* (pp. 163-194). Eugene, Kelley, L. (2002). *A Review of Findings from Research By: Cathy Ringstaff.* Retrieved October 13, 2009, from http://www.wested.org/ cs/we/view/rs/619

Jöreskog, K. G., & Sörbrom, D. (1993). *LISREL 8: Structural Equation Modelling with the SIMPLIS Command Language.* London: Lawrence Erlbaum Associates Publishers.

JSR 208. (n.d.). *JSR 000208 java Business Integration 1.0.* Retrieved August 25, 2008, from http://jcp.org/aboutJava/comm unityprocess/final/jsr208/index.html

Junaidah, H. (2008). Learning Barriers in Adopting ICT among Selected Working Women in Malaysia. *Gender in Management: An International Journal, 23*(5), 317–336. doi:10.1108/17542410810887356

Kakabadse, N., & Kakabadse, A. (2000). Critical Review – Outsourcing: A Paradigm Shift. *Journal of Management Development, 19*(8), 670–728. doi:10.1108/02621710010377508

Kakihara, M., & Sorensen, C. (2002). Mobility: An Extended Perspective. 35th Hawaii International Conference on System Sciences, Hawaii, USA.

Kaplan, R. S., & Norton, D. P. (1992). Balanced Scorecard – Measures That Drive Performance. *Harvard Business Review, 1–2,* 71–79.

Kaplan, B., & Maxwell, J. A. (1994). Qualitative Research Methods for Evaluating Computer Information Systems. In Anderson, J. G., Aydin, C. E., & Jay, S. J. (Eds.), *Evaluating Health Care Information Systems: Methods and Applications* (pp. 45–68). Newbury Park, CA: Sage Publications.

Katz, R., & Oblinger, D. (Eds.). (2000). *The "e" is for everything: Ecommerce, e-business, and e-learning in the future of higher education.* San Francisco, CA: Jossey-Bass.

Keen, P. G. W. (1981). Information systems and organizational change. *Communications of the ACM, 24*(1), 24–33. doi:10.1145/358527.358543

Kela, N., Rattani, A., & Gupta, P. (2006). Illumination invariant elastic bunch graph matching for efficient face recognition. In *Proceedings of Conference on Computer Vision and Pattern Recognition Workshop.*

Kendall, P. (1992). *Introduction to Systems Analysis and Design: A Structured Approach* (2nd ed.). USA: Wm. C Brown Publishers.

Khalil, T. M. (1993). Management of Technology and the Creation of Wealth. *Industrial Engineering (American Institute of Industrial Engineers), 25*(9), 16–17.

Khalil, T. M. (2000). *Management of Technology: The key to Competitiveness and Wealth Creation.* Singapore: McGraw Hill.

Kim, H. S., Lee, J. K., & Yoo, K. Y. (2003). ID-based password authentication scheme using smart cards and fingerprints. *ACM SIGOPS Operating Syst. Rev., 37*(4), 32–41. doi:10.1145/958965.958969

Kirchner, P. A., & Pass, F. (2001). Web enhanced higher education: a Tower of Babel. *Computers in Human Behavior, 17*(4), 347–353. doi:10.1016/S0747-5632(01)00009-7

Kiritchenko, S., & Matwin, S. (2001). *Email classification with co-training* in the Centre for Advanced Studies on Collaborative Research (pp.1-8). Ontario, Canada.

Kisku, D. R., Gupta, P., & Sing, J. K. (in press). Face recognition by fusion of invariant facial landmarks.

Kisku, D. R., Gupta, P., & Sing, J. K. (in press). Fusion of multiple matchers using SVM for offline signature identification, *International Conference on Security Technology (SecTech).*

Kisku, D. R., Rattani, A., Grosso, E., & Tistarelli, M. (2007). Face identification by SIFT-based complete graph topology, *5th IEEE International Workshop on Automatic Identification Advanced Technologies (AutoId)* (pp. 63—68).

Kisku, D. R., Rattani, A., Tistarelli, M., & Gupta, P. (2008). Graph application on face for personal authentication and recognition. *Proceedings of 10th IEEE International Conference on Control, Automation, Robotics and Vision* (pp. 1150—1155).

Kisku, D. R., Sing, J. K., Tistarelli, M., & Gupta, P. (2009). Multisensor biometric evidence fusion for person authentication using wavelet decomposition and monotonic-decreasing graph. In *Proceedings of 7th IEEE International Conference on Advances in Pattern Recognition* (pp. 205—208).

Kitasuka, T., Nakanishi, T., Fukuda, A (2003). Wireless LAN Based Indoor Positioning System WiPS and Its Simulation. *Communications, Computers and signal Processing, 1*(28), 272–275.

Klein, H., & Myers, M. (1999). A set of principles for conducting and evaluating interpretive field studies in Information Systems. *Management Information Systems Quarterly, 23*(1), 67–93. doi:10.2307/249410

Knikker R., Guo, Y., Li1, J., Kwan, A., Yip, K.,Cheung, D., & Cheung, K. (2004). A web services choreography scenario for interoperating bioinformatics applications. *BMC Bioinformatics.*

Kokiopoulou, E., & Frossard, P. (2009). Video face recognition using graph based semi-supervised learning, *International Conference on Multimedia and Expo* (pp. 1564-1565).

Kossenkov, A., Manion, F., & Korotkov, E. (2003). ASAP: Automated Sequence Annotation Pipeline for Web-based Updating of Sequence Information with a Local Database. *Bioinformatics (Oxford, England), 19*, 675–676.

Kozma, R. (2005). National policies that connect ICT-based *education* reform to economic and social development. *Human Technology, 1*(2), 117–156.

Krajcik, J., & Blumenfeld, P. (2006). Project-based learning. In Sawyer, R. K. (Ed.), *Cambridge Handbook of the Learning Sciences* (pp. 317–334). Cambridge, UK: Cambridge University Press.

Krishnan, P., et al. A System for LEASE: location estimation assisted by stationery emitters for indoor rf wireless networks. *Twenty-third Annual Joint Conference of the IEEE Computer and Communications Societies, v.2, n.7, p.1001–1011, 2004.* Retrieved March 2005 for: http://citeseer.ist.psu.edu/ krishnan04system.html

Kristoffersen, S., & Ljungberg, F. (1999). Mobile use of IT. In the proceedings of IRIS22, Jyvaskyla, Finland.

Kuppusamy, M., Raman, M., & Lee, G. (2009). Whose ICT Investment Matters To Economic Growth: Private or Public? The Malaysian Perspective. *The Electronic Journal on Information Systems in Developing Countries, 37*(7), 1–19.

Kuppusamy, M., & Shanmugam, B. (2007). Information Communication Technology and Economic Growth in Malaysia. *Review of Islamic Economics, 11*(2), 87–100.

Kushchu, I., & Kuscu, H. (2003). From e-government to m-government: Facing the Inevitable? In the proceeding of European Conference on e-government (ECEG 2003), Trinity College, Dublin.

Kuwabara, M., & Nishio, N. (n.d.). Wi-Fi based radio map for location sensing by hypothesizing existence of barriers. In *ICUIMC '09: Proceedings of the 3rd international Conference on Ubiquitous Information Management and Communication*, 2009, New York.

Labarga, A., Valentin, F., Anderson, M., & Lopez, R. (2007). *Web Services at the European Bioinformatics*, EMBL-EBI, European Bioinformatics Institute, Wellcome Trust Genome Campus, Hinxton, CB10 1SD, Cambridge, UK.

Lacity, M. C., & Willcocks, L. P. (1998). An Empirical Investigation of Information Technology Sourcing Practices: Lessons From Experience. *Management Information Systems Quarterly*, (September): 363–408. doi:10.2307/249670

Lades, M., Vorbrüggen, J. C., Buhmann, J., Lange, J., von der Malsburg, C., Würtz, R. P., & Konen, W. (1993). Distortion invariant object recognition in the dynamic link architecture. *IEEE Transactions on Computers, 42*(3), 300–311. doi:10.1109/12.210173

Lai, M. L., Siti, N. S. O., & Ahamed, K. M. (2005). Tax Practitioners And The Electronic Filing System: An Empirical Analysis. *Academy of Accounting and Financial Studies Journal, 9*(1), 93–109.

Lai, M.L., Siti, N.S.O., & Ahamed, K.M. (2004). Towards An Electronic Filing System: A Malaysian Survey. *eJournal of Tax Research, 5*(2), 1-11.

Lam, S. S. K. (1998). Organizational performance and learning styles in Hong Kong. *The Journal of Social Psychology, 138*(3), 401–403. doi:10.1080/00224549809600392

Lambrinoudakisa, C., Gritzalisa, S., Dridib, F., & Pernul, G. (2003). Security requirements for e-government services: A methodological approach for developing a common PKI-based security policy. *Computer Communications, 26*, 1873–1883. doi:10.1016/S0140-3664(03)00082-3

Lan, M., & Zhou, W. (2005). Spam filtering based on preference ranking, Fifth International Conference on Computer and Information Technology (pp.223-227). China: IEEE Computer Society.

Landow, G. P. (2006). *Hypertext 3.0: Critical theory and new media in an era of globalization.* Baltimore, MD: Johns Hopkins University Press.

Layne, K., & Lee, J. (2001). Developing fully functional e-government: A four stage model. *Government Information Quarterly, 18*, 122–136. doi:10.1016/S0740-624X(01)00066-1

Lee, A. S. (1989). A scientific methodology for MIS case studies. *Management Information Systems Quarterly, 13*(1), 33–50. doi:10.2307/248698

Lee, A. S. (1994). Electronic Mail as a Medium for Rich Communication: An Empirical Investigation Using Hermeneutic Interpretation. *Management Information Systems Quarterly, 18*(2), 143–157. doi:10.2307/249762

Lee, S. M. (2003). Korea: from the land of morning calm to ICT hotbed. [Abstract]. *Journal of the Academy Management Executive (USA), 17*(2).

Lee, J., & Kim, Y. (1999). Effect of Partnership Quality on IS Outsourcing Success: Conceptual Framework and Empirical Validation. *Journal of Management Information Systems, 15*(4), 29–61.

Lei, D., Hitt, M. A., & Bettis, R. (1996). Dynamic core competencies through meta-learning and strategic context. *Journal of Management, 22*(4), 549–569. doi:10.1177/014920639602200402

Lei, D., Slocum, J. W., & Pitts, R. A. (1999). Designing organizations for competitive advantage: The power of unlearning and learning. *Organizational Dynamics, 27*(3), 24–38. doi:10.1016/S0090-2616(99)90019-0

Leonard-Barton, D. (1992). The factory as a learning laboratory. *Sloan Management Review, 34*(1), 23–38.

Levitt, B., & March, J. G. (1998). Organizational learning. *Annual Review of Sociology, 14*, 319–340. doi:10.1146/annurev.so.14.080188.001535

Lewis, J. R. (1991a). An after-scenario questionnaire for usability studies: psychometric evaluation over three trials. *SIGCHI Bulletin, 23*, 79. doi:10.1145/126729.1056077

Lewis, J. R. (1991b). Psychometric evaluation of an after-scenario questionnaire for computer usability studies: The ASQ. *SIGCHI Bulletin, 23*, 78–81. doi:10.1145/122672.122692

Lewis, J. R. (1991c). *User satisfaction questionnaires for usability studies: 1991 manual of directions for the ASQ and PSSUQ* (Tech. Report 54.609). Boca Raton, FL: International Business Machines Corporation.

Lewis, J. R. (1992a). *Psychometric evaluation of the computer system usability questionnaire: The CSUQ* (Tech. Report 54.723), Boca Raton, FL: International Business Machines Corporation.

Lewis, J. R. (1992b). Psychometric evaluation of the post-study system usability questionnaire: The PSSUQ. In *Proceedings of the Human Factors Society 36th Annual Meeting* (pp. 1259-1263). Santa Monica, CA: Human Factors Society.

Li, S. Z., & Jain, A. K. (Eds.). (2005). *Handbook of face recognition*. New York: Springer.

Lim, S., Lee, K., Byeon, O., & Kim, T. (2001). Efficient iris recognition through improvement of feature vector and classifier. *ETRI Journal*, *23*(2), 61–70. doi:10.4218/etrij.01.0101.0203

Lin, C., Pervan, G., & Mcdermid, D. (2007). Issues and Recommendations in Evaluating and Managing the Benefits of Public Sector IT Outsourcing. *Information Technology & People*, *20*(2), 161–183. doi:10.1108/09593840710758068

Lin, W. T., & Shao, B. B. M. (2000). The Relationship Between User Participation and System Success: A Simultaneous Contingency Approach. *Information & Management*, *37*(6), 283–295. doi:10.1016/S0378-7206(99)00055-5

Lin, C. H., & Lai, Y. Y. (2004). A flexible biometrics remote user authentication scheme. *Computer Standards & Interfaces*, *27*(1), 19–23. doi:10.1016/j.csi.2004.03.003

Lin, Z. C., Lee, H., & Huang, T. S. (1986). Finding 3-D point correspondences in motion estimation. *Proceedings of International Conference on Pattern Recognition* (pp.303 – 305).

Liu, X., Hotchkiss, D. R., & Bose, S. (2008). The Effectiveness of Contracting out Primary Health Care Services in Developing Countries: A Review of the Evidence. *Health Policy and Planning*, *23*, 1–13. doi:10.1093/heapol/czm042

Liu, J., & Liu, Z.-Q. (2005). EBGM with fuzzy fusion on face. *Advances in Artificial Intelligence. LNCS, 3809*, 498–509.

LiuZ. (2005). http://www.eecs.lehigh.edu/SPCRL /IF/image_fusion.htm

Livingstone, D. W. (2001). *Adults' Informal Learning: Definitions, Findings, Gaps and Future Research*. NALL Working Paper 21. Toronto, Canada: Centre for the Study of Education and Work.

Lööf, A. (2008). *Eurostat: Data in focus* 46/2008.

Lord, P. W., Bechhofer, S., Wilkinson, M. D., Schiltz, G., Gessler, D., Hull, D., et al. (2004). Applying semantic Web services to bioinformatics: Experiences gained, lessons learned. In *Proceedings of the 3rd International Semantic Web Conference*, Springer

Lorence, D. P., & Spink, A. (2004). Healthcare Information Systems Outsourcing. *International Journal of Information Management*, *24*(2), 131–145. doi:10.1016/j.ijinfomgt.2003.12.011

Lowe, D. G. (2004). Distinctive image features from scale invariant keypoints. *International Journal of Computer Vision*, *60*(2), 91–110. doi:10.1023/B:VISI.0000029664.99615.94

Lowe, D. G. (1999). Object recognition from local scale invariant features. *International Conference on Computer Vision* (pp. 1150–1157).

Lu, Y. B., & Chu, P. L. (2000, December). Gain Flattening by Using Dual-Core Fiber in Erbium-Doped Fiber Amplifier. *IEEE Photonics Technology Lrtters, 12*(12). J. R. Qian and H. F. Chen "Gain Flattening Fiber Filters Using Phaseshifted Long Period Fiber Gratings," Electronics Letters Vol. 34, No. 11, May 1998.

Luca, B., Bistarelli, S., & Vaccarelli, A. (2002). Biometrics authentication with smartcard, *IIT TR-08/2002*, Retrieved October, 9, 2009, from http://www.iat.cnr.it/attivita/progetti/ parametri biomedici.html

Lucas, H. C. Jr. (1975). *Why Information Systems Fail*. New York, London: Columbia University Press.

Luftman, J., Kempaiah, R., & Nash, E. (2006). Key Issues for IT Executives 2005. *MIS Quarterly Executive*, *5*(2), 27–45.

Ma, L., Tan, T., Wang, Y., & Zhang, D. (2004). Efficient iris recognition by characterizing key local variations. *IEEE Transactions on Image Processing, 13*(6), 739–750. doi:10.1109/TIP.2004.827237

Machin, S. (2006). *New Technologies in Schools: Is There a Pay Off?* Germany: Institute for the Study of Labour.

MacManus, R., & Porter, J. (2005): *Web 2.0 for design: bootstrapping the social web*. Retrieved April 15th 2008, from: http://www.digital-web.com/articles/web_2_for_designers

Mallia, G. (2007). A Tolling Bell for Institutions? Speculations on student information processing and effects on accredited learning. In *Readings in Technology in Education* (pp. 24–32). Abbotsford, BC, Canada: UCFV Press.

Mallia, G. (2009). Transfer through Learning Flexibility and Hypertextuality. In Wheeler, S. (Ed.), *Connected Minds, Emerging Cultures: Cybercultures in Online Learning* (pp. 185–208). Charlotte, N.C.: Information Age Publishing.

Mallia, G. (2003). Pushing media democracy: Giving marginalized illiterates a new literacy. In K. Fernstrom (Ed.), *4th ICICTE Proceedings* (pp. 387–392). Athens: National and Kapodistrian University of Athens.

Maltoni, D., Maio, D., Jain, A. K., & Prabhakar, S. (Eds.). (2003). *Handbook of fingerprint recognition*. Springer.

Mancini, C. (2005). *Cinematic hypertext: Investigating a new paradigm*. Amsterdam: IOS Press.

Mandinach, E. B., & Honey, M. (2005). *A theoretical framework for data-driven decision making*. Paper presented at the Wingspread Conference on data-driven decision making, October 30-November 1, Racine, WI.

Marek, T., Diallo, I., Ndiaye, B., & Rakotosalama, J. (1999). Successful Contracting of Prevention Services: Fighting Malnutrition in Senegal and Madagascar. *Health Policy and Planning, 14*(4), 382–389. doi:10.1093/heapol/14.4.382

Markus, M. L. (1983). Power, politics, and MIS implementation. *Communications of the ACM, 26*(6), 430–444. doi:10.1145/358141.358148

Markus, M. L., & Benjamin, R. J. (1996). Change agentry – the next information systems frontier. *Management Information Systems Quarterly, 20*(4), 385–407. doi:10.2307/249561

Marsh, J., Brooks, G., Hughes, J., Ritchie, L., Roberts, S., & Wright, K. (2005). *Digital beginnings: Young children's use of popular culture, media and new technologies*. Sheffield: University of Sheffield. doi:10.4324/9780203420324

Masatoshi, N. (1997). A Fast Computer Algorithm for Switching Converters. *IEEE Transactions on Power Electronics, 12*(1), 180–186. doi:10.1109/63.554184

Masuda, H., & Takada, A. (1990). High Gain Two-Stage Amplification with Erbium-Doped Fiber Amplifier. *Electronics Letters, 26*(10), 661–662. doi:10.1049/el:19900432

Matthew, W. (2006). *E-File Goals too Ambitious. FWC. COM*. Retrieved on 2/11/2009, from http://fcw.com/articles/2006/02/27 /efile-goal-too-ambitious.aspx

May, P. (2001). *Mobile commerce: opportunities, applications, and technologies of wireless business*. New York: Cambridge University Press. doi:10.1017/CBO9780511583919

Mc Clure, D. L. (2000). Federal Initiatives Are Evolving Rapidly But They Face Significant Challenges. *Testimony* United States General Accounting Office, GAO/T-AIMD/GGD-00-179.

McGlasson, L. (2009). *ATM Fraud: 7 Growing Threats to Financial Institutions*. Retrieved April 2, 2010, from http://www.bankinfosecurity.com/articles. php?art_id=1523&opg=1

McIvor, R. (2000). A Practical Framework for Understanding the Outsourcing Process. *Supply Chain Management, 5*(1), 22. doi:10.1108/13598540010312945

McKay, S., Thurlow, C., & Toomey Zimmerman, H. (2005). Wired whizzes or techno slaves? Teens and their emergent communication technologies. In Williams, A., & Thurlow, C. (Eds.), *Talking adolescence: Perspectives on communication in the teenage years* (pp. 185–203). New York: Peter Lang.

McLemore, A. (2009). *Advantages and disadvantages of online instruction*. Retrieved 12 August, 2009 from http://www.americanchronicle.com

Md Nor, K., & Pearson, J. M. (2007). The Influence of Trust on Internet Banking Acceptance. *Journal of Internet Banking and Commerce, 12*(2), 2–10.

Means, B., Roschelle, R., Penuel, W., Sabelli, N., & Haertel, G. (2004). Technology's contribution to teaching and policy: Efficiency, standardization, or transformation? In Floden, R. E. (Ed.), *Review of Research in Education* (*Vol. 27*). Washington, DC: American Educational Research Association.

Means, B. (2006). Prospects for transforming schools with technology-supported assessment. In Sawyer, R. K. (Ed.), *Cambridge Handbook of the Learning Sciences* (pp. 505–520). Cambridge, UK: Cambridge University Press.

Mehrabian, H., & Hashemi-Tari, P. (2007). *Pupil boundary detection for iris recognition using graph cuts* (pp. 77–82). Image and Vision Computing New Zealand.

Menachemi, N., Burke, D., & Diana, M. (2007a). Characteristics of Hospitals that Outsource Information. System Functions. *Journal of Healthcare Information Management, 19*(1), 63–69.

Menachemi, N., Burkhardt, J., Shewchuk, R., Burke, D., & Brooks, R. G. (2007b). To Outsource or not to Outsource: Examining the Effects of Outsourcing it Functions on Financial Performance in Hospitals. *Health Care Management Review, 32*(1), 46–54.

Meskauskas, A., Lehmann-Horn, F., & Jurkat-Rott, K. (2004). Sight: Autmating Genomic Data-mining without Programming Skills. *Bioinformatics (Oxford, England), 20*, 1718–1720.

Meyers, S. (2004). ED Outsourcing: Is It Good for Patient Care? *Trustee, 57*, 12–14.

Microsoft, S. O. A. (n.d.). *Microsoft – SOA and Business Process*. Retrieved September 9, 2008, http://www.microsoft.com/SOA.

Mihyar, H., & Hayder, A. (2007). Online security evaluation process for new e-services. *Journal of Business Process Management, 13*(2), 223–246. doi:10.1108/14637150710740473

Miles, M. B., & Huberman, A. M. (1994). *Qualitative Data Analysis: An Expanded Sourcebook*. Sage Publications.

Milheim, K. L. (2007). Influence of technology on informal learning. *Adult Basic Education and Literacy Journal, 1*(1), 21–26.

Miner, A. S., & Mezias, S. J. (1996). Ugly duckling no more: pasts and futures of organizational learning research. *Organization Science, 7*(1), 88–99. doi:10.1287/orsc.7.1.88

Ming, L., Yunchun, L., & Wei, L. (2007). Spam Filtering by Stages, *International Conference on Convergence Information Technology* (pp. 2209-2213).

Mintzberg, H. (1990). Strategy formation: Schools of thought. In Frederickson, J. W. (Ed.), *Perspectives of strategic management* (pp. 105–235). New York: Harper Business.

Mislevy, R. J., Behrens, J. T., Bennett, R. E., Demark, S. F., Frezzo, D. C., Levy, R., Robinson, D.H., Rutstein D. W., & Valerie J. (2007). *On The Roles of External Knowledge Representations in Assessment Design*. CSE Report 722.

Misra, R. B. (2004). Global IT Outsourcing: Metrics for Success of All Parties. *Journal of Information Technology Cases and Applications, 6*(3), 21–34.

Monteiro, E., & Hanseth, O. (1996). Social Shaping of Information Infrastructure: On Being Specific about the Technology. In Orlikowski, W. J., Walsham, G., Jones, M. R., & DeGross, J. I. (Eds.), *Information Technology and Changes in Organizational Work* (pp. 325–343). London: Chapman and Hall.

Moraes, L. F. M., & de, Nunes, B. A. A (2006). *Calibration-free WLAN location system based on dynamic mapping of signal strength*. In MOBIWAC '06 *Proceedings Of The 4th Acm International Workshop On Mobility Management And Wireless Access, 2006*, New York.

Morrison, J. D. (2002). *IEEE 802.11 wireless local area network security through location authentication*. (Masters Thesis. Naval Postgraduate School Monterey, California). Retrieved January 2003 from: http://cisr.nps.edu/downloads/ theses/02thesis_morrison.pdf

Moschuris, S. J., & Kondylis, M. N. (2006). Outsourcing in Public Hospitals: A Greek Perspective. *Journal of Health Organization and Management*, *20*(1), 4–14. doi:10.1108/14777260610656534

Moskowitz, R., & Fleishman, G. (2003). *Weakness in Passphrase Choice in WPA Interface*. Retrieved January 2004 from: http://wifinetnews.com/ archives/002452.html

Mueller, R. O. (1996). *Basic Principles of Structural Equation Modelling: An Introduction to Lisrel and EQS*. New York: Springer.

Muller, M. J., Wildman, D. M., & White, E. A. (1993). Equal opportunity PD using PICTIVE. *Communications of the ACM*, *36*(4), 64–66. doi:10.1145/153571.214818

Myers, M. (1994). Dialectical Hermeneutics: A Theoretical Framework for the Implementation of Information Systems. *Information Systems Journal*, *5*(1), 51–70. doi:10.1111/j.1365-2575.1995.tb00089.x

Myers, M. (1997). Qualitative Research in Information Systems. *Management Information Systems Quarterly*, *21*(2), 241–242. doi:10.2307/249422

Myers, M. (1998). Interpretive Research in Information Systems. In Mingers, M., & Stowell, F. (Eds.), *Information Systems: An Emerging Discipline? London*. Maidenhead.

Myers, M., & Avison, D. (2002). An Introduction to Qualitative Research in Information Systems. In Myers, M. D., & Avison, D. (Eds.), *Qualitative Research in Information Systems: A Reader* (pp. 3–12). London: Sage publications.

Nakatsu, R. T., & Iacovou, C. L. (2009). A Comparative Study of Important Risk Factors Involved in Offshore and Domestic Outsourcing of Software Development Projects: A Two-Panel Delphi Study. *Information & Management*, *46*, 57–68. doi:10.1016/j.im.2008.11.005

Navarette, C. J., & Pick, J. B. (2002). Information technology expenditure and industry performance: The case of the Mexican banking industry. *Journal of Global Information Technology Management*, *5*(2), 7–28.

Neerincx Pieter, B. T., & Leunissen, J. A. (2005). Evolution of web services in bioinformatics. *Briefings in Bioinformatics*, *6*(2), 178–188.

NetWorld Alliance. (2003). *Timeline: The ATM's history*. Retrieved June, 20 2009, from http://www.atm24.com/NewsSection/Industry%20News/Timeline%20-%20The%20ATM%20History.aspx

Neuhaus, M., & Benke, H. (2005). *A graph matching based approach to fingerprint classification using directional variance, Audio and Video based Biometric Person Authentication* (*Vol. 3546*, pp. 191–200). LNCS.

News, B. B. C. (2009). *Shoppers are targeted in ATM scam*. Retrieved July 11, 2009, from http://news.bbc.co.uk/2/hi/uk _news/england/tees/4796002.stm

Nichols, R. K., & Lekkas, P. C. (2002). *Wireless Security Models, Threats, and Solutions*. New York, NY: McGraw-Hill.

Niederhauser, D. S., & Shapiro, A. (2003, April). Learner Variables Associated with Reading and Learning in a Hypertext Environment. Paper presented at the meeting of the *American Educational Research Association*, Chicago, IL.

Nielsen, J. (1993). *Usability Engineering*. Boston, MA: Academic Press.

Nielsen, J. (1994). Heuristic evaluation. In Nielsen, J., & Mack, R. L. (Eds.), *Usability Inspection Methods* (pp. 25–64). New York, NY: John Wiley & Sons.

Nielsen, J., & Landauer, T. K. (1993). A mathematical model of the finding of usability problems, *Proceedings of the ACM INTERCHI'93 Conference,* Amsterdam, the Netherlands, 206-213.

Noel, J., & Eric, B. (1996). *The definitive guide to using the Win32 API with visual basic 4.* Los Angeles, CA: Waite Group Press.

Nonaka, I. (1994). A dynamic theory of organizational knowledge creation. *Organization Science, 5*(1), 14–37. doi:10.1287/orsc.5.1.14

Nonaka, I., & Takeuchi, H. (1996). A Theory of Organizational Knowledge Creation. *International Journal of Technology Management, 11*(7/8), 833–846.

Norris, C., Sullivan, T., Poirot, J., & Soloway, E. (2003). No Access, No Use, No Impact: Snapshot Surveys of Educational Technology in K-12. *Journal of Research on Technology in Education, ISTE, 36*(1), 15–28.

NSO. (2008). *Nso News Release. December 15, 2008.* Malta: National Statistics Office.

O'Reilly, T. (2005). *What Is Web 2.0. Design Patterns and Business Models for the Next Generation of Software.* Retrieved November 10, 2009, from http://oreilly.com/web2 /archive/what-is-web-20.html

Odedra, M. (1991). Information technology transfer to developing countries: is really taking place? In J. Berleur & J. Drumm (Eds.) *The 4th IFIF.TC9 International Conference on Human Choice and Computers,* North Holland, Amsterdam, Netherlands, HCC 4 held jointly with the CEC FAST Program.

OECD. (2004). *Are Pupils Ready for a Technology-rich World? What PISA Studies Tell Us.* France: OECD.

OECD. (2005). E-learning in tertiary education: where do we stand? *Evaluation & Skills, 4*(1), 1–293.

O'Hara, K., & Stevens, D. (2006). Democracy, Ideology and Process Re-Engineering: Realising the Benefits of e-Government in Singapore. In Proceedings of Workshop on e-Government: Barriers and Opportunities, WWW06 (in press), Edinburgh. Huai, J., Shen, V. and Tan, C. J., Eds

Omrane, B., Norman, M., Senan, M., Ishak, A., & Taib, S. (2003). CAD System for Power Electronic Converters. *Journal of Engineering Transaction, 6,* 97–105.

Omrane, B., Norman, M., Senan, M., Ishak, A., & Taib, S. (2005). A Learning Aid Tool for Power Electronics Converters. *Journal of Electrical Systems, 1*(2), 35–62.

Omrane, B., Norman, M., Senan, M., Ishak, A., & Taib, S. (2005). Knowledge-based design aid tool for power electronic converters, Engineering Computations. *International Journal for Computer-Aided Engineering. Emerald, 22*(1), 5–14.

Ondo, K., & Smith, M. (2006). Outside IT the Case for Full IT Outsourcing: Study Findings Indicate Many Hospitals Are Turning to Full IT Outsourcing to Achieve IT Excellence. What's the Best Approach for Your Organization? *Healthcare Financial Management,* (February): 1–3.

OpenBioInformatics Projects. (n.d.). *Open BioInformatics Foundation – Projects.* Retrieved from http://www.open-bio.org/wiki/Projects

Oracle, S. O. A. (n.d.). *Oracle - Service-Oriented Architecture (SOA).* Retrieved September 20, 2008, from http://www.oracle.com/tec hnologies/soa/index.html

Orlikowski, W., & Baroudi, J. J. (1991). Studying Information Technology in Organizations: Research Approaches and Assumptions. *Information Systems Research, 2*(1), 1–31. doi:10.1287/isre.2.1.1

Ozcelik, E., & Yildirim, S. (2005). Factors influencing the use of cognitive tools in Web-based learning environments: A case study. *The Quarterly Review of Distance Education, 6*(4), 295–308.

Pandey, S., et al. (2005). Client assisted location data acquisition scheme for secure enterprise wireless networks. In *Proceedings of the ACM, 2005... v.2, p.1174–1179.*

Paul, T. J., & Kim, M. T. (2003). E-government Around the World: Lessons, Challenges and Future Directions. *Government Information Quarterly, 20,* 389–394. doi:10.1016/j.giq.2003.08.001

Péréz López, S., Montes Peón, J. M., & Vázquez Ordás, C.Managing knowledge: The link between culture and organizational learning. *Journal of Knowledge Management, 8*(6), 93–104. doi:10.1108/13673270410567657

Perry, M. (2003). Distributed cognition. In Carroll, J. M. (Ed.), *HCI models, theories, and frameworks: Toward a multidisciplinary science* (pp. 193–222). San Francisco, CA: Martin Kaufmann. doi:10.1016/B978-155860808-5/50008-3

Pettigrew, A. M. (1985). Contextualist Research and the Study of Organizational Change Processes. In Mumford, E., Hirschheim, R., Fitzgerald, G., & Wood-Harper, A. T. (Eds.), *Research Methods in Information Systems* (pp. 53–78). Amsterdam: North Holland.

Phillips, P. J., Wechsler, H., Huang, J., & Rauss, P. (1998). The FERET database and evaluation procedure for face-recognition algorithms. *Image and Vision Computing Journal, 16*(5), 295–306. doi:10.1016/S0262-8856(97)00070-X

Pieter, B., Neerincx, T., & Leunissen, J. A. M. (2005). Evolution of Web Services In Bioinformatics. *Briefings in Bioinformatics, 6*(2), 178–188.

Pirretti, M., Traynor, P., McDaniel, P., & Waters, B. (2006). Secure Attribute-Based Systems. *ACM Conference on Computer and Communications Security* (pp. 99–112). New York: ACM.

Pitman, T. (2009). Recognition of Prior Learning: The accelerated rate of change in Australian universities. *Higher Education Research & Development, 28*(2), 227–240. doi:10.1080/07294360902725082

Pittard, V., Bannister, P., & Dunn, J. (2003). *The Big pICTure: The Impact of ICT on Attainment, Motivation and Learning,* DfES Publications, UK. http://www.dfes.gov.uk/research/ data/uploadfiles/ThebigpICTure.pdf

Poh, N., & Kittler, J. (2008). On Using Error Bounds to Optimize Cost-sensitive Multimodal Biometric Authentication, *17th International Conference on Pattern Recognition* (pp. 1 – 4)

Polemi, D. (1997). *Biometric Techniques: Review and evaluation of biometric techniques for identification and authentication, INFOSEC*. Institute of Communications and Computer Systems, National Technical University of Athens.

Porter, M. F. (1980). An algorithm for suffix stripping. *Program, 14*(3), 130–137.

Post, L. J. G., Roos, M., Marshall, M. S., Driel, R. V., & Breit, T. M. (2007). A semantic web approach applied to integrative bioinformatics experimentation: a biological use case with genomics data. *Bioinformatics (Oxford, England), 23*(22), 3080–3087.

Pouget, M., & Osborne, M. (2004). Accreditation or *Validation* of Prior Experiential Learning: Knowledge and *savoirs* in France – a different perspective? *Studies in Continuing Education, 26*(1), 45–66. doi:10.1080/158037042000199452

Prensky, M. (2001). Digital Natives, Digital Immigrants. *Horizon, 9*(5), 1–6. doi:10.1108/10748120110424816

Prensky, M. (2007). *Digital Game-Based Learning*. New York: McGraw-Hill.

Quale, A. (2003). Trends in instructional ICT infrastructure. In Plomp, T., Anderson, R., Law, N., & Quale, A. (Eds.), *Cross-national information and communication technology policies and practices in education* (pp. 31–42). Greenwich, CT: IPA.

Quality Education Data (QED). (2004). *Technology Purchasing Forecast, 2003-2004*. Denver, CO: Scholastic, Inc.

Raelin, J. A. (1997). A model of work-based learning. *Organization Science, 8*(6), 563–578. doi:10.1287/orsc.8.6.563

Rama, A., Goodwin, R., Doshi, P., & Roeder, S. (2003). A Method For Semantically Enhancing the Service Discovery Capabilities of UDDI, In *Proceedings of the Workshop on Information Integration on the Web, IJCAI 2003*, Mexico, Aug 9-10, 2003

Raman, M., Stephenaus, R., Alam, N., & Kuppusamy, M. (2008). Information Technology in Malaysia: E-Service Quality and Uptake of Internet Banking. *Journal of Internet Banking and Commerce, 13*(2), 2–17.

Ramayah, T., Ramoo, V., & Ibrahim, A. (2008). Profiling Online And Manual Tax Filers: Results from An Exploratory Study In Penang, Malaysia. *Labuan e-Journal of Muamalat and Society, 2,* 1-18.

RBR. (2010). *Global ATM Market and Forecasts to 2013.* Retrieved May 7, 2010, from www.rbrlondon.com

Redaschi, N., Doelz, R., & Eggenberger, F. (1995). *HASSEL v5.* Advanced Computer Network Communications: Hierarchical Access System for Sequence Libraries in Europe.

Reychav, I., & Weisberg, J. (2009). Good for workers, good for companies: How knowledge sharing benefits individual employees. *Knowledge and Process Management, 16*(4), 186–197. doi:10.1002/kpm.335

Richardson, W. (2004). Personal mail to Stephen Downes, quoted in Educational Blogging. *EDUCAUSE Review, 39*(5), 14–26.

Riding, R., & Rayner, S. (1998). *Cognitive styles and learning strategies: Understanding Style differences in learning and behaviour.* London: David Fulton Publishers.

Ringstaff, C., & Kelley, L. (2002). *The Learning Return on our Educational Investment.* Retrieved October 6, 2009 from http://www.westedrtec.org.

Roach, S. (1987). *America's technology dilemma: A profile of the information economy. Economics Newsletter Series.* New York: Morgan Stanley.

Roberts, V. (2001). Managing Strategic Outsourcing in the Healthcare Industry. *Journal of Healthcare Management, 46*(4), 239–249.

Robey, D., Boudreau, M., & Rose, G. M. (2000). Information Technology and Organizational Learning: a Review and Assessment of Research. *Accounting. Management and Information Technologies, 10,* 125–155. doi:10.1016/S0959-8022(99)00017-X

Roggenkamp, K. (2004). Development Modules to Unleash the Potential of Mobile Government: Developing mobile government applications from a user perspective. In the proceedings of the 4th European Conference on e-Government, Dublin, Ireland.

Roode, D. (1993). Implications for teaching of a process-based research framework for information systems. In *Proceedings of the 8th annual conference of the International Academy for Information Management.* Orlando, FL.

Rosenberg, M. (2001). *E-Learning, Strategies for Developing Knowledge in the Digital Age. New York.* McGraw-Hill.

Ross, A., & Govindarajan, R. (2005). Feature Level Fusion Using Hand and Face Biometrics, In. *Proceedings of SPIE Conference on Biometric Technology for Human Identification, II,* 196–204.

Ross, A., & Jain, A. K. (2003). Information Fusion in Biometrics. *Pattern Recognition Letters, 24,* 2115–2125. doi:10.1016/S0167-8655(03)00079-5

Rottman, J. W., & Lacity, M. C. (2004). Twenty Practices for Offshore Sourcing. *MIS Quarterly Executive, 3*(3), 117–130.

Rouet, J. F., & Levonen, J. J. (1996). Studying and learning with hypertext: Empirical studies and their implications. In Rouet, J.-F. (Eds.), *Hypertext and cognition* (pp. 9–24). Mahwah, NJ: Lawrence Erlbaum Associates.

Russell, M., Bebell, D., O'Dwyer, L., & O'Connor, K. (2003). Examining Teacher Technology Use Implications for Preservice and Inservice Teacher Preparation. *Journal of Teacher Education, 54*(4), 297–310. doi:10.1177/0022487103255985

Sadeh, N. (2002). *M-Commerce: Technologies, services, and business models.* Hershey, PA: Wiley Computer Publishing.

Sahai, A., & Waters, B. (2005). Fuzzy Identity-Based Encryption.

Sakhtevil, S. (2007). Managing Risks in Offshore Systems Development. *Communications of the ACM, 50*(4), 69–75. doi:10.1145/1232743.1232750

Salonius-Pasternak, D. E., & Gelfond, H. S. (2005). The next level of research on electronic play: Potential benefits and contextual influences for children and adolescents. *Human Technology, 1*, 5–22.

Samaria, F., & Harter, A. (1994). Parameterization of a stochastic model for human face identification. In *Proceedings of IEEE Workshop on Applications of Computer Vision*.

Sandholtz, J. H. (2001). Learning to teach with technology: A comparison of teacher development programs. *Journal of Technology and Teacher Education, 9*(3), 349–374.

Sang Hyun, K., Holmes, K., & Mims, C. (2005). Opening a dialogue on the new technologies in education. *TechTrends: Linking Research & Practice to Improve Learning, 49*(3), 54–89.

SAP SOA. (n.d.). *SAP – Service-Oriented Architecture (SOA)*. Retrieved August 26, 2008, from http://www.sap. com/ platform/soa/index.epx

Sarier, N. D. (2010). *A New Biometric Identity Based Encryption Scheme secure against DoS Attacks. Special Issue on "Trusted Computing and Communications". Journal of Security and Communication Networks SCN.* Wiley Interscience.

Sarier, N. D. (2007). Identity Based Encryption: *Security notions and new identity based encryption schemes based on Sakai-Kasahara's Key Construction.* Unpublished Master's thesis. RWTH Aachen.

Sarier, N. D. (2008). A New Biometric Identity Based Encryption Scheme. *The 2008 International Symposium on Trusted Computing - TrustCom 2008* (pp. 2061-2066). IEEE Computer Society.

Sarier, N. D. (in press). Generic Constructions of Biometric Identity Based Encryption Systems. *WISTP'10.* Heidelberg, Germany: Springer.

Sasaki, M., & Shinnou, H. (2005). Spam detection using text clustering, *International Conference on Cyberworlds* (pp.1-4). Singapore: IEEE Computer Society

Sayed, A. et al. Network-based wireless location: challenges faced in developing techniques for accurate wireless location information.

Schneider, R. (2005). Hypertext narrative and the reader: A view from cognitive theory. *European Journal of English Studies, 9*(2), 197–208. doi:10.1080/13825570500172067

Schneider, K. (2003). A comparison of event models for naive bayes anti-spam e-mail filtering, *11th Conference of the European Chapter of the Association for Computational Linguistics.* Hungary: ACM

Schugurensky, D. (2000). *The Forms of Informal Learning: Towards a Conceptualization of the Field.* NALL Working Paper 19. Toronto, Canada: Centre for the Study of Education and Work.

Schwiderski-Grosche, S., & Knospe, H. (2002). Secure mobile commerce. *Electronics and Communication Engineering Journal, 14*(5), 228–238. doi:10.1049/ecej:20020506

SecurityDigest. (2010). *ATM Fraud and Security Digest News.* Retrieved April 7, 2010, from www.atmsecurity. com/monthly-digest March 2010

Selwyn, N., Gorard, S., & Furlong, J. (2006). Adults' use of computers and the Internet for self-education. *Studies in the Education of Adults, 38*(2), 141–159.

Sena, O., & Paul, P. (2009). Exploring the adoption of a service innovation: A study of Internet banking adopters and non-adopters. *Journal of Financial Services Marketing, 13*(4), 284–299. doi:10.1057/fsm.2008.25

Senaratne, R., Halgamuge, S., & Hsu, A. (2009). Face recognition by extending elastic bunch graph matching with particle swarm optimization. *Journal of Multimedia, 4*(4), 204–214. doi:10.4304/jmm.4.4.204-214

Senaratne, R., & Halgamuge, S. (2006). Optimized landmark model matching for face recognition. In *Proceedings of 7th International Conference on Automatic Face and Gesture Recognition* (pp. 120–125).

Senge, P. M. (1990). *The fifth discipline: art and practice of the learning organization*. New York: Doubleday.

Senn, J. A. (2000). The emergence of m-commerce. *IEEE Computer Magazine, 33*(12), 148–150.

Sevilla, C., & Wells, T. D. (1988). Contracting to ensure training transfer. *Training & Development, 6*(1), 10–11.

Shackel, B. (1971). Human factors in the P.L.A. meat handling automation scheme. A case study and some conclusions. *International Journal of Production Research, 9*(1), 95–121. doi:10.1080/00207547108929864

Shaffer, D. W. (2006). *How Computer Games Help Children Learn*. New York: Palgrave Macmillan. doi:10.1057/9780230601994

Shapiro, A. M. (1998). Promoting active learning: The role of system structure in learning from hypertext. *Human-Computer Interaction, 13*(1), 1–35. doi:10.1207/s15327051hci1301_1

Shapiro, A. M. (1999). The relevance of hierarchies to learning biology from hypertext. *Journal of the Learning Sciences, 8*(2), 215–243. doi:10.1207/s15327809jls0802_2

Shapiro, A., & Niederhauser, D. (2004). Learning from hypertext: Research issues and findings. In Jonassen, D. (Ed.), *Handbook of research for educational communications and technology* (2nd ed., pp. 605–620). Mahwah, NJ: Lawrence Erlbaum Associates.

Sheila, A., McIlraith, T. C. S., & Zeng, H. (2001). *Semantic Web Services*. IEEE Educational Activities Department.

Shi, W., Jang, I., & Yoo, H. S. (2009). Chosen Ciphertext Secure Fuzzy Identity-Based Encryption Scheme with Short Ciphertext. [IEEE Computer Society.]. *ICCIT, 09*, 1036–1040.

Shinkman, R. (2000). Outsourcing on the Upswing. *Modern Healthcare, 30*(37), 46–54.

Shittu, A. J. K. (2009). Information Technology Outsourcing in Developing Countries- an Exploratory, Interpretive Case study of Malaysia Suppliers' Perspective. Unpublished doctoral dissertation, University Technology PETRONAS, Malaysia.

Shittu, A. J. K., Mahmood, A. K.. & Ahlan, A. R (2009). Information Security and Mutual Trust as Determining Factors for Information Technology Outsourcing Success. *International Journal of Computer Science and Information Security IJCSIS* – July 2009.

Shneiderman, B., & Kiersley, G. (1989). *Hypertext hands on!*New York: Addison-Wesley.

Shrivastava, P. A. (1983). Typology of Organizational Learning Systems. *Journal of Management Studies, 20*, 1–28. doi:10.1111/j.1467-6486.1983.tb00195.x

Siau, K., & Shen, Z. (2003). Mobile communications and mobile services. *International Journal of Mobile Communications, 1*(1-2), 3–14. doi:10.1504/IJMC.2003.002457

Simonin, B. L. (1997). The importance of collaborative know-how: An empirical test of the learning organization. *Academy of Management Journal, 40*(5), 1150–1173. doi:10.2307/256930

Sinton, J. (1994) *Outsourcing: Why Is It So? An Exploratory Study Into Factors That Contribute To Outsourcing Information Systems*, Research Report, Curtin University of Technology, Perth, November.

Sirisanyalak, B., & Sornil, O. (2007). An artificial immunity-based spam detection system, *IEEE Congress on Evolutionary Computation* (pp.3392-3398). Singapore: IEEE.

Sivin-Kachala, J., & Bialo, E. (2000). *2000 research report on the effectiveness of technology in schools* (7th ed.). Washington, DC: Software and Information Industry Association.

Škerlavaj, M., & Dimovski, V. (2006). Study of the Mutual Connections among Information-communication Technologies, Organisational Learning and Business Performance. *Journal for East European Management Studies, 11*(1), 9–29.

Škerlavaj, M. (2003). *Vpliv informacijsko-komunikacijskih tehnologij in organizacijskega učenja na uspešnost poslovanja: teoretična in empirična analiza*. Unpublished Master's theses. Ljubljana: Ekonomska fakulteta.

Skillman, B. (1998). Fired up at the IRS. *Accounting Technology, 14*, 12–20.

Slater, S. F., & Narver, J. C. (1995). Market orientation and the learning organization. *Journal of Marketing, 59*(3), 63–74. doi:10.2307/1252120

Sloan, T. R., Hyland, P. W. B., & Beckett, R. C. (2002). Learning as a competitive advantage: Innovative training in the Australian aerospace industry. *International Journal of Technology Management, 23*(4), 341–352. doi:10.1504/IJTM.2002.003014

Smeraldi, F., Capdevielle, N., & Bigün, J. (1999). Facial features detection by saccadic exploration of the gabor decomposition and support vector machines. *Proceedings of the 11th Scandinavian Conference on Image Analysis* (pp. 39-44).

Smith, M. D., Bailey, J., & Brynjolfsson, E. (2000). Understanding Digital Markets: Review and Assessment. In Brynjolfsson, E., & Kahin, B. (Eds.), *Understanding the Digital Economy*. Cambridge, MA: MIT Press.

Smith, R. (2008). Aligning Competencies, Capabilities and Resources. *Research Technology Management: The Journal of the Industrial Research Institute*, September-October.

Snopes. (2004). *Thieves Equip ATMs with Duplicate Card Reader and Wireless Camera*. Retrieved April 20, 2010, from http://www.snopes.com/fraud/ atm/atmcamera.asp

Software and data (n.d.). *Software and data – Natural Language Processing Group*. Retrieved March 20, 2009 from http://nlp.cs.aueb.gr/software.html

Software, A. G. SOA. (n.d.). *Software AG – Service-Oriented Architecture (SOA)*. Retrieved September 11, 2008, from http://www.softwareag.com/ Corporate/products/wm/default.asp

Solow, R. M. (1957). Technical Change and the Aggregate Production Function. *The Review of Economics and Statistics, 39*(3), 312–320. doi:10.2307/1926047

Souchelnytskyi, S. (2005). Proteomics of TGFbeta signaling and its impact on breast cancer. *Expert Review of Proteomics, 2*, 925–935.

Spam Filter Reviews. (n.d.). *Spam Filter Reviews*. Retrieved January 25, 2010, from http://www.whichspamfilter.com /Reviews/ SpamFilterReviews.htm

SpiderLabs. (2009). *ATM Malware Analysis Briefing*. Retrieved May 15, 2010, from https://www.trustwave.com/ spiderLabs-papers.php

Spiro, R. J., Feltovich, P. J., Jacobson, M. J., & Coulson, R. L. (1991). Cognitive flexibility, constructivism, and hypertext: Random access instruction for advanced knowledge acquisition in ill-structured domains. *Educational Technology, 5*, 24–33.

Stake, E. (1994). *Handbook of Qualitative Research* (Denzin, N. K., & Lincoln, Y. S., Eds.). London: Sage Publications.

Stathaki, T. (2008). *Image fusion – algorithms and applications*. United Kingdom: Academic Press.

Steven, K. (2002). Testing iris and face recognition in a personnel identification application. *In The Biometric Consortium Conference*, February 2002. Retrieved October, 21, 2009, from http://www.itl.nist.gov/div895/isi s/bc/bc2001/FINAL_BCFEB02/FINAL_1 _Final%20Steve%20King.pdf

Stevens, R., Robinson, A., & Goble, C. (2003). myGrid: Personalized BioInformatics on the Information Grid. *Bioinformatics (Oxford, England), 19*(90001), 302–304.

Stoyanova., et al. Evaluation of impact factors on RSS accuracy for localization and tracking applications. In MOBIWAC '07: *Proceedings of The 5th ACM International Workshop on Mobility Management and Wireless Access*, 2007.

Sun, S. O. A. (n.d.). *Sun Service-Oriented Architecture (SOA)*. Retrieved August 28, 2008, from http://www.sun.com/ products/soa/index.jsp.

Swanton, B., & Finley, I. (2007). *SOA and BPM for Enterprise Applications: A Dose of Reality*, Report #: AMR-R-20372, AMR Research Inc., 125 Summer Street, 4th floor, Boston, MA 02110-1616.

Sweller, J., van Merrienboer, J. G., & Paas, F. G. (1998). Cognitive architecture and instructional design. *Educational Psychology Review, 10*(3), 251–296. doi:10.1023/A:1022193728205

Tachikawa, K. (2003). A perspective on the evolution of mobile communications. *IEEE Communications Magazine, 41*(10), 66–73. doi:10.1109/MCOM.2003.1235597

Taheri, A., et al. *(2004)*. Location fingerprinting on infrastructure 802.11 wireless local area networks (WLANs) using Locus. *In:* Anual Ieee International Conference - Local Computer Networks, *29*.

Tallon, P. P., Kraemer, K. L., & Gurbaxani, V. (2000). Executives' Perceptions of the Business Value of Information Technology: A Process-Oriented Approach. *Journal of Management Information Systems, 16*(4), 145–173.

Tan, C., & Sia, S. (2006). Managing flexibility in outsourcing. *Journal of the Association for Information Systems, 7*(4), 179–206.

Tanenbaum, A. S., & Van Steen, M. (2002). *Distributed Systems: Principles and Paradigms.* Upper Saddle River, N.J.: Prentice-Hall.

Tarjoman, M., & Zarei, S. (2008). Automatic fingerprint classification using graph theory, World Academy of Science. *Engineering and Technology, 47*, 214–218.

Thakar, S., Ambite, J. L., & Knoblock, C. A. (2005, September). Composing, Optimizing, and Executing Plans for bioinformatics Web services. *VLDB Journal, Special Issue on Data Management. Analysis and Mining for Life Sciences, 14*(3), 330–353.

The National ICT Association of Malaysia (PIKOM). (2008). *ICT Strategies, Societal and Market Touch.* Retrieved on June 24th, 2009. from http://www.witsa.org/news/2009-1 /html_email_newsletter_jan09_b.html

The STAR. (2009). Amount of Malaysian's choosing e-filing up by 30%. 1st May.

The, S. T. A. R. (2009). *It's Time Inland Revenue Board got Real on E-Filing.* Retrieved on June 19th, 2009. from http://thestar.com.my/news/story.asp? file=/2009/3/2/focus/3380923&sec=focus

TIBCO SOA. (n.d.). *TIBCO – Service-Oriented Architecture (SOA) Resource Center.* Retrieved September 1, 2008, from http://www.tibco.com/solution s/soa/default.jsp

Tippins, M. J., & Sohi, R. S. (2003). IT competency and firm performance: Is organizational learning a missing link? *Strategic Management Journal, 24*(8), 745–761. doi:10.1002/smj.337

Tony, M., Gavin, K., David, C., & Jan, K. (2001). Biometric product testing final report. *Issue 1.0, CESG/BWG Biometric Test Programme.* Retrieved August 17 2009, from http://www.cesg.gov.uk/technology/ biometrics/media/Biometric% 20Test%20Report%20pt1.pdf

Trauth, E. M. (1997). Achieving the Research Goal with Qualitative Methods: Lessons Learned along the Way. In Lee, A. S., Liebenau, J., & DeGross, J. I. (Eds.), *Information Systems and Qualitative Research* (pp. 225–245). London: Chapman and Hall.

Trustgate Sdn, M. S. C. Bhd. (2009). *Secure E-Filing.* Retrieved on June 24th, 2009. from http://www.mykad.com.my /Website/secureefiling.php

Turban, E., King, D., Lee, J., & Viehland, D. (2004). *Electronic Commerce 2004: a Managerial Perspective.* Englewood Cliffs, NJ: Pearson/Prentice-Hall.

Tuschling, A., & Engemann, C. (2006). From education to lifelong learning: The emerging regime of learning in the European Union. *Educational Philosophy and Theory, 38*(4), 451–469. doi:10.1111/j.1469-5812.2006.00204.x

Types of Spam Filters. (n.d.). *Types of Spam Filters.* Retrieved January 25, 2010 from http://www.whichspamfilter.com/ TypesOfFilters.htm

Ulrich, D., Jick, T., & von Glinow, M. A. (1993). High-impact learning: Building and diffusing learning capability. *Organizational Dynamics*, *22*(2), 52–66. doi:10.1016/0090-2616(93)90053-4

Underwood, J., et al (2005). *Impact of Broadband in Schools,* Nottingham Trent University, Becta, June 2005.

Underwood, J., et al. (2006). *ICT Test Bed Evaluation-Evaluation of the ICT Test Bed Project,* Nottingham Trent University, UK. Retrieved from http://www.evaluation.ictte stbed.org.uk/about

Unni, R., & Harmon, R. (2003). Location-based services: models for strategy development in m-commerce. *In proceedings of IEEE International Conference on Management of Engineering Technology*, pp. 416-424, Portland, USA.

van Liesdonk, P. P. (2007). *Anonymous and fuzzy identity-based encryption.* Unpublished Master's Thesis. Technische Universiteit Eindhoven.

Varney, S. (2008). Leadership learning: key to organizational transformation. *Strategic HR Review*, *7*(1), 5–10. doi:10.1108/14754390810880471

Varshney, U. (2002). Mobile commerce: framework, applications and networking support. *Mobile Networks and Applications*, *7*(3), 185–198. doi:10.1023/A:1014570512129

Varshney, U., & Vetter, R. (2000). Emerging mobile and wireless networks (Technology information). *Communications of the ACM*, *43*(6), 73–81. doi:10.1145/336460.336478

VISA. (2004). *Guidelines for PIN Security Requirement: Version 2.0.* Retrieved March 6, 2010, from http://partnernetwork.visa.com/st/pin/pdfs/PCI PIN Security Requirements.pdf

Voydock, V. L., & Kent, S. T. (1983). Security Mechanisms in High-level Network protocols. *ACM Computing Surveys*, *15*(2), 35–71. doi:10.1145/356909.356913

W3C. (n.d.). *URIs, URLs, and URNs: Clarifications and Recommendations 1.0.* Retrieved June 14, 2006, from http://www.w3.org/TR/uri-clarification/

W3C. (n.d.). *Web Services Description Language (WSDL) 1.1.* Retrieved October 7, 2008, from http://www.w3.org/TR/wsdl

W3C. (n.d.). *Web Services Interoperability Organization.* Retrieved October 15, 2008, from http://www.ws-i.org/)

Wagner, D., Day, R., James, T., Kozma, R., Miller, J., & Unnwin, T. (2005). *Monitoring and evaluation of ICT in education projects: A handbook for developing countries.* Washington: infoDev, World Bank.

Wall, B. (1998). Measuring the Right Stuff: Identifying and Applying the Right Knowledge. *Knowledge Management Review*, *1*(4), 20–24.

Walsham, G. (1993). *Interpreting information systems in organizations.* Chichester, UK: John Wiley & Sons.

Walsham, G. (1995). The Emergence of Interpretivism in IS Research. *Information Systems Research*, *6*(4), 376–394. doi:10.1287/isre.6.4.376

Walsham, G. (2006). Doing Interpretive Research. *European Journal of Information Systems*, *15*(3), 320–330. doi:10.1057/palgrave.ejis.3000589

Wang, S. J., & Lee, Y. S. (1996). Development of an Expert System for Designing, Analysing and Optimising Power Converters. In *Proc. of the Nineteenth Convention of Electrical and Electronics Engineers*, 359-362

Wasserman, A. S. (1989). Redesigning Xerox: A design strategy based on operability. In Klemmer, E. T. (Ed.), *Ergonomics: Harness the Power of Human Factors in Your Business* (pp. 7–44). Norwood, NJ: Ablex.

West, D. (2002). *Global E-Government.* Providence, Rhode Island: Brown University.

Wheeler, S. (2007). Learning with "e"s: Defining technology supported e-learning within a knowledge economy. In Fernstrom, K. (Ed.), *Readings in Technology in Education* (pp. 306–312). Abbotsford, BC: UCFV Press.

White, T. (2002). *Reinventing the IT Department*. Oxford, UK: Butterworth-Heinemann.

Wholey, D. R., Padman, R., Hamer, R., & Schwartz, S. (2001). Determinants of Information Technology Outsourcing Among Health Maintenance Organizations. *Health Care Management Science*, *4*(3), 229–239. doi:10.1023/A:1011401000445

Wildes, R. P. (1997). Iris recognition: An emerging biometric technology. *Proceedings of the IEEE*, *85*, 1348–1363. doi:10.1109/5.628669

Wilkinson, M., Gossler, D., Farmer, A., & Stein, L. (2003). A Bio-Moby Project Explores Open-Source, Simple, Extensible Protocols for Enabling Biological Database Interoperability. In *Proceedings of Virt. Conference Genom and Bioinformatics, 3*, 16-26.

Willcocks, K. T., & Heck, E. (2002). The Winner's Curse in IT Outsourcing: Strategies for Avoiding Relational Trauma-. *California Management Review*, *44*(2), 47–69.

Willcocks, L. P., Lacity, M. C., & Kern, T. (1999). Risk Mitigation in IT Outsourcing Strategy Revisited: Longitudinal Case Research at LISA. *The Journal of Strategic Information Systems*, *8*, 285–314. doi:10.1016/S0963-8687(00)00022-6

Willcocks, L., & Lester, S. (1997). Assessing IT Productivity: Any Way Out of the Labyrinth? In Willcocks, L., Feeny, D. F., & Islei, G. (Eds.), *Managing IT as a Strategic Resource, Ch4* (pp. 64–93). London: The McGraw-Hill Company.

Williams, K. (2003). *Why I (still) want my MTV: Music video and aesthetic communication*. Cresskill, NJ: Hampton Press.

Wiskott, L., Fellous, J. M., Kruger, N., & von der Malsburg, C. (1997). Face recognition by elastic bunch graph matching. *IEEE Transactions on Pattern Analysis and Machine Intelligence*, *19*(7), 775–779. doi:10.1109/34.598235

Wood, R. T. A., Griffiths, M. D., & Parke, A. (2007). Experiences of time loss among videogame players: An empirical study. *Cyberpsychology & Behavior*, *10*(1), 38–44. doi:10.1089/cpb.2006.9994

Yaghi, H., & Krim, H. (2008). Probabilistic graph matching by canonical decomposition. *Proceedings of the IEEE International Conference on Image Processing* (pp. 2368 – 2371).

Yang, B., Xue, T., Zhao, J., Kommidi, C., Soneja, J., Li, J., et al. (2006). Bioinformatics web services, In *Proceedings of The 2006 International Conference on Bioinformatics & Computational Biology (BIOCOMP)*, June 2006, Las Vegas, NV.

Yasat, A.-U.-H., et al. Low cost solution for location determination of mobile nodes in a wireless local area network. In ACE '06: *Proceedings Of The 2006 Acm Sigchi International Conference On Advances In Computer Entertainment Technology*, 2006, New York, NY.

Yin, R. K. (1993). *Applications of case study research*. Newbury Park, CA: Sage Publications.

Yin, R. K. (2003). *Case Study Research, Design and Methods* (2nd ed.). Newbury Park, CA: Sage Publications.

Yoon, E. J., & Yoo, K. Y. (2005). A new efficient fingerprint-based remote user authentication scheme for multimedia systems, in *9th Int. Conf. Knowledge-Based & Intelligent Information & Engineering Systems (KES 2005)*, 2005, (pp. 332–338), Paper LNAI 3683.

Young, K. (2009). Understanding Online Gaming Addiction and Treatment Issues for Adolescents. *The American Journal of Family Therapy*, *37*(5), 355–372. doi:10.1080/01926180902942191

Young, M. (2007). Qualifications frameworks: Some conceptual issues. *European Journal of Education*, *42*(4), 445–457. doi:10.1111/j.1465-3435.2007.00323.x

Young, S. (2005). Outsourcing in the Australian Health Sector: The interplay of Economics and Politics. *International Journal of Public Sector Management*, *18*(1), 25–36. doi:10.1108/09513550510576134

Young, S. H. (2003). Outsourcing and Benchmarking in a Rural Public Hospital: Does Economic Theory Provide the Complete Answer? *Rural and Remote Health*, *3*, 124–137.

Yuan, Y., & Zhang, J. J. (2003). Towards an appropriate business model for m-commerce. *International Journal of Mobile Communications, 1*(1-2), 35–56. doi:10.1504/IJMC.2003.002459

Yun, S. H., Lee, B. W., Kim, H. K., & Kim, B. Y. Y. (2000, December). Dynamic Erbium-Doped fiber Amplifier Based on Active Gain Flattening with Fiber Acousto-optic Tunable Filters. *IEEE Photonics Technology Letters, 11*(10).

Zakareya, E., & Zahir, I. (2005). E-Government Adoption: Architecture and Barriers. *Business Process Management Journal, 11*(5), 589–611. doi:10.1108/14637150510619902

Zalesak, M. (2003). *Overview and opportunities of mobile government*. Retrieved June 21, 2005 from http://www.developmentgateway.or g/ download/218309/mGov.doc

Zervas, M. N., Laming, R. I., & Payne, D. N. (1995, March). Efficient Erbium-Doped Fiber Amplifiers Incorporating an Optical Isolator. *IEEE Journal of Quantum Electronics, 31*(3). doi:10.1109/3.364402

Zhang, H., & Ma, H. (2005). Grid-based parallel elastic graph matching face recognition. [LNCS.]. *Proceedings of International Workshop on Web-Based Internet Computing for Science and Engineering, 3842*, 1041–1048.

Zhang, D. *Media structuration – Towards an integrated approach to interactive multimedia-based E-Learning.* (Ph.D. dissertation, The University of Arizona, 2002. Zhang, D., & Nunamaker, J. F. (2003). Powering e-learning in the new millennium: an overview of e-learning and enabling technology. *Information Systems Frontiers, 5*(2), 207–218.

Zhou, Y., Jorgensen, Z., & Inge, M. (2007). Combating Good Word Attacks on Statistical Spam Filters with Multiple Instance Learning. *IEEE International Conference on Tools with Artificial Intelligence* (pp.298-305). France: IEEE Computer Society.

Zorkadis, V., & Donos, P. (2004). On biometrics-based authentication and identification from a privacy-protection perspective deriving privacy-enhancing requirements. *Information Management & Computer Security, 12*(1), 125–137. doi:10.1108/09685220410518883

About the Contributors

Mubarak S. Al-Mutairi received the B.Sc. degree in systems engineering from King Fahd University of Petroleum & Minerals, Dhahran, Saudi Arabia, in 1997, the M.A.Sc. degree in industrial and systems engineering from the University of Florida, Gainesville, Florida, USA, in 2003, and the Ph.D. degree in systems design engineering from the University of Waterloo, Waterloo, Canada, in 2007. From 1997 to 2000, he was an industrial engineer with the Saudi Arabia Oil Company (Aramco). He is currently an assistant professor in the computer science and engineering department and the assistant dean of Hafr Albatin Community College, Hafr Albatin, Saudi Arabia. His research interests include decision analysis, expert systems, information security, fuzzy logic, trust, and e-commerce. He is a member of the IEEE and the recipient of the distinguished teaching award of the University of Waterloo for the year 2007.

Lawan A. Mohammed is currently an Assistant Professor in Computer Science and Engineering Technology Department at King Fahd University of Petroleum and Minerals (HBCC Campus), Saudi Arabia. His main research interests are in the design of Authentication Protocols for both wired and wireless networks, Wireless Mobility, Group Oriented Cryptography, Smartcard Security, and Mathematical Programming.

***

Syed Muhammad Ahsan is an Associate Professor at Department of Computer Science & Engineering at U.E.T., Lahore. He did his Bachelor in Engineering, Master in Computer Science and Ph. D. in Computer Science, all form U.E.T., Lahore. His area of specialization is Cheminformatics / Bioinformatics. He is the Project Director for development of ChemBank V3, a Public data sharing platform for Chemical Biology and related informatics components in collaboration with The Broad Institute of MIT and Harvard. He is also a consultant at Al-Khawarizmi Institute of Computer Science, University of Engineering and Technology, Lahore (KICS-UET) , an institute of applied research in the general area of information technology .His other areas of interest include Distribute Databases, Data Provenance and Semantic Web which has resulted in numerous publications in International books, journals and Conferences.

Tanja Arh graduated of Computer Science at the Faculty of Organizational Sciences, University of Maribor. She obtained her Master's degree at the Faculty of Organizational Sciences, University of Maribor. She is a PhD candidate at Faculty of Economics, University of Ljubljana. She works in Laboratory for Open Systems and Networks at Jožef Stefan Institute as a researcher in the field of e-learning and organizational learning. Her current research is performed mostly for European-wide research programmes (GLOBAL, iCoper, e4VET, etc.) with focus on e-learning, applications of ICT in education, education and transfer of knowledge, human resource development and organizational learning. Tanja Arh is member of Executive Board of Slovenian Project Management Association. She is Technical editor of Slovenian scientific journal Project Management Review.

Borka Jerman Blažič is working as a head of the Laboratory for Open Systems and Networks at Jožef Stefan Institute, Slovenia and as a full professor at the University of Ljubljana, Faculty of Economics in Slovenia. The main field of applications and research are computer communications, internet technologies, security in networking, privacy and internationalisation of Internet services, etc. She is a member of many professional associations and is appointed expert to UNECE UN (Economic Commission for Europe), appointed member of UNECE/CEFAT Team of specialist on Internet enterprise development, appointed member of eTEN management committee of EU, member of FP7 PC on security, chair of the Execom of the Internet Society of Europe (www.isoc-ecc.org), member of New York Academy of science 1999, IEEE, ACM, distinguished member of Slovene Society for Informatics, member of IEEE on Computers, ACM. She is also chair of Slovenian Standardisation Committee on ICT as well as chair of the Slovenian chapter of Internet Society and a member of the European ICT Standardisation Board. She is holding Plaque of appreciation of Thai branch of IFIP and ACM for her services in Internet development. She has published more than 80 papers in refereed journals, 154 communications scientific meetings, 15 chapters in scientific books, 6 books and other 142 non-classified contributions.

Omrane Bouketir is currently an Assistant Professor in Electrical and Electronics Engineering Technology Department at King Fahd University of Petroleum and Minerals (KFUPM), HBCC Campus, Saudi Arabia. Prior to joining KFUPM he has been with the Nottingham University Malaysia Campus as an Assistant Professor. Dr Omrane's main research interests include CAD in electrical engineering, power electronics systems, and renewable energy systems in addition to pedagogical issues in engineering.

Belloui Bouzid was born in Ouled Tebane, Algeria, in 1968. He received the B.S. degree from the University of Farhat Abass in Setif, Algeria, 1996 and the M.S. degree from the University of Malaya, Malaysia, 1999 and the Ph. D from University Putra Malaysia 2004. Currently he is an assistant professor at King Fahd University of Petroleum and Minerals Saudi Arabia.

Vlado Dimovski is a full professor of management and organizational theory at the University of Ljubljana, Faculty of Economics in Slovenia. He holds B.A. degrees in Economics and Philosophy, M.A. in Economics, and Ph.D. in Management and Finance. As an academician Dimovski has taught and researched at various universities and institutions, and has published numerous articles in recognized journals. His academic research interests cover learning organization, competitiveness, corporate strategy, developing knowledge-based organizations, and labor markets. Besides his university position, professor Dimovski was the State Secretary for Industry (1995–97), the president of the Center for International Competitiveness (1997–2005), and Minister for Labor, Family and Social Affairs (2000–2004).

Phalguni Gupta received his Ph.D. degree from Indian Institute of Technology, Kharagpur, India in 1986. He works in the field of data structures, sequential algorithms, parallel algorithms, on-line algorithms and image analysis. From 1983 to 1987, Prof. Gupta was in the Image Processing and Data

Product Group of the Space Applications Centre (ISRO), Ahmedabad, India and was responsible for software for correcting image data received from Indian Remote Sensing Satellite. In 1987, he joined the Department of Computer Science and Engineering, Indian Institute of Technology Kanpur, India. Currently he is a Professor in the department. He is involved in several research projects in the area of Biometric Systems, Mobile Computing, Image Processing, Graph Theory and Network Flow. He is member of ACM and IEEE. He has made many significant contributions to parallel algorithms, on-line algorithms and image processing and published many research papers in conferences and journals.

Yu-An Huang is an Associate Professor in the Department of International Business Studies, National Chi Nan University, Taiwan. He received a Ph.D. in technology management from National Cheng Chi University in Taiwan. He has been a visiting scholar at Curtin University of Technology in Perth, Australia. He has published papers in European Journal of Information Systems, European Journal of Marketing, Journal of Marketing Channels, Technovation, and numerous other journals.

Biju Issac is a senior lecturer in Information Technology at Swinburne University of Technology (Sarawak Campus), Malaysia. He holds BEng (Electronics and Communication Engineering) degree, along with MCA (Master of Computer Application) and PhD in Networking and Mobile Communication. He is an IEEE, IEEE Communication Society and IEEE Education Society member. He is also an IACSIT senior member, IAENG member etc. His research interests are mainly in computer networks and education. Specifically, his research interest is in mobility management, wireless and network security, spam detection, data-mining, education and e-learning. He is heading the network research in Swinburne. He has a number of refereed publications that includes many conference papers, journal papers and book chapters.

Tiko Iyamu is an Associate Professor of information systems and currently the Head of Department, Informatics at Tshwane University of Technology, Pretoria, South Africa. He also serves as a Professor Extraordinaire at the Department of Computer Science, University of the Western Cape, South Africa. Before taken fulltime appointment in academic, he headed several positions in both government and corporate institutions. They include Chief Architect at the City of Cape Town and Head of Architecture and Governance at MWEB (a telecommunication company), South Africa. Research interests include Mobile Computing, Enterprise Architecture, Information Technology Strategy, Actor Network Theory (ANT) and Structuration Theory (ST). Iyamu is author of numerous peer-reviewed journal and conference proceeding articles. Tiko serves on journal board and conference committees.

Geoffrey Jalleh is Associate Director in the Centre for Behavioural Research in Cancer Control at Curtin University. His primary research interests and expertise are in the areas of social marketing and health communication. He has been involved in research in a variety of health and social policy areas for government and non-profit organisations.

Dakshina Ranjan Kisku was born in Durgapur, India. He received the Bachelor of Engineering. and Master of Engineering. degrees in Computer Science and Engineering from Jadavpur University, Kolkata, India, in 2001 and 2003, respectively. Currently, he is pursuing Ph.D. in Computer Science and Engineering at the Jadavpur University. His research interests include computer vision, pattern recognition and biometrics. In the period of March 2006 to March 2007, he was a Researcher in the

Computer Vision Laboratory, University of Sassari, Italy. He also worked as a Research Associate at Indian Institute of Technology Kanpur, India from 2005 to 2006. From August 2003 to August 2005, he was a Lecturer in Computer Science and Engineering Department at the Asansol Engineering College, India. Mr. Kisku is a member of IEEE and IET. Hc has been published several research papers on biometrics in leading peer-reviewed conferences and journals. Mr. Kisku also worked as a reviewer for several conferences and journals.

Chien-Fa Li is a pharmacist in Pharmacy Division, Puli Veterans Hospital, Taiwan. He received an EMBA degree from National Chi-Nan University in Taiwan. His primary research interests and expertise are in the areas of information technology outsourcing and health informatics.

Chad Lin is a Research Fellow at Curtin University of Technology, Australia. Dr Lin has conducted extensive research in the areas of: e-commerce, e-health, health communication, health informatics, IS/IT investment evaluation and benefits realization, IS/IT outsourcing, IT adoption and diffusion, RFID, social marketing, strategic alliance in healthcare, and virtual teams. He has authored more than 100 internationally refereed journal articles (e.g. Decision Support Systems, European Journal of Information Systems, Information and Management, International Journal of Electronic Commerce, European Journal of Marketing, Technovation, Medical Journal of Australia, and ANZ Journal of Public Health), book chapters, and conference papers in the last five years. He has served as an associate editor or a member of editorial review board for 7 international journals and as a reviewer for 11 other international journals. He is currently a member of the Research & Development Committee in the Faculty of Health Sciences at Curtin University.

Ġorġ Mallia is a senior lecturer at the Centre for Communication Technology, the University of Malta. He holds a Ph.D in instructional technology from the University of Sheffield, UK. His main areas of research include Transfer of Learning, New Media Technology impact and cognitive change, and Hypertextual Processing. He has lectured in, among others, print and presentation media, the teaching of literature, graphic story telling, and personal branding. He is a member of a number of editorial boards and scientific committees. He has guest lectured at several universities, pre-eminently at Lund University, Sweden. Outside of his academic work, Dr Mallia is also a published author, particularly of books for children. He is also an illustrator and cartoonist. At present he is the chairman of Malta's National Book Council.

André Peres received his PhD in Computer Science from the Institute of Informatics at the University of Rio Grande do Sul (UFRGS) in Porto Alegre, Brazil in 2009, with a thesis on wireless location techniques regarding dynamic obstacles. He received his MSc in Computer Science in 2000 also from UFRGS with a research on fault tolerant systems in network management. In 1998 he joined the Lutheran University of Brazil (ULBRA) as a professor in network and network security. He is involved in research projects concerning network security, signal propagation behavior and wireless networks.

T. Ramayah has an MBA from Universiti Sains Malaysia (USM). Currently he is an Associate Professor at the School of Management in USM. He is an avid researcher, especially in the areas of technology management and adoption in business and education. His publications have appeared in Computers in Human Behavior, Direct Marketing: An International Journal, Information Development,

Journal of Project Management (JoPM), Management Research News (MRN), International Journal of Services and Operations Management (IJSOM), Engineering, Construction and Architectural Management (ECAM) and North American Journal of Psychology. He also serves on the editorial boards and program committees of many international journals and conferences of repute. In 2006 he was awarded the "AGBA DISTINGUISHED ASEAN SCHOLAR" for his contribution to research and publication in the ASEAN region. He was a Visiting Professor at the National Taiwan University for a month in 2007. His profile can be accessed from http://www.ramayah.com

Neyire Deniz Sarier received her B.Sc. degree in Mathematics and Industrial Engineering from Technical University of Istanbul, Turkey in 2005. She is currently a Ph.D. candidate at Cosec, B-IT Bonn, where she obtained her master degree on Media Informatics in 2007. Her research interests include Biometric security, in particular, integration of biometrics into cryptographic applications.

Abad Ali Shah is a Foreign Professor of Higher Education Commission (HEC) of Pakistan and placed in Department of Computer Science & Engineering, University of Engineering & Technology (UET), Lahore, Pakistan. He is also Director of Bioinformatics Labs., Al-Khawizmi Institute of Computer science, UET, Lahore, Pakistan. He spent 12 years at computer science department, King Saud University, Riyadh, KSA before joining HEC on July 2004. He received his B. Sc. in Mathematics and Physics from Punjab University, Lahore, Pakistan in 1967, a M. Sc. in Mathematics from Quaid-e-Azam University, Islamabad, Pakistan in 1981 with Quaid-I-Azam Award, a MS in Computer Science from Rensselaer Polytechnic Institute, Troy, New York in 1986, and Ph. D. in Computer Science from Wayne State University, Detroit, Michigan, USA in 1992. His current research interests include object-oriented databases, temporal databases, web databases, Web services, information retrieval (IR) software engineering, semantic web, web engineering and Bioinformatics. He has more than hundred (100) research articles on his credit. Currently, he is supervising many Ph.D. and MS dissertations.

Abdul Jaleel Kehinde Shittu obtained his Bachelor of Management Information Systems and Master Information Technology degrees from International Islamic University (2004) and (2007) respectively and PhD at Universiti Teknologi PETRONAS 2009. His research focuses on Information Technology Outsourcing, Shared Service and Outsourcing, Digital divide, IT/IS implementations, and IT project management, Quality assurance, Software engineering process and practices among others. He worked as a lecturer at the Department of Information Systems at the Kulliyyah of Information and Communication Technology, International Islamic University Malaysia. Currently, he is lecturing at the Department of Information Technology, University Utara Malaysia.

Nafisat Afolake Adedokun-Shittu is a PhD candidate at the Institute of Education, International Islamic University (IIUM), Malaysia. She obtained her Masters degree in Education in the field of instructional technology in the same university and has since written academic papers on Information and Communication Technology (ICT) issues in Education, Digital divide, knowledge management, among others.

Jamuna Kanta Sing was born in 1974 in West Bengal, India. He received the B.Engg degree in Computer Science and Engineering from Jadavpur University, Kolkata, India, in 1992 and M.Tech degree in Computer and Information Technology from Indian Institute of Technology Kharagpur, India, in 1994. He earned the Ph.D. degree from Jadavpur University in 2006. His research interests include image processing, medical imaging, pattern recognition, artificial neural networks, computer vision, etc. Currently Dr. Sing working as a Associate Professor in Computer Science and Engineering Department at Jadavpur University, Kolkata, India. He was a Scientist at National Physical Laboratory in 1995. He then joined as a lecturer at Jadavpur University in 1996 and was at the same position till 2002. From 2003 to 2006, he worked as a Senior Lecturer. In 2005, he was awarded BOYSCAST fellowship for pursuing postdoctoral research at the University of IOWA and he continued his research study until 2007. He has also been serving as a Chairman of the GOLD affinity group of IEEE Kolkata section since last three years. He was a Principal Investigator for many DST, AICTE sponsored research projects on diverse fields of image processing and medical imaging. He is member of IEEE. His contribution includes many significant works, which have published in many peer-reviewed conferences and journals. He has been working as a reviewer for several conferences and journals.

Zafar Singhera has been working in software industry for the past fifteen years. His areas of interest include software engineering, automated software testing, performance engineering/benchmarking, web services, and distributed system. He has been designing and architecting complex distributed systems and frameworks. He has built and led software development and quality assurance teams. He has been providing training and consulting services to the software. Dr. Singhera served as a full-time faculty for a few years, after his graduation from University of Southern California (USC), Los Angeles, CA in 1994. His graduate work focused on modeling and test automation of event-based object-oriented systems. He also has graduate degrees in Computer Science, Computer Systems Engineering, and Electrical Engineering; and bachelor degree in Economics. While working in the industry, he has been teaching as a visiting faculty at various academic institutes. He has many conference and journal publications to his credit.

Raul Fernando Weber received his PhD in Computer Science from the Institut Für Informatik IV, Universität Karlsruhe, Germany in 1986, and received his MSc in Computer Science from the Institute of Informatics at the University of Rio Grande do Sul (UFRGS) in Porto Alegre, Brazil in 1980. In 1977 he joined the University of Rio Grande do Sul (UFRGS) as a professor in network security and computer architecture. He is involved in research projects concerning network security.

Index

O

ObjectSpot 64
Ontology Migration
OOP 267, 272
Open Architecture Community System
    (OpenACS) 63
Open Biomedical Ontologies (OBO) 38
Openness 89
optical spectrum analyzer (OSA) 258, 260, 264
organisational learning (OL) 67
Organisation for Economic Cooperation and
    Development (OECD) 123
organizational learning 59, 60, 64, 65, 66, 67,
    72, 73, 74, 75, 76
Organization for the Advancement of Struc-
    tured Information Standards (OASIS) 33
outsourcing 136, 137, 138, 139, 140, 141, 142,
    143, 144, 145, 146

P

Particle Swarm Optimization (PSO) 156, 171,
    174, 175
Personal Identification Number (PIN) 213,
    214, 215, 216, 218, 219, 221, 222, 223,
    224, 225, 226, 227, 228, 229, 230, 231,
    232
philosophical assumptions 1
Phishing Scams 213, 233
PIN Cracking 213, 219, 231
porter stemmer algorithm 194, 207, 210
power electronic design aid system (PEDAS)
    268, 269, 271, 272, 278, 279, 280, 281,
    284, 286, 287, 289
pre-shared-key (PSK) 235
Prior Equal Error Rate (PEER) 169
Private Key Generator (PKG) 183, 184, 185,
    189
Project Monitoring System (SPP II) 19
public-key cryptography (PKC) 182, 183
Public Key Infrastructure (PKI) 88, 183, 184

Q

quadruple pass double stages with filter ampli-
    fier (QPDSF) 253, 261, 262, 263
Qualitative research 1, 2

R

RDF Schema (RDF-S) 36, 37
Reduced Point based Match Constraint
    (RPBMC) 158, 160, 169, 170, 171, 174,
    175, 176
Regular Grid based Match Constraint (RG-
    BMC) 158, 169, 170, 171, 174, 175, 176
Remote Method Invocation (RMI) 31
Remote Procedure Call (RPC) 31
Resource Description Framework (RDF) 29,
    36, 37, 39, 40, 43
return on investment (ROI) 81, 87
root means square error of approximation (RM-
    SEA) 71

S

SAHER 90, 91, 92
Saudi Telecommunications and Information
    Technology Commission (STITC) 79
Scalability 89
Scale Invariant Feature Transform (SIFT) 151,
    152, 157, 159, 161, 162, 164, 165, 166,
    167, 168, 170, 171, 172, 173, 175, 176,
    177, 178, 179
second generation (2G) 78, 79
Security 21, 23, 25, 26, 27
Semantic-MOBY 28, 29, 39, 40, 43
Semantic Web 28, 29, 35, 36, 37, 38, 39, 40,
    43, 44, 45
Semantic Web Browser (SWB) 37
Semantic Web for Life Sciences (SWLS) 36,
    37, 38
Semantic Web Services (SWSs) 36
service level agreement (SLA) 130, 131
Service Oriented Architecture (SOA) 40, 41,
    42, 43, 44, 45, 46
SIFT features 151, 152, 157, 161, 162, 164,
    165, 167, 168, 170, 171, 172, 175, 176,
    177
signal-to-noise ratio (SNR) 256
Simple Object Access Protocol (SOAP) 29, 33,
    35
Single Euro Payments Area (SEPA) 216
single pass single stage (SPSS) 253, 254, 261,
    262, 263
Sistem Informasi Nassional (SISFONAS) 122

Breinigsville, PA USA
15 December 2010
251398BV00001B/2/P